The Acoustic Analysis of Speech

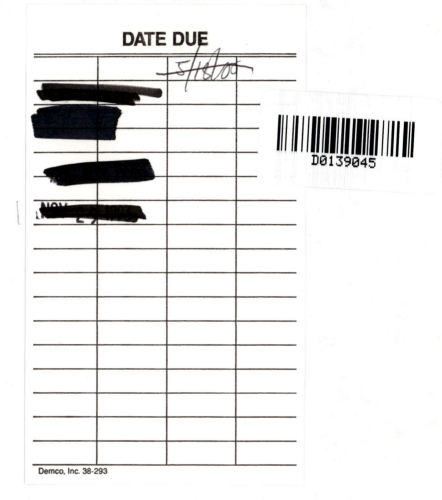

The Acoustic Analysis of Speech

Ray D. Kent, Ph.D.
and
Charles Read, Ph.D.
University of Wisconsin–Madison

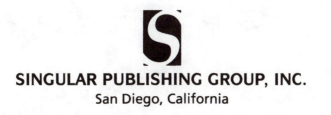

SINGULAR PUBLISHING GROUP, INC.
San Diego, California

Published by Singular Publishing Group, Inc.
4284 41st Street
San Diego, California 92105–1197

Typeset in 10/12 Palatino by So Cal Graphics
Printed in the United States of America by McNaughton & Gunn

Library of Congress Cataloging-in-Publication Data

Kent, Raymond D.
    The acoustic analysis of speech / Ray D. Kent and Charles Read.
        p.   cm.
    Includes bibliographical references and index.
    ISBN 1–879105–43–8
    1. Phonetics, Acoustic. I. Read, Charles, 1940–   . II. Title.
P221.5.K46   1992
414—dc20`   91–47740
                                                                 CIP

Contents

Dedication

To Jane and Helen

Acknowledgments

The genesis of this book was a research grant from the National Institute on Deafness and Other Communication Disorders (Grant No. DC00490; "Microcomputer systems for speech analysis: Evaluation"). A number of individuals contributed to the book's final form. We thank the students in our two courses, Acoustic Phonetics and Introduction to Experimental Phonetics, for their helpful suggestions on earlier versions of sections of this book. Dr. Eugene Buder and two anonymous reviewers offered many valuable suggestions on an initial draft of the book as a whole. We also thank the staff of Singular Publishing Group for their support and encouragement during this project.

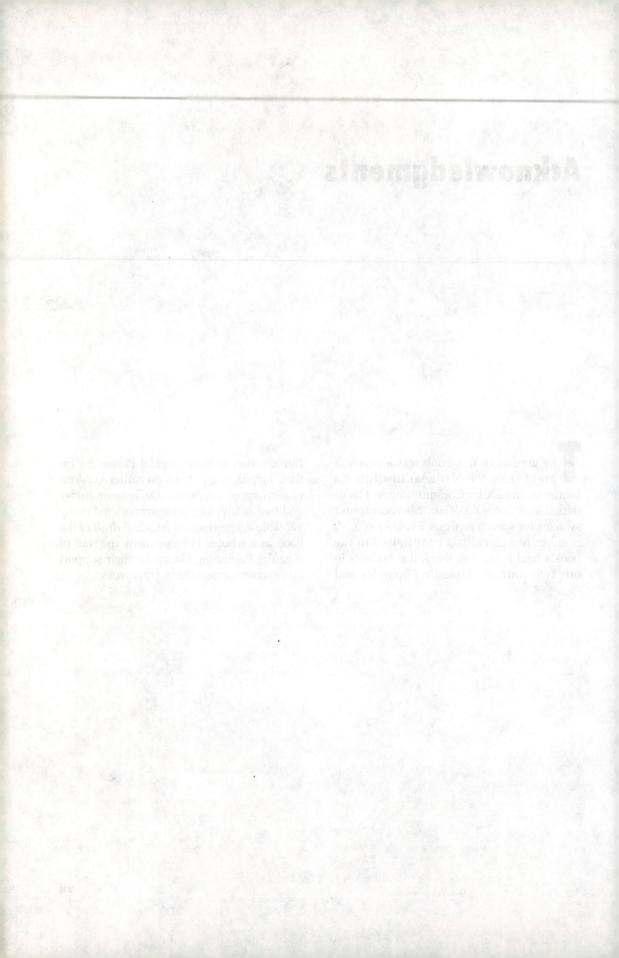

Preface

Speech is frequently cited as a most important human faculty, and sometimes as a *uniquely* human faculty. Although humans used speech long before written records of the earliest civilizations, speech itself remains an object of study, attracting the efforts of linguists, psychologists, physiologists, engineers, speech scientists, computer scientists, speech pathologists, and neurologists. To be sure, speech holds enough puzzles to occupy the concerted efforts of specialists from these disciplines. Much progress has been made in the study of speech, and this book summarizes the progress in understanding speech as an acoustic signal. In so doing, it follows the nearly 50-year-old precedent of a book entitled *Visible Speech* by Potter, Kopp, and Green (1947). The present book also endeavors to make speech visible—as patterns on paper or on a computer monitor. Remarkable progress in the study of speech acoustics has made speech visible and opened the door to diverse and exciting applications in phonetics, speech synthesis, automatic speech recognition, speaker identification, communication aids, instructional programs, speech pathology, and machine translation, to mention a few.

Our goal is to introduce readers to some closely related subjects that rarely appear together in a single book. The topics include the acoustic theory of speech production, digital signal processing of speech signals, acoustic characteristics of phonetic segments, sources of variation in the acoustic structure of speech, and speech synthesis. These topics are discussed with only a modest reliance on mathematics or engineering. Our hope is that this book will open the field of speech acoustics to a wider audience and perhaps a participatory audience. As we will try to show, modern technology places the acoustic analysis of speech within the grasp of many persons in many disciplines.

A broad base of knowledge undergirds the contemporary understanding of speech as an acoustic signal. We do not presume to have covered this base in detail. The following sources are suggested to the interested reader who seeks additional information on the topics listed.

General introductory readings on speech: Fry (1977, 1979); Ladefoged (1975); Lieberman (1972); Pickett (1980).

General readings on acoustic signals and acoustic systems: Handel (1989); Rosen and Howell (1990); Villchur (1978).

Acoustic studies of speech: Baken and Daniloff (1990); Flanagan (1972); Kent, Atal, and Miller (1991); Lehiste (1967); Pickett (1980).

Computer Speech—analysis and/or synthesis: Atal, Miller, and Kent (1991); Edwards (1991); Fallside and Woods (1985); Flanagan (1972); Flanagan and Rabiner (1973); Linggard (1985); O'Shaughnessy (1987); Witten (1982).

Perception of speech and other complex sounds: Handel (1989); Miller, Kent, and Atal (1991); Moore (1989); Prout and Bienvenue (1990); Sundberg (1987, 1991).

For those without any introduction to acoustics, we provide brief appendixes and a glossary that define essential terms and explain basic concepts. The first four chapters of this book were written to introduce the reader to basic issues in the acoustic analysis of speech. The remaining four chapters detail the acoustic characteristics of vowels and consonants, sources of variation in the acoustic signal of speech, and speech synthesis. These final four chapters are more densely referenced than the first four; as such, they summarize the literature on the acoustic characteristics of speech.

Introduction to the Study of Speech Acoustics

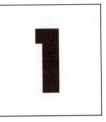

What Is Speech?

Raymond H. Stetson, a pioneer in the study of speech, wrote that *speech is movement made audible* (Stetson, 1928). The movements of the speech organs—structures such as the tongue, lips, jaw, velum, and vocal folds—result in sound patterns that are perceived by the listener. Speech therefore has three major arenas of study: the physiologic arena (or physiologic phonetics), the acoustic arena (or acoustic phonetics), and the perceptual arena (typically called speech perception). A unified understanding of speech requires the study of each of these areas in relation to the others. The discussion in this book will be concerned primarily with the acoustic arena, but references necessarily will be made to the other two arenas. Of particular importance is the need to understand how the acoustic analysis of speech can aid the study of the physiological phenomena, on the one hand, and perceptual phenomena,

on the other. Because the acoustic signal intermediates between a talker's production of speech and a listener's perception of the speech, acoustic analysis helps in the understanding of both speech production and speech perception. In many important ways, the acoustic signal helps to give a unified understanding of speech.

The Physiological Arena of Speech

The physiologic arena is identified physically with the speech apparatus, consisting of three major anatomical subsystems: respiratory (including the lungs, chest wall, and diaphragm), phonatory (larynx, or voice box), and articulatory (tongue, lips, jaw, and velum). Figure 1–1 is a simplified diagram of these subsystems. Speech articulation is a complex movement phenomenon, the understanding of which has been hindered by many obstacles, not the

1

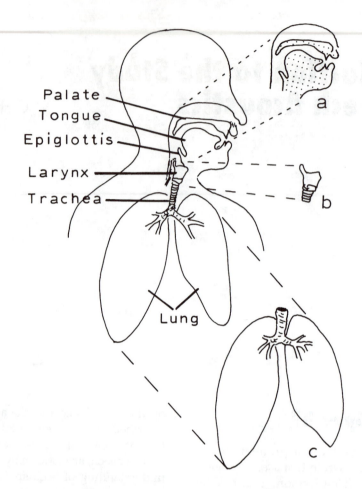

Palate
Tongue
Epiglottis
Larynx
Trachea
a
b
Lung
c

FIGURE 1-1.   Simplified illustration of the speech production system showing the three major subsystems: (a) supralaryngeal or upper airway subsystem; (b) laryngeal subsystem; and (c) respiratory subsystem.

least being the difficulty of observing the structures of interest—hidden as they are in the cavities of the mouth, neck, and thorax. The following three paragraphs give a highly simplified summary of these subsystems. The reader who is not acquainted with speech production may find it helpful to read this material before proceeding with the balance of the book.

The Respiratory Subsystem

The respiratory subsystem consists of the rib cage, lungs, diaphragm, and related tissues. Besides providing for ventilation to

support life, this system produces most of the aerodynamic energy of speech. The basic aerodynamic parameters are air volume, flow, pressure, and resistance. Volume is a measure of the amount of air and is measured with units such as liters. Flow is the rate of change in volume and is expressed in units such as liters/minute (i.e., a change in volume per unit of time). Pressure is force per unit area and is commonly expressed in Pascals, a unit which replaced earlier units such as dynes per square centimeter. In speech studies, pressure often is recorded with a different unit, such as centimeters of water (or millimeters of mercury). The reason is that manometers are a convenient way of measuring pressure as the displacement of a column of liquid. Resistance is a variable that relates flow and pressure, according to an important law called Ohm's law. This law can be expressed in the following alternative forms:

Pressure = Flow × Resistance
Flow = Pressure / Resistance
Resistance = Pressure / Flow

Speech is produced with a relatively constant lung pressure of about 6–10 cm (centimeters) of water or about 1 kPa (kPa = kiloPascal, or 1,000 Pascals.) To get an

idea of how much pressure this is, dip a straw to a depth of 6 cm in a water-filled glass (Figure 1–2). Then, blow into the straw until bubbles just begin to form at the end of the water-immersed straw. This condition corresponds to a pressure of 6 cm of water. There is only a little loss of air pressure from the tiny air sacs of the lungs up to the larynx at the top of the trachea, so that the subglottal air pressure (the pressure just below the vocal folds) is approximately equal to the air pressure in the lungs. Of course, if there were not closure at the larynx or in the upper airway of the articulatory system, air pressure developed by the respiratory system would be imme-

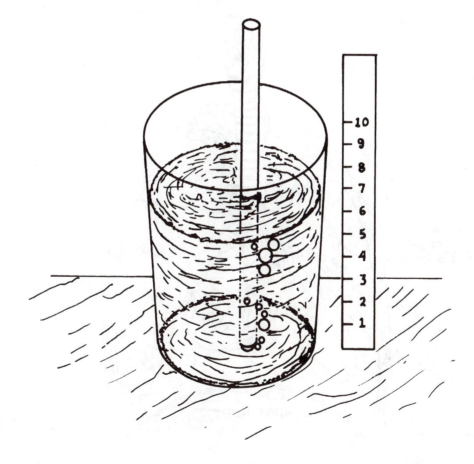

FIGURE 1–2. Sketch of materials needed to measure the air pressure requirements of speech. Place a straw into a cup of water to a depth of 6 cm. Then blow through the straw until bubbles begin to rise up through the water. This condition corresponds to a water pressure of 6 cm, which is adequate for the purposes of conversational speech.

diately released through the open tract into the atmosphere. Speech is produced by valving, or regulating, the air pressures and flows generated by the respiratory subsystem. In simple terms, the respiratory subsystem is an air pump, providing aerodynamic energy for the laryngeal and articulatory subsystems. The basic pattern of respiratory support for speech is that the talker inspires air by muscular adjustments that increase the volume of the respiratory system. Air is then released from the lungs by combinations of passive recoil and muscular activity, depending on the actual volume of air in the lungs and the aerodynamic requirements.

The essential point is that respiratory function for speech is understood in terms of aerodynamic events—air volumes, pressures, and flows. The mechanical events of speech thus begin as a speaker uses the respiratory system to generate aerodynamic energy.

The Laryngeal Subsystem

As shown in Figure 1–3, the larynx is situated on the top of the trachea. The larynx consists of a number of cartilages and muscles (the major cartilages are illustrated in Figure 1–4). Of particular importance are the vocal folds, small muscular cushions that adduct (come together) to

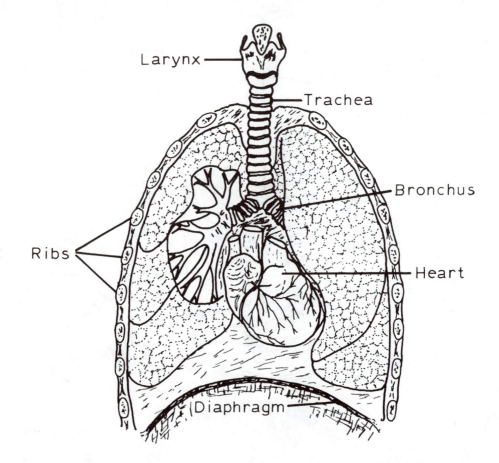

FIGURE 1–3. Sketch of the respiratory and laryngeal subsystems. Note that the larynx is located on the top of the trachea, which connects to the lungs by the paired bronchi (singular bronchus). The lungs are contained within a cavity formed by the rib cage and the muscular diaphragm.

close the laryngeal airway or abduct (separate) to open this airway. The opening between the vocal folds is called the *glottis*, and the term, *glottal*, has come to be used as a general term for laryngeal function. If the vocal folds are tightly closed, air is prevented from escaping from the inflated lungs. The vocal folds are typically tightly closed during intensive physical tasks such as lifting, defecating, and childbirth, so as to make the respiratory subsystem rigid as a foundation for pushing.

The fact that people often grunt during the lifting of a heavy object is evidence that the vocal folds are closed. The occurrence of the grunt also tells us that voiced sound is produced with adducted vocal folds. The sound results from the vibration of the folds, which alternately snap together and apart, colliding with one another in a basically periodic fashion. The rate of vibration of the vocal folds essentially determines the perception of a speaker's vocal pitch. A speaker with a high-pitched voice has a relatively high frequency of vocal fold vibration, and a speaker with a low-pitched voice has a relatively low frequency of vocal fold vibration.

The larynx is important to speech not only because it is the source of voicing energy but also because it valves the air moving into or out of the lungs. When the vocal folds are adducted tightly, no air movement will occur. Tight adduction is important for certain strenuous physical tasks, as described earlier, but it also is

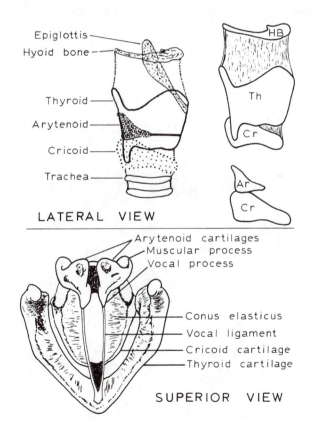

FIGURE 1–4. Lateral (from the side) and superior (from above) views of the larynx. The major cartilages are shown in the lateral view. The superior view illustrates the V-shaped opening of the glottis when the vocal folds are drawn apart or abducted. In the lateral view, the front is toward the right, and in the superior view, the front is toward the bottom.

used to interrupt the air stream for some speech sounds. Adduction with less resistance to air flow enables vocal fold vibration. A large degree of abduction allows air to move readily from the lungs into the upper airway. Voiceless sounds, such as the s in *see*, require that air pressure be impounded within the mouth as a source for noise energy. Abduction of the vocal folds satisfies this requirement by permitting the pressure in the mouth to approximate that in the lungs. Finally, a partial abduction of the vocal folds is used to generate voiceless noise energy, such as that of whispering.

As important as the larynx is, it contributes relatively little to the phonetic differentiation of speech sounds. Certainly, laryngeal action differentiates voiced from voiceless sounds. But laryngeal function is highly similar within major groupings of

sounds. For example, vocal fold vibration differs little across vowels, which gain their distinctiveness by the shaping of the articulatory system above the larynx. For this reason, the phonetic description of speech is based largely on supraglottal articulatory features.

The Articulatory Subsystem

This system extends from the larynx up through the lips or nose—that is, the two openings through which air and acoustic energy can pass (Figure 1–5). The articulators are movable structures and include the tongue, lips, jaw, and velum (or soft palate). Movements of these structures shape the vocal tract. The shape of the tract determines its resonance properties. When a speaker makes the vowel sound in

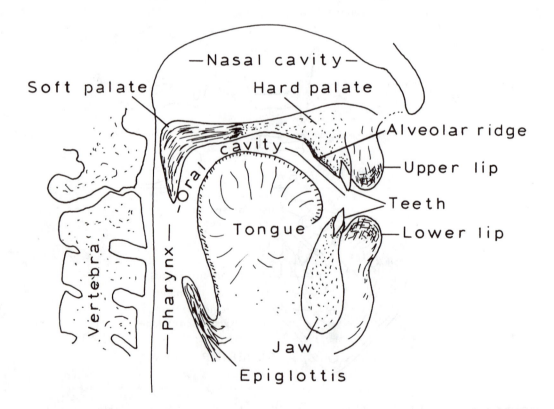

FIGURE 1–5. Simplified anatomy of the vocal tract. The major articulators are the jaw, lips, tongue, and soft palate. The major cavities are the pharynx, oral cavity, and nasal cavity.

the word *he*, the physical process can be understood as a shaping of the vocal tract to produce a particular pattern of resonance frequencies. In this process, energy from the vibrating vocal folds activates the resonance system of the vocal tract. Changing the vocal tract shape changes its resonance frequencies. The articulatory system also can be used to obstruct air flow (as in the case of the consonants in the word *pop*) and to generate noise (as in the case of the consonants in the word *seethe*).

Speech articulation typically is described in terms of articulatory contacts and positions. For example, a phonetician might describe the consonant *s* in *see* as a lingua-alveolar fricative. Lingua-alveolar denotes the place of articulatory constriction. *Lingua* means tongue and *alveolar* indicates a ridge on the bony ceiling of the mouth. *Fricative* indicates a sound that is produced with significant noise energy. The phonetician usually describes vowels with respect to the position of the tongue and the status of the lips. The vowel in *see* is termed a high-front and unrounded vowel because the tongue is relatively high and front in the mouth and the lips are unrounded. These articulatory descriptions are a convenient way to characterize the differences among speech sounds. Readers who are not familiar with phonetic descriptions should read Appendix A before moving on to the other chapters of this book. This appendix also lists the phonetic symbols that will be used in discussing speech sounds.

The Acoustic Arena of Speech

The acoustic arena is the major focus of this book but it is difficult to understand the acoustics of speech independently of speech physiology and perception. The acoustic signal of speech is the physical event that is transmitted in telecommunications or is recorded on magnetic tape, laser disc, or other mediums. That is, when we transmit or store speech, we almost always do so on the basis of the acoustic signal. This signal contains the linguistic message of speech. The listener can recover this message by hearing it. This may seem like an obvious statement. Is there any other way by which speech could be understood? To answer this question, imagine a person who is born deaf and blind. This person can neither hear speech nor see its articulation. Yet, persons with these joint disabilities can learn to produce and perceive speech. One technique used by the deaf and blind is called *Tadoma*. Users of this method place a hand over the speaker's face in such a way as to sense the actions of speech production— vocal fold vibrations, puffs of air escaping from the nose or mouth, movements of the jaw or lips, and so on. Practiced users of Tadoma can carry on conversations. That is, speech communication can be accomplished *without* perception of an acoustic signal. For these rare individuals, speech is movement only, not movements made audible. Can we ever experience speech as sound without underlying movements? In a sense, we can. Synthesized speech, or speech produced by machines, replicates the essential acoustic patterns of natural speech sufficiently well that it is intelligible. Many of the systems used for speech synthesis do not actually have anything that looks or acts like a tongue, or any other articulator for that matter. They typically work by generating a sound, either a buzz or a noise, and then modifying this sound source to give it certain acoustic properties. The synthesizer may not have a tongue, but it produces speech-like signals by performing operations that simulate the acoustic structure of natural speech.

For the great majority, speech is audible and necessarily so. Few of us can understand a televised speaker when the sound is turned off. We might guess a few words by observing the visual information (lip reading), but understanding is at best difficult and uncertain. On the other hand, if the video is faded to black while the audio signal is maintained, we continue to understand the spoken message, usually with little difficulty.

The primary objective of this book is to describe how speech sounds are carried in the acoustic signal. This objective will involve (a) an account of how the physiological events of speech production result in various types of sounds, (b) the description of speech sounds in terms of acoustic variables, (c) the description of techniques for the study of speech acoustics, and (d) a consideration of how acoustic cues are used in the perception of speech. A full understanding of speech acoustics requires that acoustic patterns be related to the physiological patterns of speech production and to the perceptual decisions that are based on the acoustic signal.

Readers who do not have at least an introductory background in acoustics should read Appendix B before proceeding with this book.

The Perceptual Arena of Speech

The study of speech perception is, in large part, an attempt to identify the acoustic cues that are used by a listener in reaching phonetic decisions. For example, what are the acoustic cues that enable a listener to decide that the consonant *b* was produced in the word *bye*? The understanding of speech perception has been advanced greatly by improvements in the acoustic analysis of speech and the synthesis of speech by machines. The ability to analyze the acoustic signal of speech and the ability to produce synthetic replicas of speech have been complementary in the modern understanding of how humans perceive speech. Although many questions remain to be answered about speech perception, the basic acoustic cues are sufficiently understood that speech synthesizers are becoming highly intelligible and sometimes even quite natural. Great progress also has been

made in machine speech recognition. As we learn how humans perceive speech, we are better able to design machines that have the capability of deriving linguistic decisions from the acoustic signal.

The Three Forms of the Acoustic Speech Signal

Progress in the study of speech and the development of speech technologies such as speech synthesis and machine speech recognition is rooted in the capabilities to record the speech signal and then play back the stored signal for analysis. Modern acoustic analysis is highly dependent on the digital computer, so much so that digital signal processing is at the heart of contemporary acoustic analysis of speech. Therefore, it is essential to understand how the acoustic signal is entered into a computer. This matter will be taken up in some detail in Chapter 3, but some background information is needed.

The Acoustic Wave

It is convenient to regard the signal of speech as having three interchangeable forms. The first of these is the airborne acoustic wave, or the signal that can be heard by the ear or sensed by a microphone. Our ears and most microphones respond to sound as pressure variations in the atmosphere. The ear converts the air pressure variations into neural impulses that are sent to the brain for interpretation. Microphones convert the air pressure variations into electrical signals. Microphones are one kind of *transducer*. A transducer is an element that converts one form of energy into another. A microphone transduces acoustic energy into electrical energy.

Technically, the airborne acoustic signal of speech is called the *propagated*, or *radiated*, acoustic signal. This signal propagates, or radiates, into space after it emerges from a speaker's vocal tract. Because this signal quickly vanishes, it is not a convenient form of speech for analysis. The acoustic analysis of speech requires stored forms of speech, or replicas of the original sound pattern, that can be examined at length.

The Stored Analog Signal

The second form of speech is the stored *analog signal*, a common example being an audiotape recording. An analog signal varies continuously in its basic properties. The analog signal of speech varies continuously in its pressure and time properties. This continuous variation is evident in the usual waveform representation of speech (Figure 1–6). Both the time and pressure dimensions can be divided into infinitely many points because of their continuous variation. Magnetic tape stores the speech signal as a magnetic field, which, like the original airborne acoustic signal, varies continuously in its properties. The advantage of the stored analog signal in a magnetic tape recording is that it can be played back for listening or analysis. Playback is accomplished by converting the magnetic energy back to electrical energy, which, in turn, is converted to acoustic energy by a loudspeaker or headphone. Each of these energy forms preserves the analog or continuous nature of the signal.

The Stored Digital Signal

The third form is another stored form, the *digital* (or *digitized*) *signal*. This form can be stored in a digital computer or on digital magnetic tapes or disks. Digital means numerical. Digital computers store information as numbers. To store a speech signal in a digital computer, it is necessary to convert the analog (continuous) signal to a series of numbers. This is accomplished by a process called *digitization*. An *analog-to-digital (A/D) converter* is a process or device that changes an analog signal to a digital one. In the reverse process, a *digital-to-analog (D/A) converter* changes the digital signal to an analog form. For example, D/A conversion would be required to play back the digitally stored signal through earphones or a loudspeaker. The abbreviations ADC and DAC are sometimes used for the two types of conversion. The digital representation of speech is very important because it permits the analysis of speech, employing the computational power of modern digital computers. Even personal computers are capable of some sophisticated speech analyses.

The three forms of speech—airborne acoustic signal, stored analog signal, and stored digital signal—are interchangeable in the sense that one form can be con-

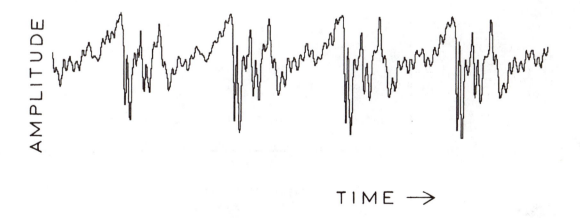

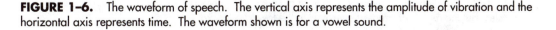

FIGURE 1–6. The waveform of speech. The vertical axis represents the amplitude of vibration and the horizontal axis represents time. The waveform shown is for a vowel sound.

verted to another form and back again. For example, the airborne acoustic signal can be recorded with a microphone, then stored in analog form on audiotape, then converted to digital form for storage in a computer, and finally converted back to analog form to drive a loudspeaker and be heard again as an airborne acoustic signal. Both analog and digital storage are virtually permanent, so that a speech signal can be held indefinitely.

With modern digital processing techniques, it is not necessary to use analog storage devices like audiotape recorders at all. The digital computer can store the signal and analyze it, and, through D/A conversion, play it back as needed. But however the speech signal is stored, it is important to recognize some basic properties of speech to be certain that the stored signal really retains the important characteristics of the airborne acoustic signal. Valuable information can be lost in the operations of transduction and storage. Unfortunately, many people have discovered that signals that were thought to be safely recorded are badly distorted on playback. For both the storage and analysis of speech, it is important to know some basic characteristics of the signal in question. This issue is taken up next.

Considerations of the Acoustic Properties of Speech

The energy of speech extends over a bandwidth of more than 10 kHz. Figure 1–7 shows the long-term spectrum of speech, that is the distribution of acoustic energy across frequencies for a long sample of speech. The long-term spectrum represents a cumulative energy distribution. Although most of the long-term energy is in the lower frequencies, energy is spread quite widely over the frequency range. In fact, the energy in speech can extend beyond 10 kHz, but for most purposes it is sufficient to consider a much smaller frequency range. In fact, the bandwidth for telephone transmission is only about 500-3500 Hz (hertz, the unit of frequency). A readily intelligible speech signal can be transmitted with a total bandwidth of less than 5 kHz (kilohertz, or 1000 x Hz). But whenever any speech is recorded or analyzed, it is important to know how frequency limitations in recording or analysis may affect the results. The frequency response of the recording or analyzing equipment should be known before quantitative analyses are performed. It should

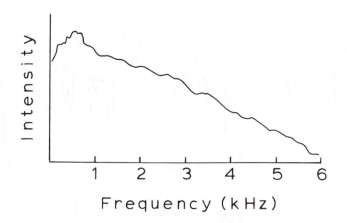

FIGURE 1–7. The long-term average spectrum of speech. The energy is spread over a range of frequencies, but the region of greatest energy is in the low frequencies.

never be simply assumed that a tape recording is faithful in its reproduction of a sound. Recorders advertised as "high fidelity" are not necessarily so. For the purposes of this tutorial, it will be assumed that a frequency range of at least 5 kHz is needed for even modest objectives in speech analysis. But a range of 10 kHz is much more appropriate for the study of various sounds produced by different speakers, including men, women, and children.

The dynamic range of speech—its range of energy—is about 60 dB (decibels). This means that the weakest sounds are about 60 dB less intense than the strongest sounds. Vowels are the most intense sounds, and the fricatives that begin the words *fin* and *thin* are typically the weakest. When a V-U (volume units) meter on a tape recorder or other instrument is used to monitor the peak intensity of a speech sample, it is responding mainly to the energy in vowels. If recording and analyzing instruments are not properly adjusted, the dynamic range of recording or analysis may not be matched to the dynamic range of the sounds of interest. As a rule of thumb, the dynamic range for a given talker can be estimated from the sounds in the word *thaw*, which consists of a weak fricative and an intense vowel. If both the fricative and the vowel are satisfactorily represented in a recording or analysis, then the procedures are at least roughly suitable. It will be assumed in this tutorial that a dynamic range of about 60 dB is appropriate for the storage and analysis of speech. Within this range, it usually is desirable that recordings be sensitive to variations of 1 dB. The human ear responds to variations of about this magnitude and it is for this reason that a 1 dB sensitivity is required.

Time also is an important dimension to consider in speech recording and analysis. The minimal time resolution for general analysis purposes is about 10 ms (milliseconds, where *milli-* means one-thousandth). This is the shortest duration of important speech events, such as the transient burst associated with the release of stop consonants. Analyses that cannot achieve this resolution may miss significant information about the temporal structure of speech.

Finally, it should be remembered that both the frequency and energy of speech sounds can change very rapidly. Storage and analysis operations should be able to follow these rapid changes with little or no distortion.

With these thoughts in mind, we can see that the study of speech acoustics involves the analysis of a signal whose energy (a) is distributed over a range of about 10 kHz for most purposes, (b) possesses a dynamic range of about 60 dB, and (c) has significant variations in time that occur in 10 ms or less. Bear in mind also that the speech signal is lost quickly as its acoustic energy dissipates into the atmosphere. We may repeat what was said but we can never retrieve the original production.

Theory, Instruments, and Measures

This book takes up issues related to the acoustic theory of speech production, the laboratory instruments suited to acoustic analysis, and measurements of the acoustic signal of speech. These three—theory, instruments, and measures—are interrelated. The use of tools and measures is influenced by the acoustic theory of speech. Test of the theory depends on the availability of laboratory instruments and measures. The application of measures requires that the signal be stored and appropriately displayed by laboratory instruments. The proper use of acoustic analysis requires an understanding of how speech is produced (the acoustic theory of speech production), a knowledge of laboratory instruments available for acoustic analysis of signals like speech, and a familiarity with various measures that can be made of the acoustic signal of speech.

Chapter 2 presents basic concepts of the acoustic theory of speech production.

Knowing what speech is—how it is generated as an acoustic signal—helps in the design and use of analysis instruments and in the selection of measures to characterize the signal. The acoustic theory of speech production summarized in Chapter 2 is a first step in understanding the acoustic analysis of speech. Chapter 3 considers the instruments used for the analysis of the acoustic signal of speech. Contemporary speech analysis relies heavily on the digital computer. Therefore, to understand speech analysis, one needs to know about the digital processing of signals. Chapter 3 is largely concerned with the procedures by which the acoustic signal, as obtained with a microphone, is converted to a form that can be stored in a digital computer. Chapter 4 describes the modern acoustic analyses used in the study of speech. These analyses are typically available on systems that run on digital computers or that are provided by stand-alone systems based on microprocessors. In both cases, digital signal processing is involved. Chapters 5 and 6 pertain to the acoustic characteristics of vowels and consonants, respectively. These two chapters define the acoustic measures that are typically used in acoustic phonetics. Chapters 5 and 6 are written more in the vein of a literature review than the preceding chapters. They consolidate the results of many investigations of the acoustic properties of vowels and consonants. Chapter 7 considers issues related primarily to phonetic context and speaker variables. Chapter 8 discusses speech synthesis, or the generation of speech by machine. The appendices and glossary may be helpful for occasional referral, so the reader may want to take a look at these materials to become familiar with the contents before continuing to the next chapter.

Acoustic Theory of Speech Production

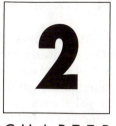

CHAPTER

This chapter summarizes a theory commonly known as the linear source-filter theory of speech production. Fant's book, *Acoustic Theory of Speech Production* (1960a) is a basic reference. This theory is useful in understanding articulatory-acoustic relationships, and it also provides a foundation for many procedures for the acoustic analysis of speech. Only broad outlines of the theory will be presented here. The reader who seeks a more complete presentation should read Fant's book, which is highly recommended to anyone interested in the acoustics of speech. The acoustic theory of speech presented here will be discussed in terms of the following major sound classes: vowels, fricatives, nasals, stops, affricates, liquids, diphthongs, and semivowels. The first three of these—vowels, fricatives, and nasals—will be discussed at length because they illustrate principles that can be applied to the other sound classes. For example, the semivowel /w/, as in *way*, can be understood as a modification of the theory for vowel production.

Some simple diagrams will help to identify the major features of interest. Vowels are sounds produced with laryngeal vibration (so that voicing is the energy source) and a relatively open vocal tract that is shaped to produce particular patterns of resonances (so that the entire vocal tract functions as a filter, or frequency-selective transmission system). A general diagram for vowels is given in Figure 2–1a. Modifications of this diagram will be used to model liquids and semivowels. Fricatives are produced with a narrow constriction somewhere in the vocal tract, as depicted in Figure 2–1b. Air passing through this constriction generates turbulence noise, so that noise is the energy source for sound production. The noise source is filtered by the vocal tract, especially by the section of the vocal tract anterior to the constriction. The model of Figure 2–1b will be modified for stop and affricative consonants, both of which involve a brief closure of the vocal tract and the generation of noise similar to that of fricatives. As shown in Figure 2–1c, nasal sounds are produced with the velopharynx open so that sound is radiated through the nasal cavity. If the mouth is closed, the resultant sound is a nasal consonant, like *m* and *n* in the word *man*. If the mouth is open, the resultant sound is a nasalized vowel. Nasals, like vowels, typically have voicing as an energy source. But nasals differ from oral vowels in that the filtering of the source energy is determined by both the oral and nasal passages.

Vowels

Tube Resonance as a Model of Vowel Production

To introduce the acoustic theory of speech production, we will begin with an apparatus that doesn't look much at all like the human vocal tract. As shown in Figure 2–2, this apparatus consists simply of a vibrator (a rubber membrane with a slit cut into it will do) and a length of straight pipe. The vibrator is stretched to fit over one end of the pipe and the other end of the pipe is left open. The vibrator is a source of acoustic energy that travels through the pipe. The pipe is a resonator, in fact, an example of a very important class of resonators—pipes closed at one end and open at the other. Such a pipe has

an infinite number of resonances, located at frequencies given by the *odd-quarter wavelength* relationship:

$$F_n = (2n-1) \, c/4l,$$
where n is an integer,
$\quad$ c is the speed of sound (about 35,000 cm/sec), and
$\quad$ l is the length of the pipe

The formula shown above gives the resonance frequencies of the pipe. If the formula is restated in words, it says that a pipe will resonate with maximal amplitude a sound whose wavelength is four times the length of the tube. In fact, such resonances occur in multiples and that is why the expression $(2n-1)$ is used to generate the set of odd numbers. Resonances occur at $c/4l$, $3c/4l$, $5c/4l$, $7c/4l$, and so on. Let us assume that the pipe has a length (l) of 17.5 cm. Then the first resonance will have a frequency given by:

$$\begin{aligned} F_1 &= c/4l \\ &= 35,000 \text{ cm/s} / (4 \times 17.5 \text{ cm}) \\ &= 500 \text{ 1/s, or } 500 \text{ Hz} \end{aligned}$$

The second resonance will have a frequency calculated as:

$$\begin{aligned} F_2 &= 3c/4l \\ &= 35,000 \text{ cm/sec} / (4 \times 17.5 \text{ cm}) \\ &= 1500 \text{ 1/sec, or } 1500 \text{ Hz} \end{aligned}$$

Higher resonances can be determined by continuing the calculations for different solutions of $(2n-1)$. Doing so results in the

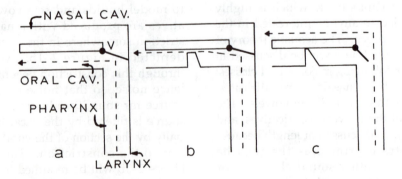

FIGURE 2–1. Vocal tract models for three classes of speech sounds: (a) vowels, (b) fricatives, and (c) nasals. Note the partial constriction in (b) and the total obstruction in (c).

Vibrating membrane

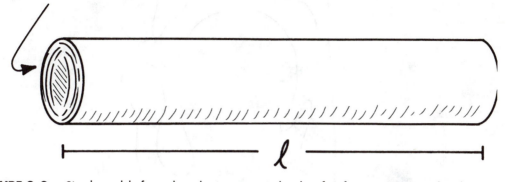

FIGURE 2–2. Simple model of vowel production: a straight tube of uniform cross section closed at one end (by a vibrating membrane to simulate the vocal folds) and open at the other (corresponding to the mouth opening).

following resonance frequencies: 500, 1500, 2500, 3500, 4500 Hz (and so on, but this is far enough for our purposes). Note that the resonance frequencies fall at intervals of 1000 Hz.

To make this example relevant to the production of human speech, we need to note two things: (1) the average vocal tract of a man has a length of about 17.5 cm running from glottis to lips, and (2) the vocal tract has approximately the same resonance frequencies as a straight tube of the same length and cross-sectional area. That is, the simple pipe apparatus shown in Figure 2–2 is a satisfactory model of one particular vowel of human speech. The vowel in question is produced with the tongue and other articulators positioned to create a uniform cross-sectional area along the length of the vocal tract. This vocal tract configuration is similar to one often used in a hesitation pause in speech, usually rendered in prose as "uhh." This vowel is depicted in Figure 2–3. As you might have guessed, the vibrating membrane in the pipe apparatus is analogous to the vibrating vocal folds. And, of course, the pipe is analogous to the vocal tract, at least for the one particular vowel shown in Figure 2–3. In a sense, the rubber membrane and pipe apparatus is a one-vowel

sound generator. It has an energy source, the vibrating membrane, and a resonator, the pipe.

Changing the length of the resonating pipe changes the resonance frequencies as indicated in the odd-quarter wavelength formula. If the pipe length is doubled from 17.5 cm to 35 cm, the resonance frequencies would assume much lower values, namely, 250, 750, 1250, and 1750 Hz for the first (or lowest) resonances. If the pipe length is halved to make a new pipe only 8.75 cm long, then the lowest four resonance frequencies would be 1000, 3000, 5000, and 7000 Hz. These results explain why the longest pipes in a pipe organ sound the lowest tones whereas the shortest pipes in a pipe organ sound the highest tones. Similarly, we have an explanation for the changes in resonance frequencies of the vocal tract as a child grows into an adult. An infant has approximately half the vocal tract length as at maturity and has much higher resonance frequencies. In fact, the resonance frequencies for an infant's vowel corresponding in vocal tract shape to Figure 2–3 are about 1000, 3000, 5000, and 7000 Hz, or the values calculated above for a pipe that is 8.75 cm in length. Obviously, then, the length of a talker's vocal tract will deter-

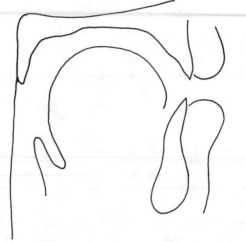

FIGURE 2–3. Vocal tract configuration of a vowel that roughly corresponds to the idealized tube in Figure 2–2. The cross-sectional area is essentially the same from glottis to lips.

mine the relative location of the resonance frequencies. The longer the vocal tract, the lower the resonance frequencies and the smaller their separation in frequency. Conversely, the shorter the vocal tract, the higher the resonance frequencies and the larger their separation in frequency.

Extending the Tube Resonance Model

But our results so far pertain to just one vowel, the so-called mid-central vowel in which the cross-sectional area is the same along the length of the vocal tract. What are the resonance frequencies for other vowels? The answer can be determined experimentally by discovering the resonance frequencies for various shapes of pipes that have the same length. As noted above, the resonance frequencies are not affected appreciably by whether the pipe is straight or curved. (The differences that occur were described by Sondhi, 1986.) But it is easier to draw a straight pipe, so straight pipes of different shapes will serve as models for this discussion. Some examples of different pipe shapes are shown in Figure 2–4. Each one of the shapes corre-

sponds roughly to the vocal tract shape of a vowel in English. Figure 2–4a corresponds to vowel /i/ (as in *he*), Figure 2–4b to vowel /u/ (as in *who*), and Figure 2–4c to vowel /ɑ/ (as in *ha*). Also shown in Figure 2–4 are spectra for each of these simple vowel models. The spectral peaks are the resonance frequencies of the pipes. Recall that, on average, the resonance frequencies are separated by about 1000 Hz, but that the individual resonance frequencies vary about the frequency locations for the mid-central vowel. For example, compared to the first resonance for the mid-central vowel, the first resonance for /i/ has a lower frequency but the first resonance frequency for /ɑ/ has a higher frequency.

Tube Resonance Summary

This is a good point to review what we have discovered so far:

1. A uniform pipe that is closed at one end and open at the other has resonance frequencies determined by the length of the pipe (assuming constant atmospheric conditions). The resonance frequencies

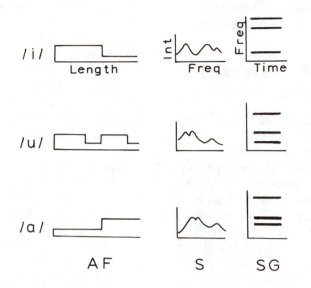

FIGURE 2–4. Shown for each of three vowels is an idealized area function (AF), spectrum (S) and spectrogram (SG). The closed end of the area function represents the glottis, and the open end, the lips. Formants are represented in the spectra by peaks and in the spectrograms by horizontal bands.

are relatively lower for long pipes and relatively higher for short pipes.

2. For nonuniform pipes (that is, pipes for which the cross-sectional area is not constant over pipe length) the individual resonance frequencies vary around the values determined for a uniform pipe.

3. The uniform pipe closed at one end and open at the other is an acoustic model for one vowel, namely the mid-central vowel.

4. In order that the pipe model can represent other vowels, the cross-sectional area must be varied as a function of pipe length in a way that approximates the vocal tract shape for a particular vowel.

At this point, you might be wondering if simple pipes like those depicted in Figure 2–4 actually do sound like vowels produced by humans. In fact, they do sound something like human vowels, provided that an appropriate source of vibratory energy is applied to them. (Remember that resonators do not generate sound energy but only respond to energy that is

delivered to them.) Moreover, all the other vowels in English can be modeled, at least roughly, by appropriate shape modifications of a straight pipe.

What is the relationship between the resonator (such as a pipe) and the source of energy (such as a vibrating rubber membrane)? To a large degree, the energy source and the resonator are independent, except for special conditions. This is an important fact, and it explains why a talker can produce a low-pitched vowel [i] or a high-pitched vowel [i] without losing the phonetic distinctiveness of the vowel. Vocal pitch is determined almost entirely by the vibrating frequencies of the vocal folds. The lower the rate of vibration, the lower the pitch. Therefore, a bass voice has a lower vibratory frequency than a soprano voice. But the frequency of vibration of the vocal folds does not affect the properties of the resonator. The resonance frequencies of a pipe resonator are determined almost entirely by just two factors: the length of the pipe and its cross-sectional area as a function of length. Changing the frequency of the energy source does not change the resonance frequencies of the pipe receiving the energy.

The Source-Filter Theory of Vowel Production

The principles introduced to this point can be summarized in a conceptualization called the *source-filter theory* (Figure 2–5). This theory, as applied to vowel production, states that the output energy (what was called the radiated speech signal in an earlier section) is a product of the source energy and the resonator (or filter). We might more accurately refer to this theory as *linear source-filter theory* because it is based on a linear mathematical model. It is convenient to think of the source energy in the form of a spectrum. The vibrating vocal folds produce a sound spectrum like that in Figure 2–6. The energy falls at discrete frequencies determined by the rate of vibration. The result is called a *line spectrum*, or a spectrum in which the energy distribution takes the form of lines. The spectrum of voicing energy can be idealized as a line spectrum in which the individual lines fall at integer multiples of the fundamental (lowest) vibratory frequency. For example, the average man's voice has a fundamental frequency of about 120 Hz, and the energy of this source spectrum will fall at the frequencies of 120, 240, 360, 480 Hz, and so on. But a man can produce much lower or higher frequencies of vibration than this average value. If a man's fundamental frequency increases to 300 Hz, then the energy in the source spectrum will fall at the frequencies of 300, 600, 900, 1200 Hz, and so on. A woman's fundamental frequency averages about 225 Hz but a large range of fundamental frequencies are possible. Similarly, a very young child may have a mean fundamental frequency of 300 Hz but a large range around this figure. These changes in vibratory frequency for a given speaker are changes in the source only and do not necessarily have any effect on the resonator or filter. Similarly, the amplitude

of vocal fold vibration can be changed. A talker can produce a soft voice or a loud voice. Such changes affect the resonator only in that they determine the level of energy which the resonator will receive. The relative independence of source and filter makes it possible for us to produce intelligible speech with a variety of energy sources, including low- and high-pitched voices, whisper, gravelly voices, and other phonatory variations.

To extend the source-filter model to the production of all vowels (and eventually to other speech sounds as well), it is helpful to make some changes in terminology. First, different kinds of sources are involved in speech production, but for the moment we are concerned with only one kind of source—the vibrating vocal folds. We will refer to this source as the *laryngeal spectrum*, which, as noted above, can be idealized as a line spectrum. It is characteristic of the laryngeal spectrum that the energy in its harmonic components (each line is a harmonic of the fundamental frequency) declines as frequency increases. This decline in the energy of the higher harmonics is shown in Figure 2–6 and means that most of the energy in voiced speech is in the lower frequencies. The rate of decline in energy is 12 dB per octave, or a drop in energy of 12 dB for every doubling of frequency. We can say, then, that the laryngeal spectrum can be regarded as a line spectrum in which the energy of the harmonics falls with frequency at a rate of 12 dB/octave.

The next terminological change applies to the filter. Instead of referring to resonances, we now will refer to *formants*. A formant is a natural mode of vibration (resonance) of the vocal tract. Theoretically, there is an infinite number of formants, but for practical purposes only the lowest three or four are of interest. Formants are identified by formant number, for example, F1, F2, F3, and F4, numbered in succession beginning with the lowest-frequency formant. Each formant can be described by two characteristics: center frequency

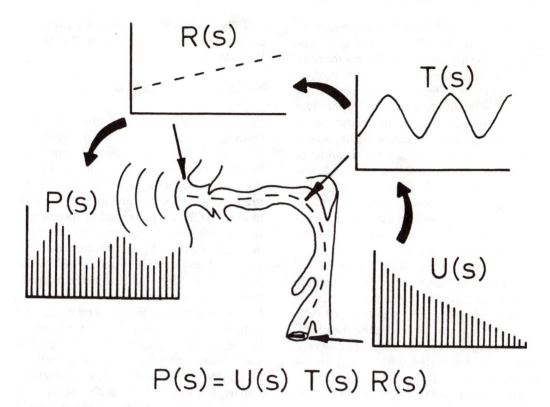

$$P(s) = U(s) \; T(s) \; R(s)$$

FIGURE 2–5.   Diagrammatic representation of the source-filter concept for vowels. The laryngeal source spectrum, U(s), is filtered by the vocal tract transfer function, T(s), and the radiation characteristic, R(s), to yield the output spectrum, P(s). Mathematically, P(s) is a coproduct of U(s), T(s) and R(s) where s = frequency.

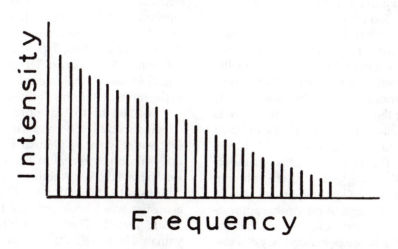

FIGURE 2–6.   Idealized laryngeal spectrum in which the energy is located at discrete frequencies which are integer multiples of the fundamental frequency. The amplitudes of the successive harmonics decrease with frequency.

(commonly called the formant frequency) and bandwidth (a measure of the breadth of energy in the frequency domain, or a measure of the rate of damping in the time domain).

The term formant is used somewhat differently by different authors. Some refer to a formant as a peak in the acoustic spectrum. In this usage, a formant is an acoustic feature that may or may not be evidence of a vocal tract resonance. In this book, formant will be used synonomously with vocal tract resonance. A formant often is associated with a peak in the acoustic spectrum, but not necessarily so. One of the goals of acoustic analysis is to estimate the formant structure of a sound segment.

Taken together, the formants constitute the *transfer function* of the vocal tract. A transfer function is the input-output relation and is one way of describing the operation of a process like filtering. Because each formant is associated with a peak in the transfer function (Figure 2–5), each formant is *potentially* associated with a peak in the output spectrum (or radiated spectrum). There would, of course, be no peak in the radiated spectrum at a given formant region if the laryngeal source didn't supply energy in the frequency region corresponding to the formant location. Formants do not supply energy; they only modify energy supplied by a source.

The final term to be introduced is *radiation characteristic*. This term refers to a filtering effect that arises when sounds escape the mouth to radiate into space. An acoustic engineer would say that that the acoustic coupling of the mouth to the atmosphere is like an infinite baffle. That is, the radiated sound spreads in all directions as it leaves the mouth. This kind of radiation characteristic acts like a high-pass filter (reducing energy more in the low frequencies than in the high frequencies). A reasonable approximation to this effect is to assume that the output sound increases in frequency at a rate of 6 dB/octave. Because this is a constant characteristic, it is sometimes combined with the 12 dB/octave drop in the laryngeal spectrum to yield a resultant 6 dB/octave.

The source-filter theory of vowel production is summarized in Figure 2–5 and in the following equation:

$$P(f) = U(f)\ T(f)\ R(f)$$

$P(f)$ is the radiated sound pressure spectrum of speech. P stands for pressure and (f) simply indicates a function of frequency. Recall from an earlier discussion that most microphones and the human ear respond to pressure variations. Therefore, it is useful to describe the output signal of speech as a sound pressure waveform (in the time domain) or a sound pressure spectrum (frequency domain). The three terms on the right side of the equation refer, respectively, to the laryngeal source spectrum, the transfer function of the vocal tract, and the radiation characteristic. The term U refers to volume velocity and is used because the vocal folds act like a source of air pulses. Of course, T represents transfer function, and R denotes radiation characteristic. Putting this equation into words, we could say that the radiated sound pressure waveform of speech is the product of the laryngeal spectrum, the vocal tract transfer function, and the radiation characteristic.

For the present, we will consider the terms $U(f)$ and $R(f)$ to be constant as different vowels are produced. That is, different vowels will be described as variations in the transfer function, $T(f)$, and the radiated spectrum, $P(f)$. Because $T(f)$ consists of the vowel formants, the discussion boils down to the formant patterns of different vowels.

A brief historical note is in order. Credit already has been given to the highly influential work by Gunnar Fant, particularly his book *Acoustic Theory of Speech Production* (1960a). Another important contribution to the understanding of vowel acoustics was a book published just before World War II. This book, Chiba and Kajiyama's *The Vowel: Its Nature and Structure* (1946), unfortunately was not widely distributed because of complications associated with the war. Although copies of the book are hard to come by, its influence should be noted in the modern understanding of speech acoustics.

Articulatory-Acoustic Relations for Vowels

Shown in Figure 2–7 is an X-ray picture of the vocal tract. This kind of picture is called a lateral X-ray because the image obtained represents a projection of X-rays through the object to be studied from one side to the other. This X-ray picture of the vocal tract corresponds anatomically to a *midsaggital section*, or a plane that runs through the head from front to back, cutting the head into right and left halves. The entire vocal tract, extending from larynx to lips, is the resonating cavity of vowel production. This cavity can be described in terms of its cross-sectional area as a function of length. Of course, the X-ray picture in Figure 2–7 provides only partial information because the vocal tract is seen in only two dimensions. Precise determination of the area over the length of the vocal tract requires information on the third dimension, the width of the

cavity over its length. However, by some simplifying assumptions, such as an assumption that the vocal tract is essentially circular along its length, we can estimate the area of the vocal tract for any given distance along its length. The result of such an estimation is sketched in Figure 2–8a and b. What we have accomplished is to determine the three-dimensional shape of the vocal tract. This is equivalent to creating a mold by filling the vocal tract with a semiliquid material that gradually hardens so as to retain the shape of the tract. As noted earlier in this chapter, the fact that the actual vocal tract is curved is not of critical significance to its function as an acoustic resonator. Therefore, we can straighten the curved model of the vocal tract in Figure 2–8a to produce the version in Figure 2–8c.

The labors described in the preceding paragraph are necessary to obtain an accurate acoustic model of the resonating cavity of the human vocal tract. But for purposes of discussion, it is sufficient to represent the vocal tract shape as a graph of its cross dimension over its length. Such a graph is depicted for four vowels in

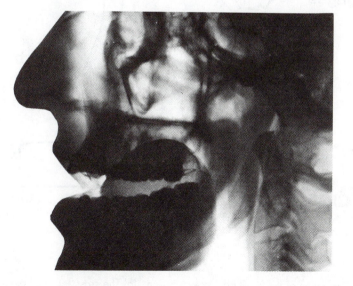

FIGURE 2–7. Lateral (side-view) X-ray of the vocal tract. (Courtesy of the Phonetics Laboratory, University of California at Los Angeles.)

Figure 2–9. In making these graphs, we have neglected the third dimension. Clearly, the vocal tract configurations for these vowels have some relatively constricted regions and other regions that are widely flared. For example, vowel /i/ (as in *he*) has a constricted region near the lip opening but a large open region near the larynx and pharynx. In contrast, vowel /ɑ/ (as in *ha*) has a constricted region in the pharyngeal portion of the model but a large open region near the lip opening. It is possible to calculate the resonance frequencies of such configurations using formulas from acoustic theory. When such calculations are carried out, the results generally conform to measured formants of the human vowels on which the models are based. The agreement between the formant frequencies of the vowel models and those of the human vowels being modeled

is evidence of the validity of the approach.

The same four vowels are shown again in Figure 2–10, this time as acoustic spectra. The spectral peaks represent the vowel formants. Notice that the high vowels /i/ and /u/ have in common a relatively low frequency of the first formant (F1), whereas the low vowels /ɑ/ and /æ/ have in common a relatively high frequency of this formant. That is, the frequency of the first formant varies inversely with tongue height of the vowel. Next, notice that the back vowels /u/ and /ɑ/ share a relatively low frequency of the second formant (F2), whereas the front vowels /i/ and /æ/ have a relatively high frequency for this formant. That is, the frequency of the second formant varies with the posterior-anterior dimension of vowel articulation. This result points to an articulatory-acoustic correspondence: the

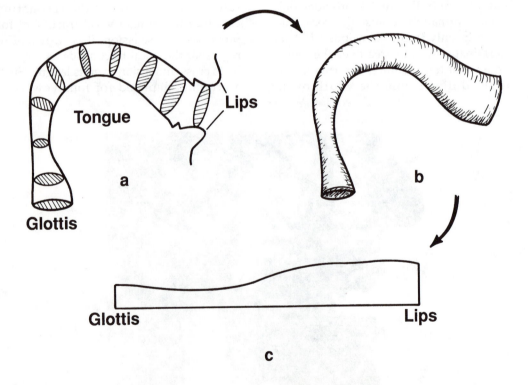

FIGURE 2–8. Derivation of the vocal tract area function. (a) The cross-sectional diameter is determined for length increments of the vocal tract, proceding from glottis to lips. The curved tube (b) can be straightened to form the straight tube in (c).

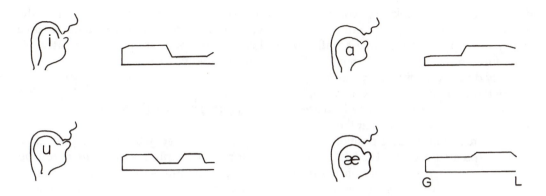

FIGURE 2–9. Vocal tract configurations and corresponding area functions (idealized) for the four vowels /i/ as in *he*, /u/ as in *who*, /a/ as in *pa*, and /æ/ as in *map*. G = glottis and L = lips.

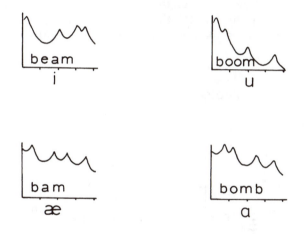

FIGURE 2–10. Spectra for the four vowels shown in Figure 2–9. The four peaks in each spectrum reflect formants. Hence, the frequency location of each peak is an estimate of a formant frequency. The frequency axis represents a range of 0–4 kHz.

frequencies of the first two formants, F1 and F2, can be related to dimensions of vowel articulation. The frequency of F1 is inversely related to tongue height (e.g., high vowels have a low F1 frequency), and the frequency of F2 is related to tongue advancement (e.g., F2 frequency increases as the tongue position moves forward in the mouth).

All of the vowels of American English can be plotted as shown in Figure 2–11 to

depict their F1 and F2 values. Note that in this F1–F2 plot, the axes can be considered to have two labels. The F1 axis has the articulatory label of tongue height, and the F2 axis has the articulatory label of tongue advancement (or posterior-anterior position). These paired articulatory-acoustic labels are consistent with the discussion in the preceding paragraph. In general, the frequency of F1 varies with tongue height and the frequency of F2 varies with tongue advancement. This articulatory-acoustic correspondence makes it possible to draw articulatory inferences from acoustic data on vowel formant frequencies. When the F1 frequency decreases, it is usually safe to conclude that the tongue has moved to a higher position. When the F2 frequency increases, it is usually safe to conclude that the tongue has moved to a more anterior position.

The lips also are involved in vowel production. Labial participation is quite simple for English vowels. Lip rounding occurs for some back and central vowels, such as the vowels in the words *who, hoe,* and *her.* Front vowels are not rounded in English. The effect of lip rounding is to lower all formant frequencies. The reason follows directly from the fact that formant frequencies depend on the length of the vocal tract. The longer the length, the lower the formant frequencies. Because lip

rounding tends to extend the length of the vocal tract, rounded vowels tend to have lowered formant frequencies relative to nonrounded vowels.

Perturbation Theory

Perturbation theory allows the prediction of formant-frequency changes resulting from perturbations (local constrictions) of a tube resonator. This is a powerful theory in acoustics and is particularly important for the acoustics of speech production as it can explain the formant frequencies of vowel sounds.

To see how this theory applies to vowel production, we will use a single-tube representation of the vocal tract, as shown in Figure 2–12. This tube model should be quite familiar by now. Such a

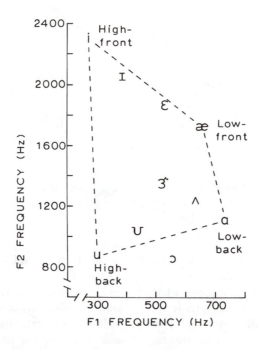

FIGURE 2–11. Classic F1–F2 chart in which a vowel is represented acoustically by its F1 and F2 frequencies. The values shown are for an average adult male. The phonemic symbols are positioned to show the F1 and F2 values for that vowel. An articulatory-acoustic relationship is suggested by the labels in the figure. Low vowels have a high F1 frequency; high vowels have a low F1 frequency; front vowels have a high F2 frequency; and back vowels have a low F2 frequency.

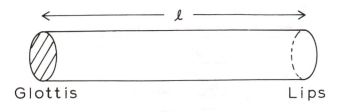

FIGURE 2–12. Straight tube model of the vocal tract for vowel production.

tube will have at each of its resonance frequencies a standing wave distribution of volume velocity or the inverse of volume velocity, pressure. Basically, volume velocity variations during resonance in the pipe reflect the way in which individual particles vibrate at various positions in the pipe. At certain positions, particle vibration is maximal (and pressure has its minimum). At other positions, particle vibration is minimal (and pressure has its maximum). Regions where the particle vibrate with maximum amplitude are regions of volume velocity maxima, or *nodes*. Regions where the particles vibrate with minimum amplitude are regions of volume velocity minima, or *antinodes*. It is characteristic of pipe resonance that volume velocity or its inverse, pressure, will have a stationary distribution along the length of the pipe. Because the pipe has an infinite number of resonances, a volume velocity or pressure distribution can be described for each resonance. We will restrict our discussion to the first three resonances, corresponding to the first three formants of vowels. Incidentally, it is possible to verify these standing wave distributions experimentally. The Nobel laureate Georg von Békésy (1960) demonstrated pressure variations within the vocal tract by slowly moving a miniature microphone into the vocal tract as the speaker phonated a vowel. The output of the microphone had maxima and minima corresponding to the standing wave pressure variations.

As shown in Figure 2–13, the first resonance has a standing wave distribution with a volume velocity maximum, or node, at the open end (the lip ending of the vocal tract) and a volume velocity minimum, or antinode, at the closed end (the glottal end of the vocal tract). For the second resonance, there are two volume velocity maxima (nodes) and two volume velocity minima (antinodes). For the third resonance, there are three volume velocity maxima and three minima. In other words, each formant, Fn , of the vocal tract has n nodes and n antinodes (where n is an integer).

Suppose that the single-tube resonator in Figure 2–12 is pliable so that it can be squeezed at various points along its length. Each local constriction of the tube produced by squeezing is a perturbation, and the effect of the perturbation on a formant frequency Fn depends on whether the constriction is proximal to a node or antinode. The general relationship is as follows:

1. A local constriction of the tube near a volume velocity maximum lowers the formant frequency.

2. A local constriction of the tube near a volume velocity minimum raises the formant frequency.

Now Figure 2–12 can be redrawn as shown in Figure 2–14 to resemble the human vocal tract with nodes and antinodes located by the symbols N and A, respectively. The subscript for each N or A indicates the formant number for which the associated region is a node or antinode. For example, N_1 is a node, or volume velocity maximum, for the first formant F1. The effect of a vocal tract constriction is to

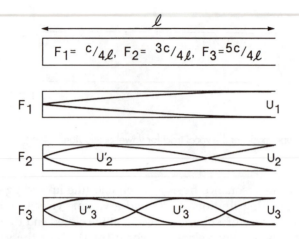

FIGURE 2–13. Straight-tube model of the vocal tract showing spatial distribution of volume velocity for each of the first three formants. U indicates a volume velocity maximum.

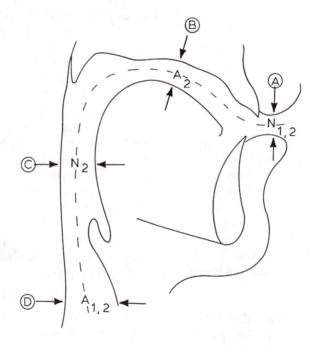

FIGURE 2–14. Drawing of vocal tract showing nodes (N) and antinodes (A) for volume velocity distribution (or the inverse, pressure distribution). Subscripts indicate formant numbers.

change the formant frequencies from those for the neutral vowel according to the relationships just described. A constriction at Node A tends to lower both F1 and F2 (in fact, all formant frequencies are lowered by lip constriction). A constriction at Antinode B raises F2. A constriction at Node C lowers F2. Consider how these relations apply to individual vowels. Vowel /i/ (*he*) has a constriction in the palatal region (near Antinode B) and therefore has a high F2 frequency. The vowel /ɑ/ (*ha*) has a constriction in the pharyngeal region (near Node C) and therefore has a low F2 frequency. The vowel /u/ has a labial constriction (near Node A) and therefore has lowered frequencies of both F1 and F2. In this way, perturbation theory allows a prediction of the effects of constriction of the vocal tract on the formant frequencies for the resulting configuration.

As a final way of showing the predictions of perturbation theory, Figure 2–15 illustrates how the location of a constriction along the length of a single-tube resonator affects F1, F2, and F3 frequencies. A positive sign indicates that the constriction at that point raises the formant frequency and a negative sign indicates that the constriction at that point lowers the formant frequency. Notice in particular the following effects:

1. All three formant frequencies are lowered by labial constriction.

2. All three formant frequencies are raised by a constriction near the larynx.

3. The curve for F2 has a negative region corresponding to the tongue constriction for /ɑ/ and a positive region corresponding to the tongue constriction for /i/.

4. The curve for F3 has negative regions corresponding to constrictions at the lips, the palate, and the pharynx. (This result is helpful in understanding the different articulations of the American English /r/, which can be rounded, is sometimes produced with a palatal constriction and sometimes with a pharyngeal constriction—all three of these constrictions are associated with a lowering of F3.)

The first conclusion deserves additional comment. It was mentioned previously that lip rounding tends to lower all formant frequencies because rounding usually lengthens the vocal tract. But some speakers accomplish a lowering of formant frequencies merely by constricting the lips without protrusion. How is this possible? Examination of Figures 2–13, 2–14 and 2–15 gives the answer: the lips are a volume velocity maximum for each formant; therefore, constriction in this region will lower all formant frequencies. In fact, there are three general ways by which a speaker can accomplish a lowering of all formant frequencies: (1) protrude the lips to lengthen the vocal tract, (2) constrict the

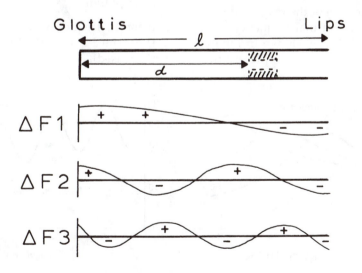

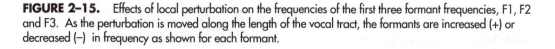

FIGURE 2–15. Effects of local perturbation on the frequencies of the first three formant frequencies, F1, F2 and F3. As the perturbation is moved along the length of the vocal tract, the formants are increased (+) or decreased (−) in frequency as shown for each formant.

lips, and (3) lower the larynx, an action that also lengthens the vocal tract.

Formant Amplitudes

Recall that the vocal tract, like all pipe resonators, has an infinite number of resonance frequencies. But because most of the laryngeal energy that activates the resonances is at frequencies below about 5 kHz, the usual discussion of vowel formants is limited to the lowest four or five formants, F1, F2, F3, F4, and F5. However, the higher formants cannot be neglected without introducing errors into acoustic analysis of the vocal tract. Following Fant, we can consider the formants of vowel production in terms of the graph shown in Figure 2–16. Each of the first four formants is shown as a resonance curve. In addition, a single curve could show the contributions from the larynx source, the vocal tract radiation, and the higher formants. The acoustic output of the vocal tract for the formant configuration shown in Figure 2–16 can be determined by algebraically adding the separate curves. That is, the output spectrum at one frequency, say 1 kHz, is the sum of the magnitudes of the separate curves at that frequency. An example of the result is shown in Figure 2–16. The first formant is typically the

most intense formant, largely because of the interaction with the amplitudes of the other formants. One way of thinking about it is to say that F1 rides on the low-frequency tails of the other formant curves, so that F1 is boosted in amplitude relative to the other formants.

Note that the vowel spectrum represented in Figures 2–16 corresponds to the neutral vowel, which has an equal spacing of its formant frequencies. According to perturbation theory described earlier, this neutral vowel may be taken as the starting configuration upon which local perturbations (constrictions) are introduced. Perturbation theory predicts the change in formant frequencies that results from a local constriction. The formant frequency changes, in turn, can be used to predict changes in the formant amplitudes. In other words, the amplitude relations among the formants depend on their frequency relations.

The general principles can be stated quite simply:

1. If the F1 frequency is lowered (raised), then higher formants decrease (increase) in amplitude.

2. If the F1 frequency is lowered (raised), then the F1 amplitude is decreased (increased).

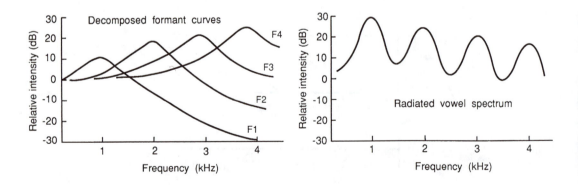

FIGURE 2–16. Decomposed formants (left) and their combination in a radiated vowel spectrum (right).

3. If two formants are moved more closely together in frequency, then both peaks increase in amplitude.

These principles follow directly from the algebraic additions performed on resonance curves such as those in Figure 2–16. For example, when the F1 frequency is lowered, the amplitudes of the higher formants are reduced because they then ride on a smaller magnitude of the F1 curve. In like fashion, F1 will itself lose amplitude because it then rides on lower magnitudes of the other formant tails.

Several examples of amplitude relations for English vowels are shown in Figure 2–17. The central conclusion is that formant amplitude relations are determined by formant frequencies. The dependency of resonance amplitudes on resonance frequencies is characteristic of resonators that are connected in series (one after the other). The output of one resonator is the input to the next, so that they interact in determin-

ing the relative amplitudes of the resonance peaks in the output spectrum.

Parametric Descriptions of Vowel Articulation

Many efforts have been made to simplify the description of the vocal tract configurations for vowels relative to their acoustic output. Stevens and House (1955) and Fant (1960) described three-parameter models of the vocal tract shape for vowels based on (a) location of the constriction, (b) size of the constriction, and (c) the ratio of mouth opening to length. Nomograms relating the first three formant frequencies with the three parameters of the Stevens and House model are illustrated in Figure 2–18. This simple description based on three parameters captures significant information about vowel articulation and predicts fairly well the acoustic signal generated by a given vocal tract shape. Fant

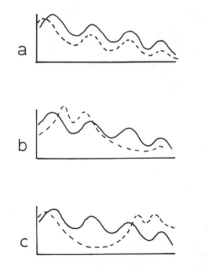

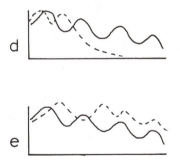

FIGURE 2–17. Effects of selected changes in formant frequency on the amplitude relations of the formants. The solid line in each drawing represents the neutral vowel. (a) As the frequency of F1 is decreased, all formant amplitudes are reduced. (b) As the frequencies of F1 and F2 draw more closely together, their amplitudes are increased. (c) As the frequency of F1 decreases and the frequencies of F2 and F3 come together, there is an overall reduction in the spectrum but a mutual strengthening of F2 and F3. (d) As the frequencies of F1 and F2 are decreased, all formants tend to lose amplitude but there is some mutual strengthening of F1 and F2. (e) As the frequency of F1 increases, all formant amplitudes increase.

(1960) generated nomograms based on variations in the three control parameters of a four-cavity model of the vocal tract. Badin, Perrier, Boe, and Abry (1990) extended this idea to identify what they called *focal points*, or regions in which formant convergences occur and where formant-cavity affiliations are exchanged. Badin and colleagues noted that the extreme cardinal vowels /i ɑ u/ are focal points.

Statistical approaches also have been taken to the problem of obtaining simplified descriptions of vowel articulation (Harshman, Ladefoged & Goldstein, 1977; Kiritani, 1977; Liljencrants, 1971; Maeda, 1990). One of the most powerful of these is the use of factor analysis to derive a small set of variables most important for describ-

ing vowel articulation. Generally, factor analytic studies indicate that vowel articulation can be described with two tongue factors, a lip factor and perhaps a jaw factor.

Another direction in modeling vowel articulation is to represent the articulatory organs as independently controllable functional blocks, or solid articulatory structures (Coker, 1976; Lindblom & Sundberg, 1971; Mermelstein, 1972; Rubin, Baer, & Mermelstein, 1981). The model developed by Mermelstein is shown in Figure 2–19. A principal aim of this work is to reduce the number of degrees of freedom in modeling vowel articulation compared to that required for an acoustic tube model of the vocal tract that is quantized into sections of 0.5 or 1.0 cm in length. In addition, such a

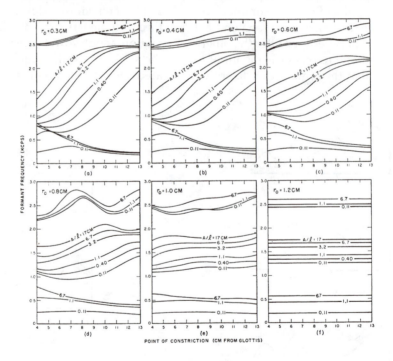

FIGURE 2–18. Nomograms relating the parameters of the Stevens and House model of vowel articulation to the output formant frequencies. The curves show the frequencies of the first three formants as a function of r_o, d_o, and A/1. In each section data are presented for a given degree of constriction (r_o) as indicated, with mouth opening (A/1) as the parameter. Three families of curves corresponding to F1, F2, and F3 are plotted in each section. The abscissa is d_o, the distance from the glottis to the point of the constriction. Reprinted from K.N. Stevens and A.S. House, "Development of a quantitative description of vowel articulation," *Journal of the Acoustical Society of America, 27,* 1955, 484–493. (Reprinted with the permission of the American Institute of Physics.)

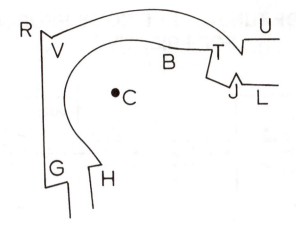

FIGURE 2–19. Components of an articulatory model for speech production. J = jaw, H = hyoid bone, C = center of tongue body, B = point where blade attaches to tongue body, T = tip of tongue, U = upper lip, L = lower lip, V = velum, R = rear-pharyngeal wall, and G = glottal region (periarytenoid area). After Mermelstein, 1973.

model has the potential of reflecting the biomechanical properties of the articulators, thereby simulating the natural process of speech.

Summary of the Source-Filter Theory for Vowels

The vibration of the vocal folds produces the energy source known as voicing. This source has a harmonic spectrum in which the energy of the harmonic components falls off roughly at the rate of 12 dB/octave. This energy activates the resonances (formants or poles) of the vocal tract. The resonances act like a filter, such that the energy in the various harmonics of the source is not transmitted equally. Although there are theoretically an infinite number of formants, we will concern ourselves primarily with the first three, F1, F2, and F3. As the acoustic energy is radiated from the lips, the output spectrum also is influenced by a high-pass filter effect known as the radiation characteristic.

Fricatives

Turbulence and the Reynolds Number

The simplified model for vowels was taken to be a straight pipe. The corresponding simplified model for fricatives is a pipe with a severe constriction (Figure 2–20). The constriction functions as a nozzle. Air exiting from a constriction in a conduit forms a jet. As this jet mixes with the surrounding air, turbulence is generated. Turbulence is associated with the generation of eddies that form in the flow in the vicinity of the contraction and expansion of the conduit. The eddies are volume elements of air that perform rotations, or irregular, high-frequency fluctuations in velocity and pressure at a given point in space. For a constriction or obstruction of given dimensions, there is a critical flow velocity above which turbulence noise is generated. The critical flow velocity at which turbulence occurs is given by the *Reynold's number*:

MODEL OF TURBULENCE NOISE PRODUCTION FOR FRICATIVES

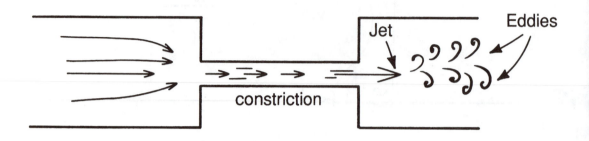

FIGURE 2–20. Model for turbulent noise production in fricatives. The vocal tract has a narrow constriction at some point along its length..

$Re = vh/v$

where v = flow velocity,

v = kinematic coefficient of viscosity (about 0.15 cm^2/s for air), and

h = characteristic dimension (for flow through an orifice, h is on the order of the diameter of the orifice)

As Re increases, an initial region of laminar flow will pass through an unstable region and finally through a condition of full turbulence.

Because volume flow, U (cm^3/s), is given by

$U = vA$ (A is cross-sectional area)

the Reynold's number can be calculated as

$Re = Uh/Av$

The volume flow U depends on the constriction size and the driving pressure (subglottal pressure), Ps:

$U = kA \sqrt{Ps}$ (where k = constant)

Then

$$Re = Uh /Av$$
$$= kA \sqrt{Ps} \, h /Av$$
$$= kh \sqrt{Ps} /v$$

Turbulence is the source of acoustic energy for various speech sounds, including fricatives, the frication portion of affricates, and the burst of stops. The random pressure fluctuations of the turbulent field generate sound. Volume velocities for fricative consonants lie in the range of 100 to 1000 cm^3/s. The critical Reynold's number for speech noise is Re > 1800.

Shadle (1990) concluded from modeling studies that there are at least two major ways in which sound is generated for fricative consonants. The first she termed an *obstacle source*. In this case, sound is generated primarily at a rigid body approximately normal to the flow. For the palatal fricative /ʃ/, the lower teeth seem to form the obstacle. In the case of the alveolar fricative /s/, the obstacle may be the upper teeth. The obstacle source may be likened to a spoiler in a duct. A spoiler is an obstruction, such as a flap in the direction of airflow. According to Shadle, an obstacle source is associated with a maximum source amplitude for a given flow velocity, by a relatively flat spectrum that falls off with increased frequency, and by a maximum rate of change of sound pressure with volume velocity.

The second source of sound is a *wall source*, which applies to situations in which sound is generated primarily along a relatively rigid wall that runs essentially parallel to the flow. Examples of this kind of sound generation are the fricatives /xç/. The wall source is associated with a high (but less than maximum) source amplitude for a given flow velocity, by a spectrum that possesses a broad peak, and by a high (but not maximum) rate of change of sound pressure with volume velocity. Shadle suggests that the wall source is really a distributed source, unlike the obstacle source, which can be modeled as a series pressure source located at the obstacle.

Ladefoged and Maddieson (1986) proposed that fricatives could be identified as either obstacle or no-obstacle cases. Obstacle fricatives were considered to be stridents (high-intensity fricatives like /s/), and no-obstacle fricatives as nonstridents (low-intensity fricatives like /θ/). Shadle (1990) cautions against the appealing simplicity of this classification, noting that many factors have to be considered in characterizing sound sources. She points out that there may be a continuum ranging from obstacle to wall source, given that the angle of the configuration relative to the airflow is the critical factor.

Modeling Fricative Production

The major steps in producing a fricative sound are to (1) make a constriction somewhere in the vocal tract, and (2) force air at high velocity through the constriction. Note that these conditions relate to the formula given for the Reynolds number. When the physical conditions are satisfied, turbulent flow is generated in the vicinity of the constriction and also at the teeth in some cases (specifically the cases that Shadle, 1990, called obstacle sources). The turbulent flow is characterized by eddies of particle motion (Figure 2–20) and is the source of turbulence noise. This noise excites the acoustic tube that forms the constriction and also the cavities anterior to the constriction. Under certain condi-

tions, there may be an acoustic coupling to the cavities posterior to the constriction, so these cavities also are excited. Figure 2–21 shows a vocal tract configuration for the fricative sound /s/ and a two-cavity model for this sound. The dot near the constriction in both the vocal tract configuration and the two-cavity model represents the location of the noise source.

In the following discussion, a different terminology will be introduced, but the concepts are basically the same as those presented for vowels. The new terms *pole* and *zero* will be used in discussing the transfer function.

Like vowels, fricatives can be described mathematically in terms of a transfer function. For fricatives, the function is

$$T(f) = [P(f)\ Z(f)]\ R(f),$$

where T(f) is the transfer function,

f is frequency,

P(f) is a function that contains the natural frequencies of vocal tract (poles or formants),

R(f) is the radiation characteristic, and

Z(f) is a function containing the zeros (antiformants), which occur at frequencies at which the source is decoupled from the front cavities

The functions P(f) and R(f) are the same as they would be for a similar vowel sound. The poles are simply the resonance frequencies (what we termed formants for the earlier discussion of vowels). The pole function P(f) for the fricative is approximately the same as that for a vowel produced with a similar vocal tract shape. Because the poles are natural frequencies of the tract, they do not depend on the location of the source of energy. The radiation function R(f) is as described for vowels. So far, the concepts are not much different for fricatives than they were for vowels. But the function Z(f) is new. The function Z(f) represents zeros. Zeros are

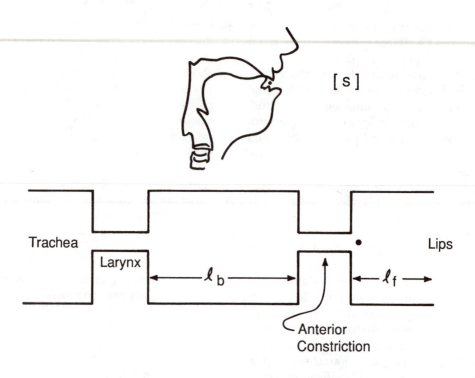

FIGURE 2–21. An idealized vocal tract model for the fricative /s/. The model has a trachea, a laryngeal constriction, a back cavity, an articulatory constriction, and a front cavity.

effective opposites of poles; they result in a loss of energy transmission. Like poles or formants, zeros have a center frequency and a bandwidth. When a pole and a zero have exactly the same frequency and bandwidth, they cancel each other. Zeros are most easily understood in terms of *impedance,* or the opposition to sound transmission. An engineer might say that zeros occur at frequencies for which the driving-point impedance of the vocal tract behind the noise source is infinite. In other words, the opposition to energy transmission through the front cavity is so great compared to that in the back cavity that the energy is short-circuited in the back cavity. Another way of putting it is that the back cavity traps all of the energy in the frequency region of the zero. As a result, the sound is not radiated into the atmosphere.

What causes zeros to occur in speech production? Basically, zeros arise for two reasons: (1) the vocal tract is bifurcated, or split into two passages (such as an oral passage and a nasal passage), or (2) the vocal tract is radically constricted at some point. It is for the second reason that fricatives involve zeros in their transfer function.

For the average male vocal tract, the poles occur at an average of 1 kHz separation, determined by the length of the vocal tract from glottis to lips. But because the noise source (articulatory constriction) usually is posterior to the mouth opening, the average spacing of the zeros is greater than 1 kHz. If a long narrow constriction is formed near the mouth opening, some of the poles and zeros tend to move together in pairs, so that their effects cancel. Recall that a pole and zero of the same frequency and bandwidth cancel one another.

However, the average spacing of the zeros is greater than that of the poles, and therefore the cancellation is not complete over the frequency range. The poles and zeros tend to cancel at frequencies less than the frequency for which the constriction length is a quarter wavelength. Above this frequency is a region containing more poles than zeros and in which the poles and zeros are separated. Normally, the first pole is heavily damped and therefore does not affect the output spectrum to a great degree.

Another way of stating matters is that cancellation occurs because the coupling between source and back cavities is small. Therefore, the influence of the back cavities can be neglected, and the zeros are determined only by the constriction. This rule breaks down under certain conditions such as when the back cavity has a tapered shape leading into the constriction. In this condition, the back cavity is not decoupled from the source.

The effect of the front cavity is largely determined by its length (l_f) as shown in Figure 2–21. When the front cavity is very short, as in the case of the labiodental fricatives /f v/, its lowest resonance frequency is too high to offer appreciable shaping of the noise energy. Consequently, the spectrum for these fricatives is flat or diffuse, lacking prominent peaks or valleys. But as the place of articulation moves backward in the oral cavity, the length of the front cavity increases, and its lowest resonance frequency decreases. In the case of the fricative

/s/, the lowest resonance frequency is around 4 kHz for a man. This value can be calculated from the assumption that the front cavity for /s/ is about 2 cm in length. Then, using the odd-quarter wavelength relationship discussed at the opening of this chapter, the first (lowest) resonance of the front cavity should be c/4l or 35,000 cm/s divided by 4×2 cm, or about 4 kHz. Spectral shaping for the /s/ is such that prominent regions of noise energy contrast with regions of much weaker energy. The relations between fricative articulation and fricative spectra are shown in Figure 2–22 for labiodental (or bilabial), linguadental, lingua-alveolar, and, linguapalatal fricatives. The caption for each illustration describes the relationships between the vocal tract configuration and the spectral pattern of each sound. Additional spectral characteristics are described more fully in a later chapter.

As noted earlier, there are conditions in which the back cavity is coupled to the front cavity, in which case the resonances of the back cavity cannot be neglected. The back cavity can be likened to a tube closed at both ends. For this kind of tube, the resonances are given by

$$Fn = (n) \ (c/2l)$$
$$e.g., c/2l, c/l, 3c/2l,...$$

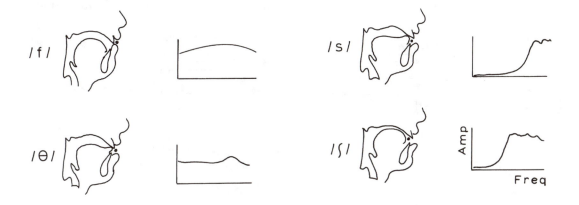

FIGURE 2–22. Articulatory-acoustic relationships for the four fricatives /f/ (fin), /θ/ (thin), /s/ (sin), and /ʃ/ (shin). The dot indicates the approximate location of the noise source. The length of the front cavity is a major determinant of the resonant shaping of the frication noise.

If the back cavity has a length of 10 cm, then it would have resonances of about 1750 Hz, 3500 Hz, and so on.

We have seen that fricatives can be modeled as a pressure source of either the obstacle or wall type that activates the resonances and antiresonances of a simple two-cavity model. When the two cavities are uncoupled, then the major filtering effects are exerted by the front cavity, which has resonance frequencies that can be approximated as those of a tube closed at one end and open at the other (i.e., the odd-quarter wavelength relationship, $f_n = (2n-1) c/4l$). When the two cavities are coupled, as is likely to happen if the constriction is gradually tapered, then the back cavity also contributes to the filtering effects. This cavity can be modeled as a tube closed at both ends, therefore having resonance frequencies at integer multiples of $c/2l$.

Nasals

The nasal sounds include nasalized vowels and the nasal consonants (English /m/, /n/, and /ŋ/). The essential articulatory property of a nasal sound is that the velopharyngeal port is open so that sound energy can pass through both the nasal tract and the oral tract (for nasal vowels) or through only the nasal tract (for nasal consonants). These two vocal tract configurations can be modeled quite simply, as shown in Figure 2–23. Both models involve a side-branch resonator, meaning that one resonator is coupled to another at the velopharyngeal port. In the case of the nasal vowel, both resonators open to atmosphere. In the case of the nasal consonant, the nasal resonator opens to atmosphere while the oral resonator is closed.

For both nasal vowels and consonants, the transfer function consists of poles and zeros. As noted earlier, a bifurcation or splitting of the resonating system introduces zeros into the transfer function. The zeros interact with poles in various ways depending on their frequencies and bandwidths. When a pole and zero have exactly the same frequency and bandwidth, they cancel. When poles and zeros have different frequencies, then they can contribute to a spectrum that reflects their combined influence. Generally, a spectral peak reflects a pole and a deep valley reflects a zero. However, this generalization has exceptions and should be used as only a rough rule of thumb in interpreting spectra for sounds known to have poles and zeros in their transfer functions.

As was the case with fricatives, nasals can be understood in part through a consideration of the average spacing of formants and antiformants. It was discussed earlier that the formants for oral sounds

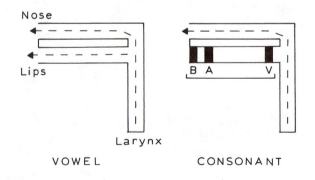

FIGURE 2–23. Simplified vocal tract models for a nasalized vowel and nasalized consonants. The nasalized vowel has open oral and nasal cavities. The nasalized consonant has an oral closure — B(ilabial); A(lveolar) or V(elar)—and an open nasal cavity.

such as vowels, depend on the tract length from glottis to lips, or $(l_p + l_o)$, which has a value of about 17.5 cm for adult males. For this vocal tract length, the formants have an average spacing of about 1 kHz. The formants of the nasal cavity depend on the length of the cavity extending from the uvula to the nares (l_n in Figure 2–23), which is about 12.5 cm in adult males. These formants have an average spacing of $c/2l_n = 1400$ Hz. The antiformants of the nasal cavity also depend on the length of the nasal cavity and have an average spacing of $c/2l_n = 1400$ Hz. Taking these various resonance phenomena together, we see that the combined oral-nasal system has a set of oral formants, a set of nasal formants, and a set of nasal antiformants. Fant described nasalized vowels as being like oral vowels with the effects of nasalization added like a distortion. That is, the nasal formants and antiformants are added to the oral formants of the original nonnasal vowel to yield a complex output spectrum. Additional details on the differences between nonnasal and nasal vowels will be provided later; it is sufficient here

to note simply the general model by which nasalization can be understood.

A somewhat more technical explanation is needed to understand the frequencies of the formants and antiformants of nasal sounds. As shown in Figure 2–24, the configuration for a nasal consonant can be considered as three cavities: a pharyngeal cavity, a nasal cavity, and a mouth cavity. Each cavity can be associated with a susceptance, its capacity to draw energy. Susceptance is the reciprocal of reactance, or opposition to energy. An internal susceptance B_i is defined as the sum of the pharyngeal susceptance, B_p and the nasal susceptance B_n. Formants occur when $B_i = -B_m$ (where m = mouth). At these frequencies, energy is passed effectively through the system and radiated outside. Antiformants occur when $B_m = \infty$ (infinity). At these frequencies, the mouth cavity acts as a short circuit, effectively trapping the energy and preventing its radiation through the nasal cavity.

That is, when the oral cavity is closed at some point for a nasal consonant, the frequencies of the antiformants are the fre-

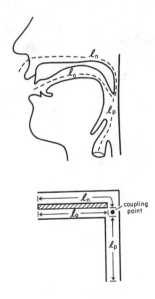

FIGURE 2–24. Illustration of the major dimensions that determine the transfer function for a nasalized vowel: l_n is the length of the nasal cavity; l_o is the length of the oral cavity; and l_p is the length of the pharyngeal cavity.

quencies at which the mouth cavity short-circuits transmission through the nose. Energy at these frequencies does not pass through the nasal cavity. The nasals /m/, /n/, and /ŋ/ are characterized by low (750-1250 Hz), medium (1450-2200 Hz), and high (above 3000 Hz) antiformant positions, respectively. The general rule is that as the place of oral articulation moves back, the frequency of the antiformant increases. A low-frequency formant, the so-called *nasal formant*, occurs at about 250-300 Hz. Higher formants are densely packed, have large bandwidths, and vary with place of articulation. To a first approximation, formants occur at about 250, 1000, 2000, 3000, and 4000 Hz. Specific details on nasal consonants will be presented in Chapter 6.

Stops

A stop involves a complete closure of the vocal tract and, depending on its phonetic context, a release of the closure and a movement toward another vocal tract configuration. The closure is associated with acoustic silence (although weak voicing energy might be detected if the stop is voiced). During the closure interval, air pressure is impounded in the mouth. Upon release of the constriction, the pressure is abruptly released. The acoustic evidence of this release is a burst or transient. The burst is a noise segment similar to the

noise segment for a fricative but much briefer. For example, the burst for the alveolar stop /t/ as in *tea* is similar to a brief version of the frication segment for the alveolar /s/ in *sea*. Particularly if the stop is followed by a vocalic sound, the burst is followed by another acoustic interval, the transition. During this interval, the vocal tract is adjusted from its closure state to another configuration. Most of the change in vocal tract configuration is accomplished within about 50 msec. In the case of a voiced stop, this transition interval is characterized by a rapidly changing formant pattern. The exact nature of this change will be discussed at length in Chapter 6.

These events in stop production can be modeled as shown in Figure 2–25 as a vocal tract closure, a burst, and a rapid transition to the configuration of the following sound. Some acoustic features of these three phases are:

Vocal tract closure: The primary acoustic correlate is silence, except for voiced stops, for which voicing energy may extend for part or all of the closure interval. When voicing is present, it is associated with low-frequency energy in the lower harmonics of the voice source, especially the first harmonic or fundamental frequency. Theoretically, for a hard-walled tube the F1 frequency is zero during a period of vocal tract closure. But because the vocal tract is not really hard-walled, the F1 frequency does not actually

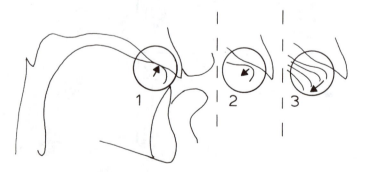

FIGURE 2–25. Major events in the production of stop consonants: (1) interval of vocal tract obstruction; (2) release of obstruction; and (3) articulatory transition into following sound.

reach zero but a value close to zero. Consequently, the F1 frequency associated with any severe constriction of the vocal tract is of very low frequency. As the constriction is released, the F1 frequency rises to a value appropriate for the following sound.

Burst: The transient noise is shaped spectrally in accord with the resonance properties of the vocal tract. To a first approximation, the noise resembles that of a homorganic fricative. Therefore, the burst for /t/ is somewhat like the frication for /s/. As will be discussed in Chapter 6, the burst spectrum reflects place of articulation for the stop.

Transition: Because the articulatory movement from a stop to another sound (such as a vowel) usually is completed within about 50 ms, the transition is associated with a brief interval of changing formant pattern. The intepretation of formant-frequency changes is a major topic in acoustic phonetics and will be reviewed in Chapter 6.

Affricates

Affricates are similar to stops in having a two-phase production of vocal tract closure followed by a noisy release. However, affricates have a frication segment that is intermediate in duration between the burst for stops and the frication interval for fricatives. The diagram in Figure 2–25 therefore applies to the production of affricates as well as to stops. The basic theory of affricate production is a modification of that presented for stops and fricatives. That is, an affricate can be modeled in two phases, first as a stop and then as a fricative.

Liquids

The liquids in English are the lateral /l/ and the rhotic /r/. They combine features of other sounds discussed so far. Both are sim-

ilar to vowels in that they have well-defined formant patterns and voiced energy.

Lateral consonants, such as English /l/, have both formants and antiformants and are therefore similar to nasal consonants. Laterals usually involve a splitting of the vocal tract around a midline constriction. The /l/ is produced with a midline apical constriction, which allows sound to radiate through openings at the sides. This midline bifurcation causes the formation of antiformants. The /l/ is acoustically similar to nasals in having a relatively low acoustic energy with a predominantly low-frequency concentration.

Rhotic consonants, like English /r/, have well-defined formant patterns but are typically less intense than surrounding vowels. The most consistent acoustic characteristic of English /r/ is a very low F3 frequency. More will be said about this feature in Chapter 6.

Diphthongs and Glides

Diphthongs and glides (semivowels) are similar to vowels, differing mainly in the presence of a dynamic characteristic, a change in vocal tract configuration. As the articulatory configuration changes, so does the acoustic pattern. Diphthongs and glides are associated with a gradually changing formant structure. The acoustic theory developed earlier for vowels applies in general form to any given configuration in the dynamic complex. For example, the diphthong /aɪ/ involves a series of vocal tract configurations running from the onglide [a] to the offglide [ɪ].

Nonlinear Theories

The linear source-filter theory has dominated the acoustic understanding of speech production for more than 30 years. It should be understood that the linear theory is an approximation, but this approximation has been remarkably successful. A great deal of progress in acoustic analysis and speech synthesis has been based on linear source-filter theory. But this is not to say that linear source-filter theory as described in this chapter will be sufficient to model all acoustic events in speech. Limitations of the theory must be evaluated in various applications. One important limitation is the assumption of independence of source and filter. In reality, source and filter do interact, and the nature of these interactions is an important area of current research. Linearity also may be questionable for some phenomena. Muscle and other tissues are inherently nonlinear, so that as biomechanical properties are modeled, nonlinear solutions may be the rule. It also should be recognized that the one-dimensional (longitudinal) propagation of sound waves in the vocal tract is expected for frequencies below about 5 kHz. At higher frequencies, cross-mode vibrations may occur when the wavelength approaches the cross-dimension of the vocal tract.

Teager and Teager (1990) argue that sound production in the vocal tract is neither linear nor passive. In fact, they assert that it is not even acoustic. In their view, important nonlinear sources of sound production have been neglected in the standard linear theory. The details of their argument go beyond the scope of this book. Suffice it to say that nonlinear processes of sound generation are thought to result from the interaction of sheet flows and flow vortices within the vocal tract. Nonlinearity also characterizes the newer theories of chaos and fractals, which are now being applied to accounts of long-term spectra (Voss & Clark, 1975), irregularities in vocal fold vibration (Baken, 1990) and turbulence (Frisch & Orszag, 1990).

Linear source-filter theory has been a highly productive theory, but its limitations and assumptions should be carefully evaluated for specific applications. Nonlinear theories may be more appropriate to certain phenomena and the development of these theories should be interesting to observe.

Summary

An understanding of the acoustic theory of speech production prepares the way for a discussion of speech analysis. Knowing the ways in which speech sounds are formed helps to determine appropriate analysis methods and measurements. For example, if a vowel segment is adequately characterized in terms of its formant pattern, then the analysis task is to determine the frequencies and bandwidths of the main formants for that segment. The acoustic theory also helps in relating acoustic measures for a sound segment to the underlying articulation of that segment. The object is to interpret a particular acoustic property with an articulatory correlate. In this sense, the acoustic theory of speech production is central to the analysis of speech. Certainly, one can make acoustic measures of speech without knowing theory, but the interpretation of these measures would be limited at best. Ideally, measurement and theory are closely coordinated.

Looking Ahead

The reader may wonder why reference is made so often in this chapter to the vocal tract of the adult male. The primary reason is that the early work on speech acoustics emphasized the male vocal tract, and much of the theoretical development was based on men's speech. Although occasional references were made in early studies of speech to women and children, it was only relatively recently that the effective scope of speech acoustics has broadened to include speakers of either gender and a range of ages. This matter will be taken up in Chapter 7 with a discussion of the differences among men's, women's, and children's speech.

Introduction to the Acoustic Analysis of Speech

3

CHAPTER

This chapter introduces the basic techniques for the acoustic analysis of speech, beginning with older nondigital, or analog, methods and concluding with a discussion of digitization. Chapter 4 continues the discussion of digital signal processing with a consideration of contemporary analysis procedures.

A Short History of the Acoustic Analysis of Speech

The power of modern computer methods in analyzing speech can be appreciated by taking a brief historical look at the acoustic analysis of speech. The historical review could begin well before the 20th century, but it is sufficient for our purposes to begin with the 1930s and 1940s. Figure 3–1 summarizes the developments since that time up to the present.

The Oscillogram

What might be called the modern history of the acoustic analysis of speech began with oscillograms (waveforms, or graphs of amplitude over time) of speech sounds. The sounds selected for analysis were often vowels, because they are relatively easier to analyze than most consonant sounds. The sounds to be analyzed were represented oscillographically as pressure variations over time. This first step was an important advance. Because speech sounds are perishable acoustic events of relatively short duration, representing these sounds in a permanent manner is a technical challenge. With the development of oscillographs based on string galvanometers, it became possible to derive fairly accurate waveforms of sustained vowels. The waveforms indicated certain regularities in these sounds, but were not in themselves sufficient to describe some of the important dif-

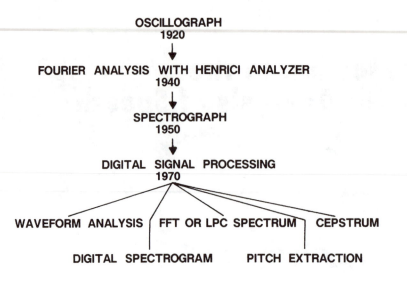

FIGURE 3-1.   Some historic developments in the acoustic analysis of speech. The approximate date of each development is noted.

ferences among vowels. Observation of these differences required the generation of spectral representations—that is, plots of signal energy versus frequency.

The Henrici Analyzer

The advantage of spectral analysis in studying speech is quite like the advantage of spectral analysis in studying light. In optical analysis, light is broken into components of different wavelengths. In the acoustic analysis of speech, sound is broken into components of different frequencies. Analysis is a matter of decomposition, or breaking the complex sound pattern into simpler constituents.

One of the earliest tools for spectral analysis was the Henrici Analyzer, a mechanical device consisting of five rolling integrating units (glass spheres). The procedure of analysis is as follows:

1. Obtain the oscillogram of the waveform.

2. Select a representative portion, typically in the middle of the wave, and enlarge it with a projector.

3. Trace the enlargement on a plain white surface.

4. Trace the enlarged waveform with the Henrici Analyzer.

5. Calculate the values of the amplitude and phase relationships from dial readings associated with the glass spheres.

6. Plot the pressure (in dB) against frequency to obtain spectral (harmonic) analysis.

As the operator traced the acoustic waveform with the analyzer, each sphere integrated a different partial or component of the wave. With each tracing, five harmonic components could be determined. This procedure performs a harmonic analysis and assumes that the sound to be analyzed is essentially periodic. But speech is not truly periodic. Rather, it is quasiperiodic (meaning almost periodic). Departures from true periodicity cause the Henrici Analyzer to give an inaccurate picture of the energy distribution in speech sounds. In addition, the analysis procedure was tedious. Nonetheless, the Henrici Analyzer played a significant role in the development of the modern understanding of speech acoustics. It foreshadowed the general approach of spectral analysis of speech. In addition, data derived from this technique contributed to ideas about distinctive energy concentrations in vowel sounds.

Filter Bank Analysis

Another approach to speech analysis was filtering. A filter is a frequency-selective transmission system. That is, a filter passes energy at certain frequencies but not at others. A filter is like an acoustic window that allows some energy to pass while blocking other energy. Figure 3–2 shows the application of a bank of filters to the analysis of speech. The energy of the signal is effectively divided into frequency bands by the filter bank. Each filter passes only the energy in its frequency band. Indicating devices at the output of each filter can be used to display the energy in

specific frequency regions. By analogy, in a pile of gravel a series of screens of different mesh size can be used to separate particle sizes. The largest pieces will be separated by the coarsest mesh, the next largest pieces by a somewhat finer mesh, and so on until the pile has been redistributed into several smaller piles according to particle size. Details of filter operation will be discussed in following chapters. For the present, it suffices to say that a filter allows a selective look at the energy in various frequency regions.

A filtering analysis of speech determines the amount of energy in specific frequency regions. Therefore, it results in a kind of spectral analysis. The detail of the analysis depends on the number of filters used and their bandwidths. The bandwidth of a filter is the frequency range in which it passes energy. For example, a filter centered at 100 Hz with a bandwidth of 10 Hz would pass only the energy at freqencies between 95 Hz and 105 Hz (105–95

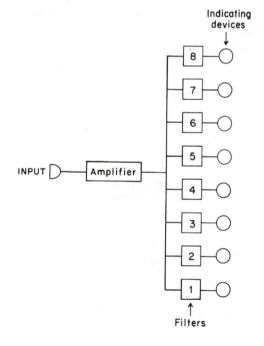

FIGURE 3–2. Schematic diagram of a filter bank for acoustic analysis. The filters numbered 1 through 8 pass successively higher frequency bands. Indicating devices at the output of each filter show the energy present in each band.

= 10 Hz). Usually, much larger bandwidths would be used, so that the entire frequency range of interest (say, 0–5 kHz) could be analyzed with fewer than 25 filters. Using a filter bandwidth of 500 Hz for all filters, a 5-kHz range could be analyzed with 10 filters. Figure 3–3 shows how such an arrangement of filters might analyze different vowels produced by an adult male speaker.

Another analysis technique is a variable band-pass filter (Figure 3–4). The idea is to use an adjustable filter that can act like any of the filters shown in Figure 3–2. The signal to be analyzed is fed repetitively through the variable band-pass filter as its settings are adjusted to different frequency regions. Practically, it is easier to modulate a variable carrier frequency with the signal to be analyzed and use a fixed filter for analysis (a process called heterodyning). In this case, the filter is not adjusted but the signal is effectively swept past it.

The Spectrograph

The variable band-pass filter was incorporated in the sound *spectrograph*, a machine developed in the 1940s. The spectrograph provided major advantages to the study of speech. Because it afforded a relatively fast analysis, the spectrograph made it possible for scientists to collect more extensive data. As a result, the pooling of data across subjects became more common. With earlier analysis techniques, data usually were obtained on a very small number of speakers, frequently one. The spectrograph also provided a better delineation of the energy concentrations in speech. Finally, the spectrograph produced a running short-term spectrum, enabling the scientist to visualize how energy concentrations changed in time. The display of the running short-term spectrum is called a *spectrogram*. Because of the strong impact that the spectrograph had on speech research, it is important to understand its essential features. These will be briefly reviewed below. The spectrographic analysis of various types of speech sounds is discussed in detail in later chapters.

The basic components of a spectrograph are shown schematically in Figure 3–5. A photograph of a spectrograph appears in Figure 3–6. The signal to be analyzed is recorded on a magnetic drum that allows a continuously repeating playback of the signal. The magnetic drum can be likened to a tape loop. The signal then modulates (multiplies) a variable carrier

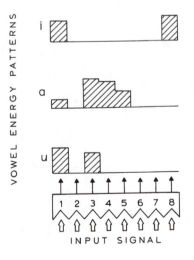

FIGURE 3–3. Hypothetical output of a simple filter bank when the three vowels /i/ (he), /a/ (ha), and /u/ (who) are presented as input. Each vowel has distinctive bands of energy.

frequency in a process called heterodyning (as mentioned earlier in reference to filter analysis). Heterodyning is used because it is more practical to sweep the signal to be analyzed past a fixed filter than to analyze the original signal with a variable filter. The end result is the same as if the signal were repeatedly played back through a filter that was continuously adjusted to act like a filter bank. In conventional spectrography, two filter bandwidths are used. The wide-band filter has an analyzing bandwidth of 300 Hz, and the narrow-band filter has an analyzing bandwidth of 45 Hz. Some spectrographs have other bandwidth selections, such as 90 Hz and 600 Hz. The selection of analyzing bandwidth is discussed in a later section.

The output of the analyzing filter is fed to a marking amplifier that provides an increase in the current. At any frequency region in the analysis, the current from the marking amplifier is proportional to the acoustic energy in the signal. The current flows through a stylus held in close contact with a piece of special paper that is wrapped around the spectrograph drum. As the drum and attached paper rotate, the stylus gradually moves up the drum in coordination with the analysis frequency. The coordination is accomplished by a mechanical linkage between the moving stylus and a variable oscillator. In this way, the vertical position of the stylus is associated with a particular frequency of analysis. The bottom of stylus travel is the lowest frequency (around 80 Hz) and the top of stylus travel is the highest frequency (around 8 kHz).

The current flowing through the stylus burns the special paper as it turns on the drum to produce a blackened region. The paper is treated so that the extent of burning is limited. In effect, the paper is charred locally as the current passes through it. Therefore, the blackness of the paper corresponds to the energy at that point in the analysis. Although controlled burning to produce a pattern may sound crude compared to modern high-technology visual displays, the idea was quite ingenious. The burning achieved two essential operations: (1) rectification of the electrical signal, so that both positive and negative parts of the waveform were represented in the analysis, and (2) a low-pass filtering (smoothing). The burning process produced an odor rarely described as fragrant and an accumulation of a fine black soot over the workspace.

The complete process, from recording to analysis, involves these steps:

1. The speech sample is transduced by a microphone so that air pressure variations of the acoustic signal are put into the form of voltage variations.

2. The electrical signal is then converted to an electromagnetic signal for storage on the magnetic drum of the spectrograph.

3. The stored magnetic pattern is converted back into an electrical signal for analysis as a spectrogram.

4. The signal is filtered so that the energy in various frequency regions can be determined.

5. The current of the electrical signal is amplified and fed to a marking stylus.

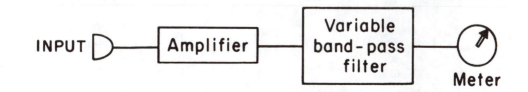

FIGURE 3–4.   Acoustic analysis using a variable band-pass filter. The filter is swept across the input signal to indicate the energy at various frequencies.

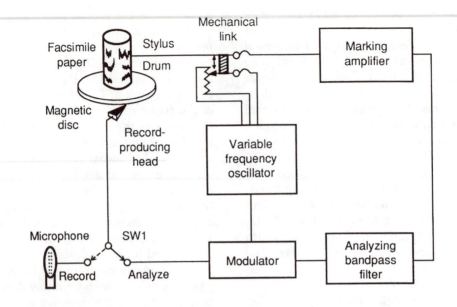

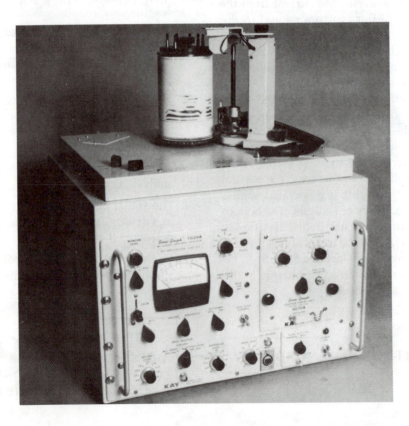

FIGURE 3–5. Schematic drawing of the components of a conventional sound spectrograph.

FIGURE 3–6. Photograph of a sound spectrograph produced in about 1980. Courtesy of Kay Elemetrics Corporation.

6. As the current flows from the stylus through the specially treated paper, a localized burning of the paper occurs. The burning produces a blackening of the paper in proportion to the current flowing through the stylus.

A sample of the finished product, the spectrogram, appears in Figure 3–7. The conventional spectrogram is a three-dimensional display of time, frequency, and intensity. Time appears on the horizontal axis, running from left to right. Frequency is plotted on the vertical axis, increasing from bottom to top. Intensity is represented by the blackness of the pattern (the so-called "gray scale"). Figure 3–8 shows spectrograms of three simple acoustic signals. Shown in Part A is the spectrogram of a sinusoid ("pure tone"). Because the sinusoid contains energy at a single frequency, the spectrogram displays a single narrow band running horizontally. The location of this band on the frequency (vertical) axis indicates the frequency of the sinusoid. Part B illustrates the spectrogram for a hissing noise. Because the noise contains frequency components at many different frequencies, most of the spectrogram is blackened to some degree. Part C shows a spectrogram

for a rapping noise made by knuckles on a table top. Each rap is a brief acoustic event (a transient) having energy over a fairly wide frequency range. Notice that each rap is distinctly represented on the spectrogram. The three spectrograms in Figure 3–8 show the usefulness of this form of analysis in determining how acoustic signals vary in time, frequency composition, and intensity.

Speech consists of a variety of sounds. The variations in acoustic properties can occur quite rapidly and it is for this reason that a running spectrum is a desirable form of display and analysis. The spectrogram shows how spectral energy changes over relatively brief intervals of time. The details of this analysis will be considered in Chapters 5 and 6, but it is appropriate to take an early look at the way in which a spectrogram reveals the acoustic features of some speech sounds. A sample spectrogram is shown in Figure 3–9. On the one hand, the spectrogram can depict the very brief energy associated with the explosive release of air in a stop consonant (the point labeled A in Figure 3–9). On the other hand, the spectrogram displays the prominent and often lengthy bands of energy that typify vowel productions (point B). When no sound is produced, as during the oral

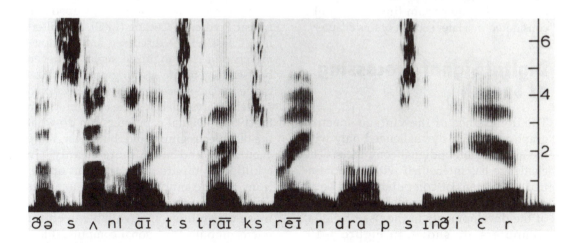

FIGURE 3–7. Sample spectrogram of the utterance "The sunlight strikes raindrops in the air." A phonetic transcript of the utterance appears at the bottom of the spectrogram.

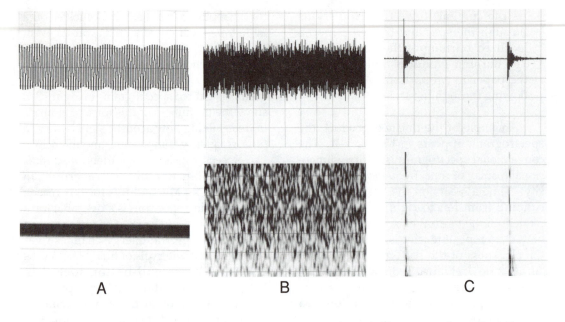

A   B   C

FIGURE 3–8. Sample spectrograms and corresponding waveforms for three types of sounds: (A) a sinusoid or pure tone with a frequency of 4 kHz; (B) a computer-generated noise; and (C) knuckles rapping on a table top.

closure for a stop consonant, the spectrogram reveals the silence (point C). And, when the vocal tract changes in its configuration during a gliding sound, the spectrogram portrays the corresponding acoustic change (point D). The spectrogram contains a great deal of acoustic information and it quickly became the standard for speech analysis, despite certain limitations to be considered in a later section of this chapter.

Digital Signal Processing of Speech

The dominance of the vintage spectrograph was seriously challenged only with the introduction of digital computers. The challenge has intensified with the continued refinement of computers (hardware) and analysis programs (software). Some of the developments in the use of digital computers are shown in Figure 3–10. These developments will be taken up in various chapters in this book. Once the speech signal has been put into a form suitable for storage and analysis by a computer, several different operations can be performed. The waveform can be displayed, measured, and even edited (for example, deleting one portion and connecting the remaining pieces together to make an entirely new sound). Spectra can be computed using methods such as the Fast Fourier Transform (FFT), Cepstrum, Linear Predictive Coding (LPC), and filtering. These will be discussed in the following chapter. The digitized signal can even be used to generate spectrograms like those made by the spectrographs that occupied speech analysis laboratories beginning in the 1950s. Digital computers can do what the old spectrographs did, but faster, more accurately and much more cleanly. In addition, computers can perform operations that go much beyond the analysis capabilities of the spectrograph. Many of these capabilities are available even for microcomputers (personal computers) like the Macintosh and the IBM PC-AT (and its clones). The rapid developments in speech analysis with microcomputers is a major

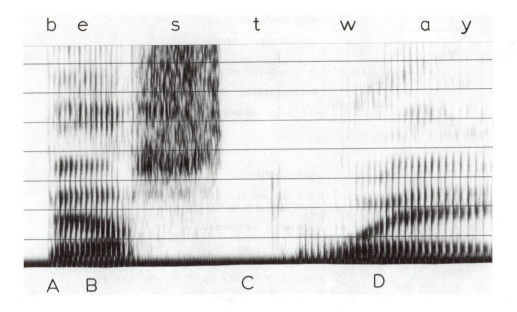

FIGURE 3–9. A spectrogram of the phrase, "best way," with labeled points corresponding to discussion in text.

reason for the preparation of this tutorial text. Although speech analysis systems are readily available for microcomputers, many users do not have sufficient background in digital processing to understand the capabilities and limitations of these systems. Both—capabilities and limitations—are significant.

Filtering, sampling, and quantization are the basic operations in digitizing a speech signal. Each operation has important consequences for the nature of the signal that is eventually stored in the computer. Consequently, the user of a digital processing system should have a good grasp of these operations. Many speech analysis systems allow the user to specify variables such as filter settings and sampling rate. Careful consideration should be given to these variables whenever a speech signal is digitized. In addition, the user of such systems may encounter a variety of issues related to amplification, cabling, and interfacing. A basic understanding of these issues can help to avoid problems and to ensure that a signal of suitable quality has been obtained.

The basic process in digitization is to convert a continuous (analog) signal to a digital (discrete) representation. The digital representation is a series of numbers. When an analog signal such as an acoustic waveform is digitized, two operations are performed simultaneously. The first is a discretization in time, meaning that the analog waveform is *sampled* at certain time points, usually periodically spaced. The periodic spacing is reflected in the *sampling rate*, which specifies the regularity of the sampling process. A sampling rate of 10 kHz means that the original analog signal is sampled 10,000 times per second. The second operation is a discretization of signal amplitude. This operation, called *quantization*, represents the continuous amplitude variation of the original signal as a series of levels or steps. Each level is a quantum, and the process of amplitude discretization is therefore one of quantization. Sampling and quantization are the essence of digitization.

The principal steps of the digital processing of speech are shown in Figure 3–11. The original acoustic signal of

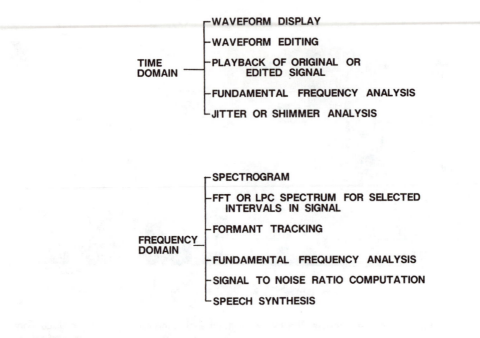

```
                  ┌─WAVEFORM  DISPLAY

                  ├─WAVEFORM  EDITING

    TIME          ├─PLAYBACK  OF  ORIGINAL  OR
    DOMAIN ───────┤            EDITED  SIGNAL

                  ├─FUNDAMENTAL  FREQUENCY  ANALYSIS

                  └─JITTER  OR  SHIMMER  ANALYSIS




                  ┌─SPECTROGRAM

                  ├─FFT  OR  LPC  SPECTRUM  FOR  SELECTED
                  │       INTERVALS  IN  SIGNAL

                  ├─FORMANT  TRACKING
    FREQUENCY ────┤
    DOMAIN
                  ├─FUNDAMENTAL  FREQUENCY  ANALYSIS

                  ├─SIGNAL  TO  NOISE  RATIO  COMPUTATION

                  └─SPEECH  SYNTHESIS
```

FIGURE 3–10.   Some developments in the use of digital methods for speech analysis.   These topics will be covered in the following chapters.

speech is represented by the function x(t), which is simply the speech waveform as might be obtained directly from a microphone or played from a tape recorder. The notation x(t) indicates a variable in time, specifically the amplitude by time variation of the acoustic signal. As noted previously, this waveform is an analog signal. Its amplitude varies continuously with time. To store this signal in a modern digital computer, the analog signal must be converted to a series of numbers. The numbers are then stored as a representation of the analog signal. This chapter considers the steps that are taken to convert the analog signal to a digital representation. The process is called *analog-to-digital conversion* and it is typically performed by an *analog-to-digital converter,* or A/D converter. The reverse operation of *digital-to-analog conversion* is the process by which the series of numbers stored in a computer are converted to an analog signal. This operation is performed by a D/A converter. Typically, systems for the acoustic analysis of speech use both A/D and D/A

converters. The A/D converter is used to convert an original analog signal to digital form. The D/A converter then is used to derive analog signals from the stored digital files, as is required if we wish to hear a digitally stored signal.

Filtering Operations

The first step in digital processing is a *preemphasis filtering* in which the high-frequency components of the signal are boosted in amplitude relative to the low-frequency components. Preemphasis is desirable, and often necessary, because most of the energy in speech is in the lower frequency range. This energy will tend to dominate the analysis unless some equalization of energy across frequency is attempted. There are two usual ways by which preemphasis is accomplished. One is the use of a filter (usually a hardware filter) that provides a 6 dB/octave increase to the speech signal above some breakpoint frequency, f_b, where f_b usually is

DIGITAL SPEECH PROCESSING

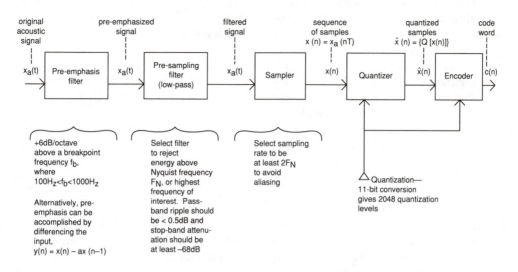

FIGURE 3–11. Major stages in the digital signal processing of speech. See text for discussion.

chosen to be above 100 Hz but less than 1000 Hz. The specification of 6 dB/octave means that for every doubling of frequency (octave) above the breakpoint, the energy increases by 6 dB. For example, a 6 dB boost would be given to energy at 2000 Hz compared to energy at 1000 Hz. The second way to achieve preemphasis is by *differencing* the input. This operation can be performed by the computer and is expressed by the following formula:

$$y(n) = x(n) - ax(n-1)$$
where $x(n)$ is a sample of the signal at time n,
$y(n)$ is the first-differenced signal,
and a is a constant of multiplication

Differencing depends on digital operations to be explained later. For the present, it is sufficient to realize that preemphasis can be accomplished either by operations on the analog acoustic signal $x(t)$ or by operations on the digitized signal $x(n)$. The two methods yield comparable results. There is a caution to be observed in the use of speech analysis systems. A system that accomplishes preemphasis by a differencing

computation should not be coupled to a hardware preemphasis filter, or the signal would be preemphasized twice—once by the hardware filter and again by the differencing operation.

The preemphasized signal is then fed to a *presampling filter*. This is a low-pass filter designed to reject energy above the highest frequency of interest. This filtering procedure is based on Nyquist's sampling theorem (Nyquist, 1928), which states that the number of samples needed to represent a signal is twice the highest frequency of interest in the signal. For example, assume that we are interested in analyzing the speech signal only to 10 kHz. This frequency is the upper limit of analysis and the low-pass filter would be selected to reject energy above this frequency. Filters have various characteristics that define their operation and two of these characteristics to be noted here are the *pass-band ripple* and the *stop-band attenuation*. As shown in Figure 3–12, the pass-band is the band of frequencies in which energy is passed with minimal loss. Many filters have a detectable ripple, or variation in transmission with frequency, within the pass-band. If the ripple is too large, it can distort the analysis of the signal. A useful rule of thumb is that the ripple should be less than 0.5 dB. The stop-band attenuation is a measure of the energy that remains in the region of the filter where energy transmission is minimal. This is the frequency band where energy transmission is most reduced, or filtered out. Filters usually do not succeed in rejecting all of the unwanted energy, however, and filters can be compared as to their ability to minimize the energy in the stop-band. For general applications in speech analysis, it is desirable to have a stop-band attenuation of at least –68 dB, meaning that the energy that remains in the stop band after filtering will be at least 68 dB below the energy peak in the pass-band. For the example under consideration, this means that the energy peaks within the pass-band of 0–10 kHz will be at least 68 dB more intense than any energy found within the stop-band.

Sampling

The signal, which is now preemphasized and low-pass filtered, is ready for digitization. Digitization really consists of two processes, sampling and quantization.

Sampling is the operation by which the analog signal is converted to a series of samples. This conversion can be expressed with the following notation:

$$x(n) = x(NT)$$
where $x(n)$ is a sequence of samples and T is the sampling interval

The basic process is to convert a continuously varying signal to a series of numbers that can be stored in a digital computer. As shown in Figure 3–13, the term sampling is descriptive of the actual operation. The original analog signal is sampled at regular intervals. The energy between the sampling points is discarded. It may seem strange that this operation occurs with no loss of information. After all, it appears that the original signal, with its infinite values along the time axis, is now reduced to a finite number of samples. But Nyquist's sampling theorem states that if the sampling rate is properly selected, the sampled signal contains the same information as the original analog signal. In other words, analog-to-digital conversion can be done without loss of information. This is a fundamental concept in the application of digital computers to the processing of speech or any signal originally in analog form.

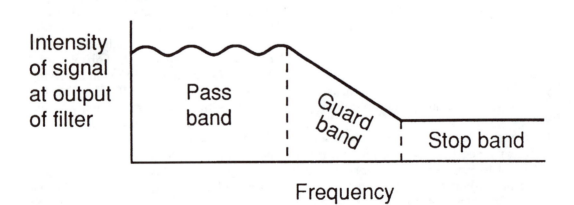

FIGURE 3–12. Frequency response of a low-pass filter. The passband is the frequency region in which energy is passed most effectively. The stop band is the region of maximum opposition (blockage) to signal transmission, and the guard band is an intervening region sometimes called the "skirt" of the filter.

How is the sampling rate selected to ensure that information is not lost? The guideline is quite simple: *The sampling rate should be at least twice the highest frequency of interest, which we will denote by F_S*. In our example, the highest frequency of interest is, $F_S = 10$ kHz. Therefore, the sampling rate should be 2×10 kHz > 20 kHz. If an analog signal that is low-pass filtered at 10 kHz is sampled at a rate of at least 20 kHz, the digitized signal will be equivalent in information to the original signal. It is important to remember this relation between the presampling filter and the sampling rate of digitization because serious errors can result if this relation is neglected. Now there is nothing really wrong about sampling at a *higher* rate. For instance, we could sample our 10-kHz low-pass filtered signal at 40 kHz or four times the value determined by Nyquist's sampling theorem. However, this high rate is usually unnecessary and will use twice as much computer memory.

But there *is* something wrong with sampling at a rate lower than twice the highest frequency of interest. When this happens, serious errors can develop in the analysis. These errors are called *aliasing*. The presampling filter is sometimes called an *anti-aliasing filter* in recognition of the need to prevent the errors of aliasing. In common usage, an alias is an assumed or false identity, and this is the essence of the error that can occur in digital processing when the sampling rate is too slow in relation to the frequency range of analysis. By way of illustration, let's consider an example from motion pictures. You probably have seen movies in which the wheels on a wagon or stage coach appeared to be moving *slowly backward* even as the horses were pulling forward at a considerable speed. The effect is most apparent with wheels that have spokes. Now, of course the wheels aren't really turning backward. Nor is this effect a visual illusion. The apparent slow, backward motion is an example of aliasing—an error in the sampling of the original event. In this case, the sampling rate is determined by the film rate of 30 frames per second, the usual rate in the motion picture industry. The spokes on the rotating wagon wheel alter their positions over time, but the relatively slow frame rate of the motion picture camera simply can't register the actual spoke positions during wheel rotation. As a result, the wheel may appear to be moving slowly in the wrong direction. What you see in the motion picture is an aliased, or false, identification of the actual dynamic event. The problem could be corrected by increasing the frame rate of the motion picture. However, increased frame rate isn't important for most of what we see on the screen, so the aliasing of stage coach wheel rotations is simply tolerated as a minor nuisance. But aliasing is not just a minor nuisance in digital signal processing. It can cause a seriously erroneous analysis.

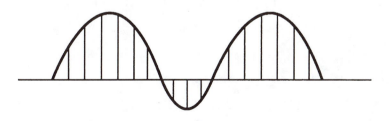

Sampled waveform

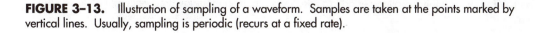

FIGURE 3–13.   Illustration of sampling of a waveform. Samples are taken at the points marked by vertical lines. Usually, sampling is periodic (recurs at a fixed rate).

Aliasing occurs if frequencies at greater than half the sampling frequency are sampled. For example, if a sampling frequency of 5 kHz is used to digitize signal components at greater than 2.5 kHz, aliasing can occur. The effect of aliasing is illustrated in Figure 3–14. The original signal—the signal to be sampled—is shown at the top of the illustration, and a sampled version of the signal is shown below. At the sampling rate represented by the vertical lines, the signal is undersampled. As a result, the sampling operation yields a false, or aliasing, signal shown at the bottom of the illustration. (Note that at half the sampling frequency, each cycle of a periodic signal is represented by two samples, which is the minimum number of samples that can represent the positive and negative portions of the sinusoidal waveform.)

One kind of aliasing error is the generation of *foldover frequencies* (Figure 3–15). This false frequency information occurs at a frequency given by:

$$F_f = S - F_n$$

where F_f is the foldover frequency,
S is the sampling rate, and
F_n is a frequency higher than half
the value of S

To avoid aliasing, these steps should be followed:

1. Determine the highest frequency of interest in analysis; this is F_s

2. Filter the energy above F_s; and

3. Sample the signal at a rate of at least $2F_s$

Other aliasing products can occur as well, but it is sufficient to note here that the entire problem of aliasing usually can be avoided if the sampling rate is carefully chosen in relation to the frequencies of interest in the original signal and if energy above the highest frequency of interest is filtered out. The major reason for the qualifier *usually* in the preceding sentence is

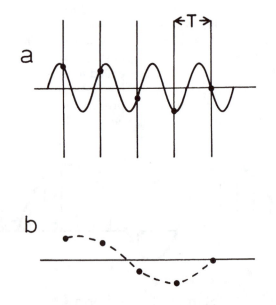

FIGURE 3–14. Graphic representation of aliasing due to undersampling of a signal. (a) Sampling at a rate of 1/T where T is the sampling period. (b) Generation of a spurious low-frequency signal, the aliasing signal.

that aliasing can also occur under another condition which results in something called granulation noise. Discussion of this issue will have to be postponed until the following discussion of quantization.

Quantization

Let's review what has happened so far. We began with a continuously variable acoustic signal denoted by x(t). Because this signal cannot be used in its original form by a digital computer, it has to be converted to a digital form—a sequence of numbers (samples). The sampling operation essentially chops the analog signal into a number of equal intervals. The size of the interval depends on the sampling rate. The higher the rate, the smaller the interval. For instance, at a sampling rate of 5 kHz, the interval between sampling points is 0.2 ms. At this rate, then, the analog signal is converted to a sequence of 5,000 samples in each second. We now have discrete entries appropriate for use by a digital computer except for one thing—the amplitude or energy level of the samples also must be converted to digital form. Sampling accomplished only part of the digitization operation, namely,

the conversion from continuous time to sampled or discrete time.

The remaining operation in digitization is called quantization. A signal is quantized when the samples determined by the sampling operation are chopped into a discrete number of amplitude levels. The term quantization is descriptive of what is done. A quantum is an increment of energy. When an analog signal is quantized, the continuous amplitude variations are converted to discrete values, or increments. The operation is illustrated in Figure 3–16 for various levels of quantization. Notice that if quantization is performed with only a few steps or levels, the quantized signal has a stair-step shape that only roughly resembles the original analog signal. However, as the levels of quantization are increased, the similarity between the quantized signal and the analog signal also increases. That is, the higher the number of quantization levels, the more accurately the quantized signal represents the analog signal. Of course, as the number of quantization levels increases, so does the need for memory to store the data. As a general rule of thumb, speech should be quantized with at least a 12-bit conversion, which provides 4,096 quantization levels. If too few levels of quantiza-

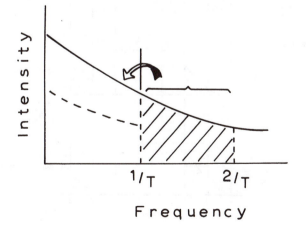

FIGURE 3–15. Graphic representation of aliasing as a "fold-over" frequency. Energy sampled at less than 2/T can appear as low-frequency energy.

tion are used, the signal will have a distortion called quantization noise. Note that with each additional bit of amplitude conversion, there is a doubling of levels of quantization, for example,

8 bits	256 levels
9 "	512 "
10 "	1,024 "
11 "	2,048 "
12 "	4,096 "

Conversion at 8 bits, as is sometimes done with low-cost systems, will produce a low-quality signal. For all but the crudest purposes in speech analysis, 8-bit conversion is inadequate. To understand what quantization means in terms of the original analog signal, the size of one level of quantization can be estimated by dividing the voltage range of the signal by 2 raised to the power N, where N is the number of levels of quantization. Suppose, for example, that the analog signal had a peak-to-peak voltage of $+/-5$ volts, or a total of 10 volts. If this signal is to be

quantized with 8 bits, then the voltage increment, v, for each level would be calculated as:

$$v = 10 \text{ volts} / 2^N$$
$$= 10 \text{ volts} / 256$$
$$= 0.039 \text{ volts, or } 39 \text{ millivolts}$$

This calculation assumes that the quantization levels are uniform (that is, of the same size).

The operation of quantization can be expressed fairly simply as a process of discretizing the continuous variations in signal energy that remain after the sampling operation:

$$x(n) = x(n) + e(n)$$
where $x(n)$ is the quantized sample,
           $x(n)$ is the unquantized
           sample, and
           $e(n)$ is the error or noise in
           quantization

The object is to minimize $e(n)$—that is, to make it small enough that it doesn't cause

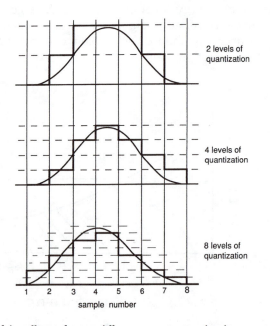

2 levels of
quantization

4 levels of
quantization

8 levels of
quantization

1   2   3   4   5   6   7   8
sample number

FIGURE 3–16.   Illustration of the effects of using different quantization levels to represent a smooth waveform. As the number of levels increases, the fit to the smooth curve improves.

problems in analysis or signal quality.

Several choices of quantization are available. Perhaps the simplest is uniform quantization in which the steps or increments are of equal size across the range of signal energy. One disadvantage to this approach is that the speech signal has a large dynamic range (the range from lowest to highest signal energy in a sample) and speakers vary considerably in their use of this range. If the dynamic range of analysis is adjusted to the most intense portion of a speech sample, while employing a uniform quantization the quantization steps for the weaker portions of the sample may be too coarse. Therefore, preference may be given to a nonuniform quantization in which the quantization increments are smaller in the low-energy range of the signal. In addition, the signal can be transformed in various ways before quantization is accomplished. For example, one might use a logarithmic transformation of the signal to achieve finer increments for weaker components. But it should be noted that quantization is inherently a nonlinear operation. Unlike sampling, which is securely based on the sampling theorem, quantization is a very difficult concept mathematically.

After the operations of sampling and quantization, the signal has been digitized as a series of quantized samples. Mathematically, we can express this process as follows:

$$x(n) = \{Q[x(n)]\}$$

where $x(n)$ are the quantized samples corresponding to the original waveform $x(t)$,

Q is the quantization operation, and

$x(n)$ is the sequence of samples

The signal is now in a form that can be encoded for storage in the computer. The original time-varying waveform of speech now takes the form of a series of quantized samples. Analog-to-digital conversion is completed.

When the amplitude of the signal is about the same as one quantization increment, the effect of quantization is to produce either a dc signal (a dc shift or change in baseline) or a square wave. The square wave is rich in odd harmonics that can reach far beyond the highest frequency of interest, F. Even the use of an anti-aliasing filter cannot prevent aliasing in this situation, which results in a gritty sound called *granulation noise*. The point to remember is that very low-amplitude signals are vulnerable to the generation of a noise distortion. Quantization level should be chosen carefully if very weak signals are to be processed. Amplification of the signal may be required, and this will be considered next.

As a quick review, let's consider a practical problem in A/D conversion. Suppose that a speech signal is to be analyzed for information that is contained within the frequency range below 3 kHz. Because the total sample of speech is very long, it is important to use as little computer memory as possible to store the signal. What are the appropriate settings for sampling rate, presampling filter, and quantization? First, the sampling rate should be at least twice the highest frequency of interest in the analysis, F. This highest frequency is 3 kHz, which means that the sampling rate should be at least 6 kHz. Because filter settings sometimes are approximate and because signal energy may be appreciable in the reject band, it is wise to choose a cut-off frequency for the low-pass, presampling filter that is slightly below the sampling rate. Therefore, this filter should have a low-pass characteristic with a cut-off frequency of slightly below 3 kHz, let us say, 2.8 kHz. Finally, an 11-bit quantization should provide a sufficiently accurate amplitude conversion, unless there is an interest in small variations in signal amplitude.

Is it ever desirable to *oversample*, that is, to use a sampling rate higher than that derived from the sampling theorem? Yes, it is. First, it may be desirable to oversample when the anti-aliasing filter has a shallow guard band. If the rejection rate of the guard band is shallow, then some undesired signal energy above F may be digitized and would result in aliasing. It is usually a good procedure to select a low-pass frequency of the anti-aliasing filter that is less than half the value of the sampling rate. Oversampling also is used to gain analytic resolution. One example is in the determination of vocal fundamental frequency (f0). Whalen, Wiley, Rubin, and Cooper (1990) note that when a file is sampled at 10 kHz, the accuracy of fundamental frequency determination will be $+/-0.5\%$ for a man with a f0 of 100 Hz, $+/-1.0\%$ for a woman with a f0 of 200 Hz, and $+/-2.5\%$ for an infant with an f0 of 500 Hz. The issue becomes especially important for the determination of irregularities (perturbations) in the voice. One such perturbation is called *jitter*, which is the cycle-to-cycle variation in the fundamental period. Another perturbation, called *shimmer*, is the cycle to cycle variation in the peak amplitude of the laryngeal waveform. Measurement of these perturbations, or departures from true regularity, can be intolerably imprecise at low sampling rates or low levels of quantization.

For additional information on A/D and the issues briefly considered below, see Lang (1987) and Gates (1989). What follows are some highly condensed comments on issues related to A/D.

Amplification (Gain)

Generally, commercially available A/Ds require an input signal in the range of –10 to +10 volts. It is desirable to adjust the input signal to this range to take full advantage of the levels of quantization afforded by the A/D. If a signal has a range of only –2 to +2 volts, many potential levels of quantization would be lost as the signal is digitized. Because the analog output of instruments such as tape recorders often does not correspond to the signal range of an A/D converter, amplification frequently is needed. Let us take as a simple example the output of a tape deck that provides a signal range of –1 to +1 volt. If this signal is to be fed into a A/D that requires a signal range of –10 to +10 volts, then the tape deck output should be amplified by a factor of ten.

Amplification usually is accomplished by one of two means: (a) using an external amplifier, or (b) using the built-in amplifier provided with some A/Ds. On-board amplifiers come with various features, one of which is programmable gain, or the capability to change the gain in software according to the needs of data conversions. An advantage of an external amplifier is that it can be placed very close to the equipment providing the signal to the A/D. Proximity is particularly important in the case of weak signals. When a weak signal is passed along a long cable, it is vulnerable to noise and further diminution because of the resistance of the connecting cable. Noise may arise, for example, because the cable can serve as an antenna, picking up 60 Hz hum from sources such as transformers and fluorescent lights. Signal diminution is possible because the wire in cables, even though it is a conductor, presents some resistance to the flow of electrical energy. The resistance is proportional to the length of the wire. The rule is simple: keep the connection between the signal instrument and the A/D as short as practical.

Cabling

Connecting instruments together may seem a trivial matter but this is, in fact, a very important consideration. Incorrect choices or faulty procedures can greatly impair the performance of a speech analysis system. One factor to consider is the type of cable used to make the connections. The cost of a cable increases with its ability to keep noise out of the signal. The least expensive are single wires and flat cables. The major difference between these two pertains to the number of connections that must be made. When many connections are made with single wires, the result can be a confusing jumble. Flat cables reduce the confusion because they may contain several wires. For applications involving a high-frequency signal or a signal with a low signal-to-noise ratio, single wires or flat cables are not the connections of choice. It is preferable to use one of the following: twisted-pair, coaxial, or triaxial cable. These connections protect the signal from environmental contamination. Finally, as noted, it is always desirable to keep cable lengths to a minimum.

Interface

Cables require connectors so signals can be passed from one device to another. For digital signals, the problem of interface arises. *Interface* refers to the communication scheme that allows devices to exchange signals. There are two main types of interface—

serial and parallel. There are many issues that arise in interfacing, most of which are not directly relevant to the applications in this book. Readers who need information in this area might consult Lang (1987) or general references for computer systems.

Summary

This chapter began with a brief review of the history of the acoustic analysis of speech. The history is largely one of analog instrumentation. The dominant equipment today is digital. Anyone using modern methods of acoustic analysis therefore should understand the basic principles of digital signal processing. This chapter discussed basic operations of digitization as a prelude to a larger discussion of digital signal processing for the analysis of speech. The next chapter presents information on modern (digital) methods for acoustic speech analysis.

Modern Analytic Techniques

CHAPTER

"Modern analytic techniques" means *digital* techniques, that is, computing with samples of speech represented as numbers. *Analog* devices, which deal with continuous data, are still used in amplifying, recording, and playback, but rarely in analysis. Instruments for speech analysis are now basically of two types: "dedicated" devices specifically designed for speech, such as digital spectrographs, and general-purpose computers running programs for analyzing speech. The similarities are more basic than the differences: both are, in fact, digital computers, operating on speech which has been sampled as described in Chapter 3. They perform similar computations and typically produce similar monitor displays, which the user may choose to print.

The difference is that in the dedicated device, the hardware and the analysis programs have been selected and optimized to work together in analyzing speech, and the programs have been written (semiperma-

nently) into the machine's memory. As a result, the dedicated device may operate faster or display results more perspicuously, but in principle, a general-purpose computer can be programmed to do the same analyses. Instructions for using a dedicated device deal solely with analyzing speech, whereas the user of a general-purpose computer typically confronts at least two manuals: one for the basic machine and one for the speech-analysis program.

Typically, a disadvantage of a dedicated device is that the user cannot modify or add to its programs. By contrast, for some micro- and minicomputers, users may choose from several programs available for various combinations of analyses. Some programs even make it relatively easy for a user to add her own analyses. Some programs are in the public domain, such as those developed with government support, and can be obtained for a small copying fee. Because of the fundamental similarities between dedicated and general use computers, we will not usually need to distinguish between them in discussing analytic techniques. With either type, it is up to the user to determine that a particular analysis is appropriate to his purposes and his data. A sophisticated user also starts with some known data in order to check whether the analyses are performed accurately.

Waveform Display

In Chapter 3, we began our brief history of acoustic analysis with the oscillograph, which traced on paper the changes in voltage from a microphone, representing the changes in air pressure which pass from speaker to listener. Displaying such a *sound pressure waveform* is one basic function of most devices for speech analysis. From such a display, one can determine duration and relative amplitude. One can judge periodicity, and from the duration of periods one can estimate fundamental frequency. Typically, one can select portions of the waveform for closer inspection and for editing. We will review each of these functions below. Figure 4–1 shows the waveform of one utterance of "we" as displayed by a program named CSpeech running on an IBM-PC.

Measuring Duration

Note the left and right cursors in Figure 4–1: the user set them around "we," using both visual and auditory cues. The next word in the utterance was "show," and the thicker waveform beyond the right cursor results from the noise of the [ʃ]. By moving the cursors and playing back the sound between them, the user could judge at what point the sound quality changed from vowel to fricative. The sampling rate at which the sound was recorded was 22 kHz (22,000 samples per second). Thus, the time between samples was 0.045 ms, that is, 45 μs (microseconds), the *potential* time resolution of a recording at that rate. CSpeech reports (line 1 of the display) that the time between the cursors is 263.273 ms, so the user might conclude that the syllable "we" was precisely that long.

However, there are two hidden limitations. The main one is the difficulty of judging exactly where a speech segment begins and ends. In this case, is the left cursor precisely at the beginning of the vowel? How much difference would it make if the user decided that the vowel begins later, where the waveform becomes periodic or where it first exceeds some voltage (amplitude) threshold? Should the

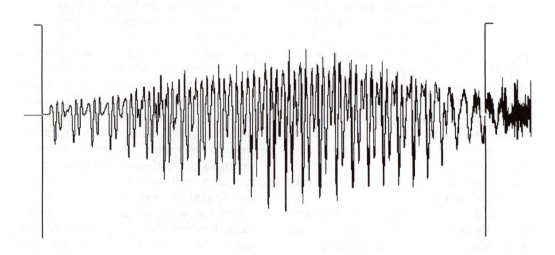

FIGURE 4–1. Speech waveform of the beginning of "We show speech." Cursors mark "we."

right cursor be moved inward to the last regular period of the vowel? Such questions become critical in attempting to make reliable measurements, especially of different types of speech sounds or sounds in different contexts. To say that the potential resolution is 0.045 ms is misleading, because no one can locate boundaries of speech units that precisely. Articulation takes time, so speech sounds begin and end gradually. The second limitation is that while the *potential* resolution is 0.045 ms, the smallest cursor movement may be larger than that, depending on the duration of sound displayed. In this case, one cursor movement was 0.4 ms, so that was the effective resolution. If we had displayed several seconds of speech, the resolution would have been coarser. For both of these reasons, we cannot always take (or offer) duration measurements at face value.

Resolution is an issue in the amplitude dimension as well. "Twelve-bit quantization" means that the input voltage is represented by a number which can take on 4,096 different values. Thus, if the input voltage ranges from +10 volts to –10 volts, that 20-volt range will be divided into 4,096 steps, or 5 mv (millivolts) per step. That resolution is normally adequate for speech analysis, but you should know the resolution of your equipment. Some inexpensive sampling devices use only 8-bit resolution (256 different values), which makes a considerable difference to the quality of the recorded speech and to subsequent analysis. The greater the resolution, the stronger will be the signal, as compared with the noise introduced by the quantization process. Table 4–1 shows the relationship between amplitude resolution (in bits, steps, and millivolts) and this signal-to-quantization noise ratio, for a few commonly used levels of resolution.

Bear in mind that this signal-to-noise ratio is a theoretical maximum for a signal of constant energy, which speech never is. In Table 4–1, it looks as if even 8-bit resolution equals the signal-to-noise ratio of an ordinary cassette tape recorder, but several other factors operate to reduce the actual ratio and to introduce other kinds of noise. To name just one example, if the sampling hardware is set for a 20-volt range of input, but the actual input spans only two volts (+1 to –1), which many preamplifiers provide, the amplitude resolution is only one-tenth of the potential, and noise will be much louder in relation to the signal.

Editing

Because we can select portions of digitized speech (usually with cursors on a screen) and play them back, we can edit speech. For example, suppose that you have recorded an utterance of "team." You can hear that the [t] is aspirated ([tʰ]), and for a perception experiment, you would like to remove the aspiration and play the result. Figure 4–2 shows such an utterance, with the cursors marking the aspiration. In "the old days" (a few years ago), you would have cut the recording tape with a razor blade and spliced it back together. Today, we have an electronic equivalent: cutting at the cursors and rejoining the digitized sound. The precise way in which you do this depends on the program or device;

TABLE 4–1
Amplitude resolution and signal-to-noise ratio

Bits	Steps	Step size (if 20v range)	Signal-to-Noise Ratio
8	256	78 mv	41 dB
12	4096	5 mv	65 dB
16	65536	0.3 mv	89 dB

some have a "splice" command, some require you to transfer segments to another channel or to label and list the segments to be spliced. In any case, the operation will be cleaner, faster, and more accurate than tape splicing, mainly because you can locate the cutting points more accurately by viewing the waveform and listening to the portions before, after, and between the cursors.

However, some tips from expert tape splicers still apply. Most basically, no splice will be completely natural because of coarticulation. If you cut a consonant from a vowel, the vowel will still contain transitions which suggest that consonant, or at least its place of articulation. Vowels before nasals will be nasalized, those before /r/ will be rhotacized, those before voiceless consonants will be shortened, etc.

Almost all speech sounds contain effects of their contexts. Second, a splice where the waveform is strongly positive or negative will probably produce a popping noise. Skilled splicers make their cuts at moments when the waveform is at or near the zero line, or at least join two ends at the same amplitude. Fortunately, with electronic tape splicing you can easily experiment with different splices.

Measuring Amplitude

The speech waveform also provides information about relative amplitude. The top channel in Figure 4–3 shows the waveforms of "import," the noun with stress on "im," and "import," the verb with stress on "port." One can see that the amplitude of

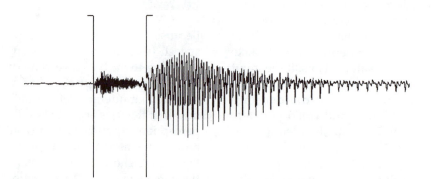

FIGURE 4–2. Speech waveform of "team," with the cursors marking the aspiration of the [tʰ].

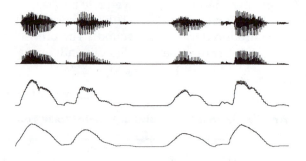

FIGURE 4–3. Speech waveform of "import" (noun) "import" (verb), with three representations of amplitude. Channel 2 is the waveform rectified; channels 3 and 4 are rms amplitude contours, calculated with a 20 ms and an 80 ms sliding window, respectively.

the first syllable ("im" with primary stress) is greater than that of the third, and that the amplitude of the fourth syllable ("port" with primary stress) is greater than that of the second.

Such comparisons of the raw waveform can be difficult, however, because the viewer must somehow combine the negative (downward) half of the waveform with the positive half. Both represent changes in air pressure which move the eardrum of a listener. Channel 2 in Figure 4–3 shows the same waveform rectified, that is, with negative pressures changed to positive — the effect is that the lower half of the waveform in channel 1 has been "folded up." This makes it easier to compare not only the overall amplitude of syllables but also the shape of amplitude change during each syllable. We can infer, for example, that within each "im" (syllables 1 and 3), the greater amplitude is in the first half of the syllable, that is, the vowel rather than the nasal.

The waveform in channel 2 still has all the jaggedness of the original, however. To obtain a smooth amplitude curve, we must somehow average the signal over time. In effect, we did that informally, "by eye," when we assessed the shape of each syllable. Such smoothing can be done arithmetically, and one way is known as *rms* amplitude, for "root-mean-square" averaging. The name identifies three of the steps, in reverse order. To calculate rms amplitude:

- Select a "window" length, the number of samples of speech to be averaged;

- Square the value of each sample in the first window, thus eliminating negative numbers and exaggerating differences;

- Calculate the arithmetic mean, or average, of the squared values in the window;

- Take the square root of the resulting mean, bringing it back to the original scale;

- Move on to the next window, that is, the next set of samples.

The waveform in channel 3 of Figure 4–3 is the rms amplitude of the original waveform, calculated with a 20 ms "sliding" window, that is, one that advanced by just one sample with each rms calculation. Now much of the jaggedness is gone, and the average has been calculated precisely.

To create an even smoother curve, we lengthen the window, averaging over longer stretches. The rms amplitude curve in channel 4 is exactly like that in channel 3 except that it was calculated with an 80 ms window. However, note that the window length has an effect: if we were trying to locate the exact peak of each syllable, we would get slightly different answers from channels 3 and 4.

Amplitude and English Stress

This discussion of Figure 4–3 may leave the impression that syllable stress, or prominence, in English is signaled mainly by amplitude. Indeed that is also our intuition. Most speakers of English would report that the main difference between the noun "import" and the verb "import" is in which syllable is louder. However, duration is also a factor. In Figure 4–3, the second (stressed) syllable of the verb is longer than that of the noun. In fact, duration is actually a more consistent cue to stress than amplitude is; in Figure 4–3, the "im" syllables are atypical, in that they do not differ in length. Notice also that we do not compare "im" with "port" with respect to stress; because they are made up of different speech sounds, they are inherently different in both amplitude and duration.

Measuring Fundamental Frequency

One can easily "see" that some parts of the waveform are periodic, that is, they consist of similar patterns of change repeated over time. For example, in Figure 4–1 ("we"), most of the waveform between the cursors

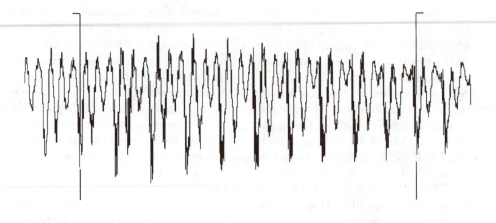

FIGURE 4–4. Speech waveform of "we," with the cursors marking 10 glottal periods. The duration of that portion is 95.8 ms (top line), so the average f0 is 104 Hz.

is *periodic*. The largest patterns (longest periods) result from the vibrations of the vocal folds and correspond to the frequency which we perceive as pitch; as those patterns become more frequent, the perceived pitch increases. Because we are very good at recognizing visual patterns, it seems easy for us to judge periodicity in a waveform display. To program a computer to make the same judgments turns out to be quite difficult. However, even human judgments are usually unclear about where periodicity begins and ends. At the right side of Figure 4–1, for instance, just where does the vowel *stop* being periodic? Likewise, after the left cursor in Figure 4–1, the sound is rapidly changing in amplitude and quality; that is the nature of /w/. Is there an aperiodic portion at the beginning? Answers to such questions are partly arbitrary, because the vocal folds move and change their modes of vibration gradually. Precisely because we can now see the effects of vocal fold activity (and of articulation) on an expanded time scale, we realize that speech does not change instantaneously. Technically, speech is only *quasi*periodic, because it is constantly changing in frequency and quality.

Within these limitations, we can use a waveform display to measure the duration of periods and therefore the fundamental

frequency of voiced speech. Figure 4–4 displays a vowel, with the cursors surrounding 10 periods. The interval between the cursors is 95.9 ms ("Length ="; line one), so the average duration of one period is 9.59 ms. Since duration and frequency are inverses, the fundamental frequency, on average, is 104 Hz ([1/9.59] × 1000), or 10 times the frequency shown at the end of line one. Averaging over 10 or 20 periods in this way is usually desirable for two reasons. First, the error, or uncertainty, in setting the cursors is reduced by a factor of 10, and second, we usually want to know the average pitch in some *region* of the waveform, not the absolute frequency of one particular vocal period. Of course, this method of measuring fundamental frequency can be tedious if you have many measurements to make. The next-to-last section of this chapter will discuss several other methods, but there are no perfect ones.

Filters

Basic Terms

We saw in Chapter 2 that a filter is a system that passes (or enhances) some frequencies

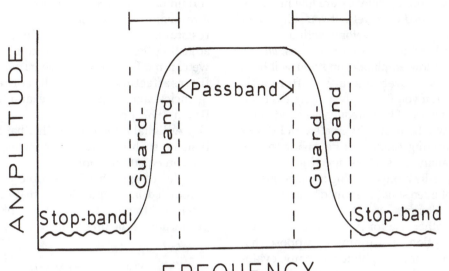

FIGURE 4–5. Response curve of a band-pass filter, identifying the pass band, stop bands, and guard bands.

but attenuates others. Thus, a filter has a *response curve* that varies across the frequency spectrum. As shown in Figure 4–5, a filter's response curve will have one or more *pass bands*, and one or more *stop bands*. The filter may be a *high-pass* or a *low-pass* filter (if the pass band is above or below the stop band), or in the general case, as in Figure 4–5, it may be a *band-pass* filter, with stop bands on both sides. The frequency at which the filter's response starts to change is called the *corner frequency*. Because the change actually occurs over a range of frequencies, the corner frequency is only nominal, however. If the change in response is abrupt, the filter is said to have *sharp cut-offs* or *steep skirts*. Real filters do not have perfectly flat response in the pass band or the stop band; instead, they have some *ripple* in their response, as in Figure 4–5. Figure 4–5 turned upside-down would be the response curve of a *band reject* filter, with a stop band in the middle and pass bands on either side. A band reject filter with a narrow stop band is called a *notch* filter.

Uses of Filters in Speech Science

Two common applications were introduced in Chapter 3: preemphasis and anti-aliasing. A preemphasis filter for speech is a high-pass filter, usually with a response that increases at 6 dB per octave above a corner frequency of a few hundred hertz. Such a filter enhances higher frequencies, which are of lower amplitude in speech, on average. In fact, as noted in Chapter 2, the radiation characteristic at the lips approximates a +6 dB per octave high-pass filter.

An anti-aliasing (presampling) filter is a low-pass filter which sharply attenuates frequencies above half the sampling rate. As explained in Chapter 3, such a filter is necessary for digital recording and analysis but not for analog processes, such as a conventional tape recording.

Another use of filtering is to focus an analysis on a frequency range of interest. For example, suppose that you wish to study two types of [s] sounds, such as those in Korean. All [s]s consist primarily of high-frequency sound, and they are low in amplitude compared to vowels. If you simply plot a sound-pressure waveform with an amplitude scale wide enough for vowels, *all* [s]s will be of low amplitude, and you will have difficulty discerning any differences. However, if you first apply a high-pass filter, the amplitude of high-frequency sounds such as [s]s will be relatively greater, and differences among them will be easier to see. Other analyses, such as spectrograms, are also typically more revealing if the frequency range of interest has been made more prominent by filtering.

Another use for filters is in the study of perception. For example, suppose that you work for a telephone company, evaluating possible improvements to the transmission systems. Such systems now transmit a *bandwidth* of only about 300 to 3000 Hz; in effect, they are band-pass filters. Suppose that some projected improvement to the system would widen that bandwidth to 5000 Hz. You might undertake a series of perceptual studies to determine whether the effect on people's perception is worth the increase in cost.

A fifth major use for filters in the study of speech is in spectrographic analysis. As noted in Chapter 3, a spectrograph breaks speech into its frequency components by filtering it, with either analog or digital filters. The bandwidth of these filters makes a crucial difference to the resulting spectrogram, as discussed below and illustrated in Figure 4–11.

These are only some examples of how filters are used in the study of speech. A central part of speech science is concerned with the frequencies that make up speech, and whenever one focuses on a certain range of frequencies, one is using filters. Filtering is also an essential part of producing speech, as we saw in Chapter 2.

Analog vs. Digital Filters

Filters can be constructed in two forms: analog and digital. An analog filter is an electronic circuit, tuned to respond to a certain range of frequencies—in short, it is a resonator. Such a circuit is made up of resistors, capacitors, and inductors. By adjusting the values of these components, we can modify the response curve of our filter, affecting bandwidth, corner frequencies, and ripple. (For examples, see Baken, 1987, pp. 21–26.)

A digital filter, on the other hand, contains no such physical components; it is a rule, an equation, applied to a sequence of samples of speech. The simple example introduced in Chapter 3 was that of *differencing*, subtracting from each sample some proportion of the preceding sample.

$$y(n) = x(n) - ax(n-1)$$

where $x(n)$ is a sample in the original
signal at time n
$y(n)$ is the corresponding sample of
the differenced signal
and a is a constant multiplier, usually
between 0.9 and 1.0.

In other words, we step backwards through a digitized signal, sample by sample, subtracting from each sample some large proportion of its predecessor, so that the resulting samples represent mainly the changes. Why does such an operation act as a high-pass filter? Basically because differences from sample to sample are high-frequency variation, assuming that the sampling rate is high. These variations are relatively well preserved by differencing, but low-frequency (slow) variation is attenuated at each step. In fact, when $a = 0.9$, differencing yields a response curve close to a 6 dB per octave preemphasis.

Of course, there are other kinds of digital filters. In fact, any function of frequency may be considered a filter. Of particular interest in speech science are filters based on linear predictive coding (LPC), discussed below. The parameters of LPC analysis represent formant frequencies and bandwidths, so one can filter a signal by altering those parameters.

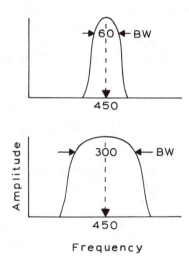

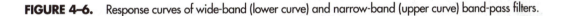

FIGURE 4–6. Response curves of wide-band (lower curve) and narrow-band (upper curve) band-pass filters.

The Time/Frequency Tradeoff

Whether analog or digital, filters share a crucial property with all other resonators, namely that there is a tradeoff between frequency resolution and time resolution. One aspect of this tradeoff is fairly obvious: a wideband filter will "smear" a range of frequencies by responding to any frequency within its bandwidth. As shown in Figure 4–6, a filter with a 300 Hz bandwidth centered on 450 Hz will respond efficiently to any frequency between 300 and 600 Hz; it will fail to distinguish between them. Conversely, a filter with a 60 Hz bandwidth (narrow-band), also centered on 450 Hz, will respond efficiently only to frequencies between 420 and 480 Hz, giving us finer-grained information about frequency.

What is less obvious is that the reverse is true for the filters' response over time. The wideband filter responds *quickly* to signals within its frequency range, while the narrow-band filter responds more *slowly*. That is why a narrow-band spectrogram (that is, one produced with narrow-band filters) provides fine-grained frequency information but smears it over time, obliterating brief events, while a wide-band spectrogram

smears information across frequency but displays brief events more clearly. Figure 4–11 illustrates this difference.

In an analog filter the bandwidth is the range of frequencies to which the tuned circuit resonates. A digital filter does not literally resonate. How then can it have a bandwidth? A digital filter cannot filter one sample (one number), of course; it can find variation (i.e., frequencies) only in a series of samples. The counterpart to bandwidth in a digital filter is the number of samples (often called "points") which the filter takes as a unit of analysis. A small difference in frequency takes a long time to manifest itself: for instance, two frequencies that are only 10 Hz apart take 1/10 s (second) to differ by a full cycle, but differences of 100 Hz show up ten times faster. If our filter operates on a long interval (many samples), it can detect small differences in frequency, but its response will change only after that interval — slow response in time. In other words, we have exactly the same tradeoff between time and frequency resolution in digital filtering that we had with hardware filters. Either way, if you want to respond to small differences in frequency, you have to operate on long intervals of time, or if you want to work with short intervals of time, you can see only large differences in frequency. Neither resonators nor equations can be highly selective in both time and frequency, because time and frequency are inversely related.

Whenever we filter a signal, we lose some information about changes over time. In fact, this effect can be quantified: the *time constant* of a filter (analog or digital) is the time required for its response to decay to about 37% of its peak value. More precisely, the proportion is $1/e$, where e is the base of the natural logarithms. It is the filter's response to its highest *pole*, its most resonant frequency, which is measured. Some computer programs allow you to construct filters that meet various specifications; the time constant is one such variable, along with corner frequencies and bandwidth. Sometimes the time constant for a digital filter is stated in terms of number of samples. For example, a time constant of 100 samples at a 10 kHz sampling rate means that the response decays to $1/e$ in 10 ms. Such a filter would distort the most rapid changes in speech, such as stop bursts and vowel transitions.

Although filters have many practical applications in the study of speech, perhaps their greatest importance is as models of the vocal tract, since as we saw in Chapter 2, the vocal tract is a complex and changing filter. Given excitation from the vibrating vocal folds or a fricative constriction, the vocal tract enhances some frequencies while suppressing others. It can be described as a set of resonators, each with a center frequency and a bandwidth. This view of speech has permitted speech science to apply the known properties of filters to the analysis of speech production.

Types of Filters

There are some classic types of filters which illustrate the tradeoffs that a filter designer must make. These types were originally analog filters, but they can be mimicked by digital filters.

- *Butterworth filter:* maximally flat; that is, minimal ripple in either pass band or stop band. The tradeoff is gradual transitions between stop and pass bands.
- *Chebychev filter:* sharper transitions than Butterworth, but ripple in the pass band.
- *Chebychev II filter:* the opposite; ripple in the stop band, but flat pass band.
- *Elliptic filter:* ripple in both the pass and the stop bands, but sharpest transitions between bands ("steep skirts").

As these descriptions illustrate, in addition to the tradeoff between frequency and time resolution, there is a tradeoff between ripple and sharp transitions. The choice depends on the application. For example, sharp transitions are not desirable in pre-emphasis, but they are essential in anti-aliasing; any frequency components above half the sampling rate will add distortion to a digitized signal.

Spectral Analysis

Fourier Analysis

Fourier analysis takes its name from the mathematician Jean Baptiste Joseph Fourier, who was made a baron by Napoleon in 1808 for his government service, not his mathematics. Fourier showed that periodic waveforms, no matter how complex, can be analyzed as the sum of an infinite series of sinusoidal components, varying in amplitude and phase. Each component is an integer multiple of the fundamental. This proof is essential to speech science, because we often deal with complex periodic waveforms whose strongest component frequencies are the resonances of the vocal tract and are essential to production and recognition. Thus, Fourier analysis can tell us a great deal about speech sounds. Essentially, it transforms a periodic amplitude by time waveform into a frequency waveform, known as a *spectrum*, a graph of the amplitude of the various frequency components.

However, as usual in applying mathematics to the physical world, there are a few "catches." First, Fourier's theorem applies to periodic waves, whereas speech sounds are only quasiperiodic, as we have seen. For instance, any sound which dies out is not truly periodic. Second, Fourier was talking about continuous waveforms, whereas in digital analysis we are dealing with discrete samples from such a waveform. Third, carrying out Fourier's analysis as he developed it is computationally difficult, even though we settle for a finite number of components, of course. However, it turns out that there are solutions to all of these problems. We can adapt Fourier analysis to a quasiperiodic waveform by *windowing* (gradually increasing and decreasing the amplitude of the signal, rather than turning it on and off abruptly). There are Discrete Fourier Transforms (DFTs) which apply to sampled data, and one type of DFT is a Fast Fourier Transform (FFT), which desktop computers can do rapidly.

Even before the computational improvements, Fourier's theorem was essential, because it guarantees that a complex waveform has component frequencies which a bank of filters, for example, could find. As we saw in Chapter 3, that was in fact the form that analysis took in analog devices. Now digital analysis consists of an FFT of samples from a waveform. It yields a spectrum showing the amplitude of each harmonic of the fundamental. (Theoretically, it ought to indicate the relative phase of each component, too, but phase is not nearly as important as frequency and amplitude for specifying speech sounds.)

Figure 4–7 shows such a spectrum for a portion of the vowel [i] in "we." The horizontal axis is frequency, from 0 to 5000 Hz (the filter cut-off). The vertical axis is amplitude, from a zero dB reference level at the top down to –80 dB at the bottom. Each peak in the graph is a harmonic (integer multiple) of the fundamental. The cursor (vertical line) points to the thirteenth harmonic, which is a local maximum because it is near a resonant frequency of this vocal tract articulating this vowel: the second formant. As the side panel indicates, the frequency of this harmonic is 2051 Hz, and its amplitude is 44 dB below the reference level. The first formant is near the second harmonic, at approximately 300 Hz. This wide separation between first and second formants is a distinguishing characteristic of the vowel

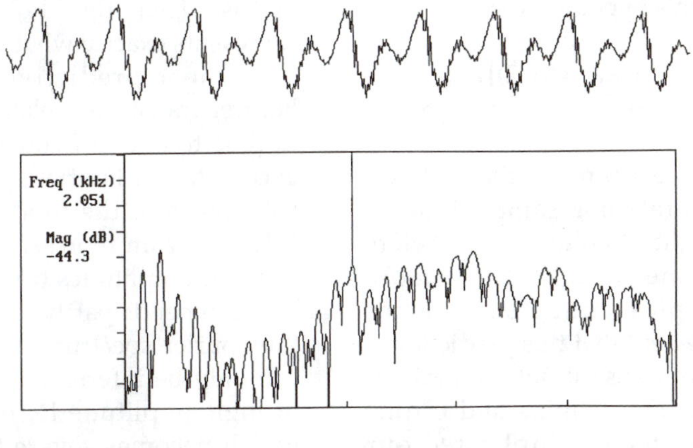

Freq (kHz)
2.051

Mag (dB)
-44.3

FIGURE 4–7. Speech waveform and Fourier spectrum of [i]. The cursor in the spectrum points to the 13th harmonic, which is near the peak of F2.

/i/. Fourier analysis makes it possible for us to identify such essential properties of speech sounds.

Linear Prediction

Fourier analysis is basic to the study of speech, but it is not the only way of determining a spectrum nor the best for all purposes. A more recently developed method of analysis is *linear prediction* or *linear predictive coding* (LPC). LPC comes from two sources: the branch of statistics known as time-series analysis, which aims to identify regularities in time-varying data, and the branch of engineering concerned with transmitting signals. Time-series analysis applies not only to speech but also to birthrates, electroencephalograms, sunspots, and stock market prices — any stream of data over time.

A classic problem in transmitting signals is that the capacity of any channel is limited. Intercontinental telephone channels via satellite, for example, are expensive, and so engineers try to find ways of compressing the signals. One way is linear predictive coding. LPC builds upon the fact that any sample in digitized speech is partly predictable from its immediate predecessors; speech does not vary wildly from sample to sample. Linear prediction is just the hypothesis that any sample is a *linear* function of those that precede it. Expressed as an equation, this hypothesis is:

$$x(n) = a_1[x(n-1)] + a_2[x(n-2)] + ... - e(n)$$

which means: "the sample at time n [$x(n)$] is equal to the preceding sample [$x(n-1)$] times some weight [a_1] plus the one before that times some weight plus more weighted samples minus some error [$e(n)$]." To the extent that this prediction is accurate, one can transmit not the individual samples but the weights and errors. This appears to have complicated our transmission, not simplified it; the simplification is that the weights do not change

as rapidly as the samples themselves. That is, if we sample a signal 10,000 times per second, we have a new sample every 100 μs. But while the signal remains in one pattern (e.g., a steady-state vowel), the LPC weights tend to remain the same. It turns out that they need to be updated only every 10 or 20 ms in order to transmit intelligible speech, a saving of about one hundredfold. Of course, the prediction is not completely accurate, so the transmitted speech is not perfect. One variable is the number of preceding samples included in the prediction, usually on the order of 10 to 20 for speech analysis.

As discussed so far, linear predictive coding is a model of the sequence of samples that make up a signal, a representation of the signal over *time*. However, a set of linear prediction coefficients has an equally valid interpretation in terms of *frequency*. It is the frequency response of a digital filter derived from those coefficients. (The derivation is beyond the scope of this book; for an overview, see Makhoul, 1975.) In its frequency interpretation, the weighted terms in the equation represent the frequencies and amplitudes of the resonances of the vocal tract, and the error term, known as the *residual*, represents that which remains unaccounted for. If the model of the resonances is a good one, what remains is just the input: the excitation of the vocal tract by the signal at the glottis. Thus, the LPC model as a whole represents exactly what we want to know!

Linear predictive analysis, like a Fourier transform, relates a representation in time to one in frequency. A key difference is that a Fourier spectrum represents harmonics of the fundamental, while an LPC spectrum represents formant frequencies and amplitudes (resonances). Which is better depends partly on your purposes. In the Fourier spectrum, formant frequencies can only be inferred from the frequencies of high-amplitude harmonics, a problem which becomes severe for speech with a high fundamental frequency. Monsen and Engebretson (1983) compared LP analysis with spectrographic measurement, using experienced readers of spectrograms. For samples with f0 between 100 and 300 Hz, those readers could measure the center frequency of F1 and F2 to within ± 60 Hz; spectrographic measurements were less accurate for F3. Both methods proved much less accurate when the fundamental frequency exceeded 350 Hz. The choice also depends on the sample; Fourier analysis assumes that there is a harmonic (periodic) structure; the LP analysis does not. However, the LP analysis makes assumptions of its own: most LP analyses today are models of resonances only, not antiresonances. But the vocal tract does introduce antiresonances, especially in the production of nasal and lateral speech sounds. For this reason, linear predictive analysis (at least an "all-pole" model) is not a good choice for analyzing such sounds.

For sounds which fit both models, we would like to see both representations of the spectrum. Figure 4–8 shows a linear predictive spectrum superimposed on the Fourier spectrum of Figure 4–7 (same vowel, same axes). The LP spectrum shows no harmonics; it is a *spectrum envelope*. Note

that in general it fits the peaks of the Fourier spectrum well. In this case, the two analyses yield highly similar spectra, partly because the speech being analyzed fits both models: it is voiced (periodic) and non-nasalized. However, note also that from the Fourier analysis alone, one would have difficulty in inferring the precise frequency of F2, measured as 2012 Hz on the LPC spectrum. From the Fourier spectrum, an expert can infer that F2 is centered between the 12th and 13th harmonics, but it is difficult to interpolate exactly where. In the Fourier spectrum, f0 is the difference in frequency between two harmonics. In the LP spectrum, there is no indication of fundamental frequency, although f0 can be derived from LP analysis because the glottal source should be the main component of the error term.

Real-time Spectrographs

Digital spectrographs now on the market carry out Fourier and other analyses and display a spectrogram in real time. "Real time" simply means the duration of the

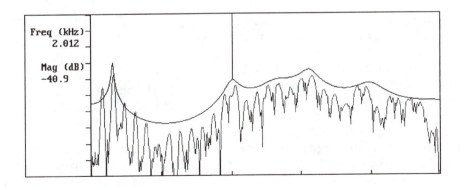

FIGURE 4–8. The same waveform as in Figure 4–7, but with an LPC spectrum overlaid on the Fourier spectrum. The cursor points to the peak of F2.

signal itself; a real-time analysis is one conducted as the signal arrives, with no delay. (Make an allowance for the hyperbole of advertising, however.) In this section, we will use the Kay DSP 5500 Sona-Graph™ as our example. (For those who like technical details, the Kay actually uses three microprocessors: one to manage the display and respond to commands from the user, and two which are specially designed to analyze signals like speech.)

From the user's point of view, perhaps the principal advantage of current spectrographs is that the analysis is always displayed first on a monitor, like that of a computer. The user then chooses whether to print that display. Previously, the printer was the only display, so a user had to wait a minute or two for each analysis to be printed — even if it turned out to be a poor one. The monitor display saves a great deal of time and money. Another difference is the great flexibility in selecting analyses and displays. One chooses from menus of analysis types, frequency ranges, time scales, effective bandwidths, and other parameters. Most of these choices are not new. Previously, one could select a frequency range and print a waveform or an amplitude contour above a spectrogram, for example; but the range of possible combinations is now much greater. A third major difference is in measurement. One measures time or frequency by moving cursors on the screen, which is easier, faster, and more accurate than measuring a printed spectrogram. One prints spectrograms to document one's work, not to make measurements. In short, the main advantages are in the way one interacts with the device, not in the nature of the analysis itself.

Figures 4–9 and 4–10 show one of the many possible combinations: Figure 4–9 is the documentation and Figure 4–10 the graphic display. In Figure 4–10, the spectrogram has the traditional three dimensions; it represents the utterance, "We show speech" (not the same utterance as in earlier figures). Above the spectrogram is a power spectrum (left) and a waveform

(right) for the interval bounded by the vertical cursors in the spectrogram, that is, the steady-state portion of [i] of "we." The frequency cursors on the spectrum mark the first and second formants of this vowel, at 260 Hz and 1980 Hz. (Only the lower frequency cursor appears on the spectrogram.) We can answer several questions from these two displays:

- *How long is the portion of vowel between the two time cursors?*
  117 ms. In the text, under cursor readings, see ^T, the difference between the two time cursors.

- *How many periods are there in that portion of vowel?*
  About 15. In the spectrogram, count the vertical striations between the two time cursors.

- *What formant transitions precede the vowel?*
  In the spectrogram, trace F2, for example, in the vowel of *show*, between the two fricatives.

- *What is the effective bandwidth of the analysis?*
  300 Hz in the spectrogram [wide band] and 29 Hz in the spectrum [narrow band]. In the text, under Analysis Settings, see Transform size.

- *Were the high frequencies boosted before the analysis?*
  Yes for the spectrogram; no for the spectrum. In the text, under Input Settings, see Input Shaping.

- *What analysis window was applied to the sample?*
  A "Hamming" window, a particular gradual onset and offset. In the text, under Analysis Settings, see Analysis Window.

- *At what rate was the speech sampled?*
  Not answered in the display. With this spectrograph, the effective sampling rate is always 2.56 times the highest frequency displayed (8 kHz), so it was 20.48 kHz.

```
            KAY ELEMETRICS CORP. MODEL 5500
               SIGNAL ANALYSIS WORKSTATION
UW PHONETICS LABORATORY
Date: JANUARY   22 1989   Time:   2:17:29 PM
Analysis by:

INPUT SETTINGS       Channel 1            Channel 2
Source               LEFT CONNECTORS      LEFT CONNECTORS
Frequency Range      DC - 8 KHz.          DC - 8 KHz.
Input Shaping        HI-SHAPE             FLAT
Buffer Size          4.0  SECONDS         4.0  SECONDS

ANALYSIS SETTINGS    Lower Screen         Upper Screen
Signal Analyzed      CHANNEL 1            CHANNEL 2
Analysis Format      SPECTROGRAPHIC       POWER AT CURSORS
Transform Size       100 pts. ( 300 Hz)  1024 pts. ( 29 Hz)
Time Axis            50ms    (1sec)       12.5ms   (250ms)
Frequency Axis       FULL SCALE           FULL SCALE
Analysis Window      HAMMING              HAMMING
Averaging Set Up     NO AVERAGING         NO AVERAGING

DISPLAY SETTINGS     Lower Screen         Upper Screen
Time Divisions        .05000 Sec.          .01250 Sec.
Freq. Divisions       500.0 Hz.            500.0 Hz.
Dynamic Range        42 dB                72 dB
Analysis Atten.      20 dB                0 dB
Set Up Options Set to:   #00

CURSOR READINGS:
FC1:  260.0 Hz. , FC2:  1980. Hz. , ^F:  1720. Hz.
FC1: -33 dB,  FC2: -49 dB,  ^F: 16 dB
^R1:  2.728 Sec.              ^R2:  2.845 Sec.
^T:  .1172 Sec.
PITCH    TC1:       Hz.  TC2:       Hz.
AMPLITUDE TC1:       dB   TC2:       dB

SUBJECT MATTER
           "We show spee(ch)"
```

FIGURE 4–9.   The textual printout which accompanies Figure 4–10. Both were produced by the Kay Elemetrics model 5500 digital spectrograph.

For many purposes, a wide-band spectrogram and narrow-band spectrum, as in Figure 4–10, is a good combination. After all, the special value of a spectrogram is to show us the dynamic changes in speech over time, so time resolution is often important. However, one can just as easily select other combinations on a digital spectrograph. For versatility, speed, and convergence of information, it seems hard to beat today's digital spectrographs. Some offer both Fourier and LPC analysis, with the ability to alter LPC parameters and resynthesize utterances, as well as to pass data to and from computers. Basic research on speech will develop even better analysis models.

Determining Fundamental Frequency

By Hand and by Eye

One of the principal goals of speech analysis is to determine fundamental frequency, which listeners perceive as pitch. On a sound pressure waveform display such as Figure 4–4, one can measure the duration of periods and thus determine f0, either period-by-period or as an average over time. This method can be quite accurate, but it is slow, and more important, it is not precisely reliable (repeatable). Because it

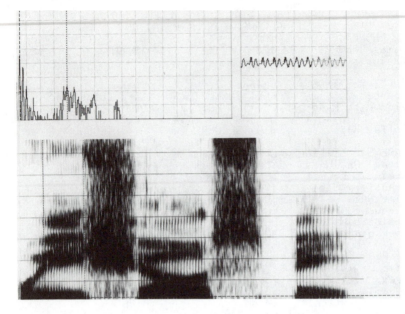

FIGURE 4–10. Spectrogram of "We show speech," produced by an adult male. The two windows above the spectrogram show a Fourier spectrum of the vowel of "we" and the waveform at the beginning of that vowel.

depends on placing the cursors around perceived patterns, two researchers may get different results from the same data. Filtering out higher frequencies may make the fundamental periods easier to identify, but the basic problems of speed and reliability remain.

Similarly, one can measure the frequency of the fundamental on a Fourier spectrum or a spectrogram with methods discussed below. These are the frequency-domain counterparts of measuring duration by hand, and they suffer from the same defects, plus that of poor resolution in some cases. Researchers have developed many devices and programs for tracking fundamental frequency automatically, seeking one which is fast, accurate, and reliable. So far, no method has all of these virtues, especially across varied speech samples.

Spectrographic Methods

A spectrogram displays the frequency components of speech over time, and one com-

ponent is the fundamental frequency. Displaying f0 on a spectrogram goes back to early publications about the spectrograph (Koenig, Dunn, & Lacy, 1946). However, the fundamental is shown quite differently in wide-band and narrow-band spectrograms. Consider again the wide-band spectrogram in Figure 4–10, specifically the vowel [i] of "we," between the cursors. We would expect to find the fundamental frequency displayed like a formant: as a dark horizontal line but at a low frequency, and indeed there is a dark line at the bottom of the spectrogram of this vowel. However, the digital filter which produced this spectrogram had a bandwidth of 300 Hz; that is, it resonated to excitation over that range of frequency. In this case, that filter responded to both the fundamental and its second harmonic at the same time; they have been smeared together. Worse yet, this vowel has a low first formant (F1), which also affects that lowest 300 Hz bandwidth. Thus the dark bar at the bottom of the spectrogram includes these three sources of sound; we cannot identify f0 within it.

However, the fundamental is reflected in the voiced segments of Figure 4–10; note the vertical bars in the three vowels of "We show speech." Since darkness on a spectrogram represents the amplitude of the spectrum, a dark vertical striation represents a moment of relatively great amplitude across a range of frequencies. In fact, each of these striations represents the resonating of the air in the vocal tract in response to a glottal pulse. (The resonation actually starts at each closure of the glottis.) These striations gradually become farther apart in the vowel of "speech," indicating the falling pitch at the end of this utterance. In the vowel of "we," there are fifteen striations between the cursors: fifteen glottal pulses. The time between the cursors (^T in Figure 4–9) is 0.117 seconds. The number of pulses divided by the time in seconds yields the number of pulses per second. In this case 15/0.117 = 128 Hz, the average pitch during this vowel.

This method of determining fundamental frequency has the same problems of speed and reliability as measuring glottal periods in the time domain. It is only as precise as our ability to count the vertical bars and to place the cursors at their edges, the boundaries of glottal periods. In this case, we could have achieved greater precision by expanding the time scale, separating the striations further. We can best obtain an average f0 over time, spreading the measurement error over several periods. Fortunately, an average is often just what we want.

Narrow-band Spectrograms

We can't see the fundamental directly in Figure 4–10 because the analyzing filter has too great a bandwidth, so let us narrow the bandwidth. Figure 4–11 shows two spectrograms of "yes" spoken with a rise-fall intonation. The upper one is a *narrow-band* spectrogram. Having separated each span of 59 Hz, we can now see the fundamental and its harmonics as equally-spaced horizontal lines within the broader formants. The rising-falling pattern is especially clear in the mid-frequency harmonics. A narrow-band spectrogram is particularly good for seeing a pattern of pitch change over time.

We can quantify f0 from this display by measuring the frequency of the fundamental or one of its harmonics, each an integer multiple of the fundamental. If possible, we choose one of the harmonics, such as the tenth. In Figure 4–11, the lowest bar is the fundamental, with a peak at 160 Hz, and its tenth harmonic has a peak at 1600 Hz, just above the fourth horizontal grid line (1500 Hz). We measure its frequency (by moving a horizontal cursor) and divide by 10 to obtain f0. Our measurement errors are also divided by 10, so they will be one-tenth as large as if we measured f0 itself. Being multiples of the fundamental, the harmonics change more rapidly: H10 changes 10 times as much as f0 in the same period of time. If we look only at the harmonics, changes in pitch appear more dramatic than they really are, but after we divide, the measurements are correct.

For measuring f0 or one of its low harmonics, the higher frequencies are irrelevant. One can change the frequency scale displayed on a spectrograph in order to "zoom in" on the relevant lower frequencies. Figure 4–12 shows the same word and the same intonation pattern as in Figure 4–11, but limited to 0–250 Hz and with an even narrower-bandwidth analysis. With the fundamental (and parts of the second harmonic) filling the screen, we can both visualize and measure the change more precisely.

The digital spectrograph on which these figures were created also has a program for computing and plotting fundamental frequency. In Figure 4–13 a wide-band spectrogram of "yes" is in the bottom half, while a sound-pressure waveform is centered in the top half. Under the waveform are three intersecting lines. The dashed line that is lowest during the vowel but rises high during the fricative is a count of zero crossings (the number of times that the waveform crosses the zero point). The dotted line that falls almost to zero during the fricative is amplitude. The dashed line that appears only during the loudest part of the vowel (rising, falling, and finally rising a bit) is the fundamental frequency.

Dedicated Devices

Some stand-alone devices graph fundamental frequency and amplitude in "real time" (that is, as fast as the speech is produced). Two well known ones are the Kay Visi-Pitch™ and the Voice Identification PM Pitch Analyzer™, both of which measure f0 period-by-period. Such devices are speedy, portable, and relatively easy to use, but they are not entirely accurate. A typical error is to double the true f0; this error is often easy to detect, because it produces a few points that are substantially out of line with the rest. Precisely because these devices are independent, it can be difficult to align and integrate their displays with those from a spectrograph or a computer. Figure 4–14 shows the pitch

and amplitude contours of an utterance as displayed by a PM Pitch Analyzer.

Computational Methods

In addition to using spectrographs and other devices designed specifically to analyze speech, researchers are now programming ordinary computers to track fundamental frequency in a speech signal. There are many types of such programs, for the simple reason that none of them is perfect. Like the dedicated devices, these programs make characteristic errors, such as confusing F1 with f0, doubling the frequency of f0, finding a fundamental frequency in unvoiced parts of the signal, or failing to find it in voiced portions. In this section, we will survey just three approaches, as examples: cepstral analysis, autocorrelation analysis, and pattern recognition, a more general alternative.

Cepstral Analysis

A method of f0 analysis developed since the mid-1960s is known as *cepstral* analysis, pronounced /'kɛpstrəl/. This tech-

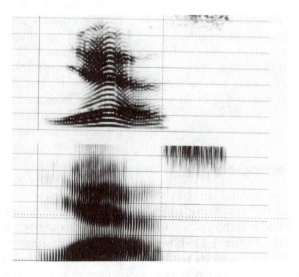

FIGURE 4–11. A wide-band (lower) and narrow-band spectrogram of "yes," spoken with a rise-fall intonation. The analysis bandwidths are 300 Hz and 59 Hz, respectively.

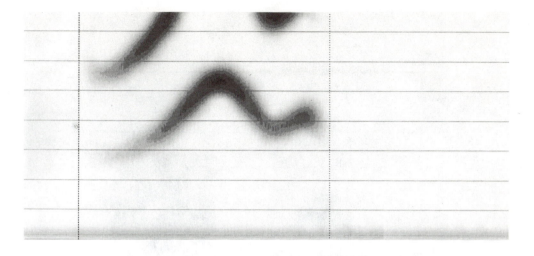

FIGURE 4–12. A narrow-band spectogram of the same intonation contour as shown in Figure 4–11, but for the frequency range from 0 to 250 Hz only. The result shows the contour of f0 and parts of the second harmonic.

nique starts with a speech signal and applies a Fourier transform to yield a spectrum such as that in Figure 4–7. The harmonics displayed in such spectra are periodic; that is, they recur at a regular interval. In fact, that interval is the fundamental frequency, since the harmonics are at multiples of the fundamental. We could measure that interval by hand, moving the cursor to each harmonic. In Figure 4–7, we would find that the harmonics are 127 Hz apart: f0 is at 127 Hz, H2 at 254 (as shown), H3 at 381, and so on. Cepstral analysis is primarily a way of recovering that interval precisely and automatically.

Consider the spectrum in Figure 4–7. Its units (amplitude vs. frequency) are different from those of Figure 4–4 (pressure vs. time), but it is certainly a periodic waveform, so the Fourier theorem is applicable. To separate the frequency components of the pressure waveform in Figure 4–4, we applied a Fourier transform, producing Figure 4–7, its spectrum. If we now apply a Fourier transform again to the periodic waveform in Figure 4–7, we will separate *its* components, of which the main one is the fundamental period. (Actually, we apply the Fourier transform

to a *log power spectrum*, that is, a spectrum of the logarithms of the squared and summed complex numbers that make up a basic Fourier spectrum.) The result of such a transformation (on a different sample) is shown in Figure 4–15, and sure enough, there is a spike at one component.

We suspect that this component corresponds to the fundamental period, but what are the units of Figure 4–15? Well, a Fourier transformation moves between the time domain (a time axis) and the frequency domain (a frequency axis). By applying the same transformation again, cepstral analysis reverses that: we start with a time axis (the sound pressure waveform), transform to a frequency axis (the Fourier spectrum), and then transform back to a time axis (the cepstrum). Thus the horizontal axis of Figure 4–15 is measured in milliseconds. The spike is at about 8.5 ms, the period of a fundamental frequency of 118 Hz.

To indicate that these units are those of cepstral analysis, they have been given their own names. "Cepstrum" is just "spectrum" with the first syllable read backwards (because cepstral analysis reverses a spectrum, in a sense). The cor-

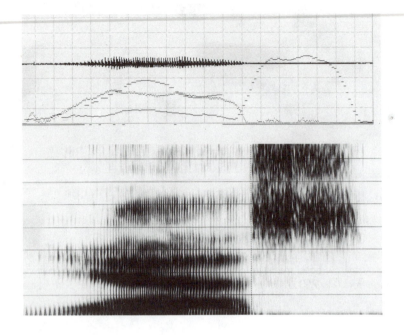

FIGURE 4–13. The "combination" display of the Kay 5500 spectrograph. The lower channel is a wideband spectrogram of "yes," spoken with rise-fall-rise intonation. The upper channel shows the speech waveform above traces which represent zero crossings, amplitude, and fundamental frequency. These traces are distinguished by color on the monitor of the spectrograph.

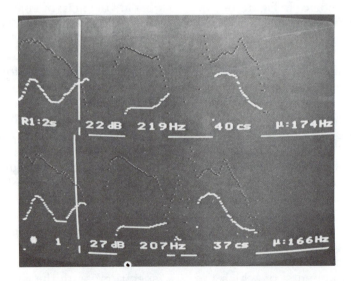

FIGURE 4–14. Fundamental frequency (white) and amplitude (black) contours on the display of a Voice Identification PM Pitch Analyzer™. The numbers represent amplitude, f0, and time at the points marked by the cursors.

responding time unit is "quefrency," that is, "frequency" with the first two syllables reversed (because it is the Fourier inverse of the frequency axis of a spectrum). Other units in cepstral analysis are named similarly: "harmonics" become "rahmonics," which are the low-quefrency components in Figure 4–15. The names may be an excess of cleverness, but the result is clear: the *quefrency* peak in Figure 4–15 represents the fundamental period in the original speech.

Cepstral analysis requires quite a lot of computing: taking the Fourier transform of a log power Fourier spectrum of the original signal, to obtain just one f0 measurement. However, with Fast Fourier Transforms and more powerful but inexpensive computers, it has become practical to perform cepstral analysis of longer stretches of speech data, plotting the changes in fundamental period over time automatically and accurately.

Autocorrelation

Two series of numbers are said to be highly correlated if they increase and decrease together. Such a series of numbers might

be the hourly temperatures for yesterday and today, for example. If the temperature followed the same pattern of increases and decreases from hour to hour, the two lists of numbers would be highly correlated, even if yesterday was, say, much colder than today. When we sample a speech signal digitally, we get a series of numbers, each one representing the amplitude of the sound pressure waveform at a particular moment, as graphed in the upper channel of Figure 4–16.

To say that this waveform is periodic is to say that there is a repeated pattern of increases and decreases. If we were to compute the correlation between this waveform and an exact copy of the waveform (thus *auto*correlation), the two copies would, of course, be perfectly correlated. But what if we computed the correlation of this signal with a slightly delayed copy of itself, as between the top and middle channels in Figure 4–16? The correlation would be highest when the delay, known as the *lag*, was close to one pitch period, as between the top and bottom channels in Figure 4–16. If we compute the correlations at lags which range over probable pitch periods (say, from 20 ms to 3 ms, cor-

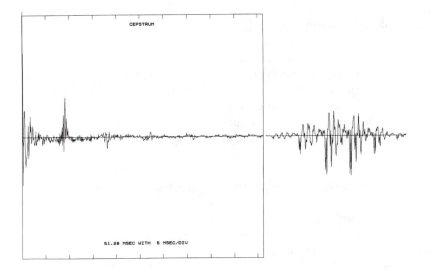

CEPSTRUM

51.20 MSEC WITH 5 MSEC/DIV

FIGURE 4–15. Cepstrum and the windowed waveform on which it was calculated. The peak is at the fundamental period.

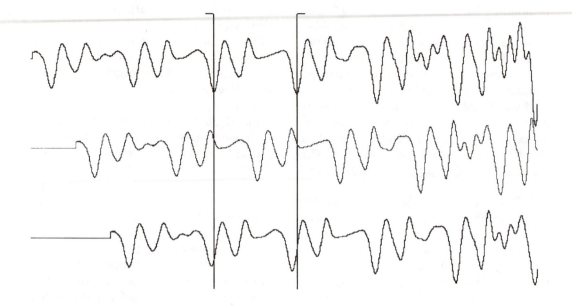

FIGURE 4–16.   Vowel waveform (top channel) with two lagged copies of itself. The cursors mark one fundamental period in the top channel and approximately one period in the lower channels.

responding to 50 to 300 Hz in f0), we would see peaks in the correlations at the actual pitch period (and its multiples). This is the essential idea of autocorrelation pitch analysis. It works because in voiced speech, formant structure does not change drastically within a few milliseconds, so that successive periods resemble each other. In unvoiced sounds such as [f] or [s], on the other hand, the quality does change rapidly because of the aperiodic noise source, so autocorrelation over a short term will normally yield no regular peaks. Of course, even voiced speech is only *quasi*periodic; it does change somewhat in quality (and pitch) from period to period. Relatively slow change does not disturb autocorrelation analysis, however, because of the remaining overall similarity from period to period.

Unfortunately, autocorrelation in this simple form applied to a "raw" speech signal does not work particularly well. The formants also affect the location of correlation peaks, so that a common error is to find, not the glottal period, but the glottal period plus the period of the first or second formant. Research since the 1960s has been devoted to preprocessing the signal to reduce the influence of the formants. A simple method is low-pass filtering to effectively eliminate formants at frequencies higher than the highest expected f0. Much more sophisticated techniques, beyond the scope of this introduction, are also used. Any adaptation must confront two basic problems: formant structure does change over time (sometimes rapidly), which disrupts autocorrelation analysis by changing the shape of the waveform, and the frequency of F1 is in some instances lower than f0, so that simply filtering the signal will not always work. Despite these difficulties, autocorrelation is one of the more reliable methods of determining fundamental frequency.

Pattern Recognition

All of these relatively elaborate methods have limitations. We are tempted to return to the basic observation with which we started: that the periodicity of voiced speech is evident in repeated patterns in the sound-pressure waveform. Consider, for example, Figure 4–17: its four channels display the waveforms of [i], [æ], [ɔ], and [u], the vowels of "bead," "bad," "baud," and "booed," respectively. In each, we see a shape that is repeated from five to seven times across the screen; that shape varies from vowel to vowel. Can we not somehow find such periods automatically from the waveform alone, without first finding a spectrum, a cepstrum, or an autocorrelation? Can't computers learn to recognize the pattern that our "eye" sees at once?

This is a case of pattern recognition, a process which is central to research in artificial intelligence. We begin to see the difficulty when we try to state an explicit procedure, such as: "Put the cursors at two successive peaks," (or "two successive valleys"). There are many peaks and valleys in a speech waveform; how do we state which

ones? If we said, "two peaks that *match*," we would have to state a criterion for *matching*, which is exactly the difficulty. If we said, "two successive *major* peaks," we would have to distinguish the "major" ones without relying circularly on the notion we are trying to explicate — that of "pattern."

Most approaches to this problem first simplify the waveform. One way is to low-pass filter it at several hundred hertz, higher than any likely fundamental frequency, unless our speaker is an infant. That removes many of the local peaks by removing the effects of higher formants. Figure 4–18 displays a vowel waveform (top channel) and that same waveform filtered at 850 Hz (middle channel). An alternative simplification is to "peak-clip" the waveform, leaving only the peaks or valleys, as in the bottom channel of Figure 4–18. (Just reduce all values to zero unless they exceed a certain threshold.) Another

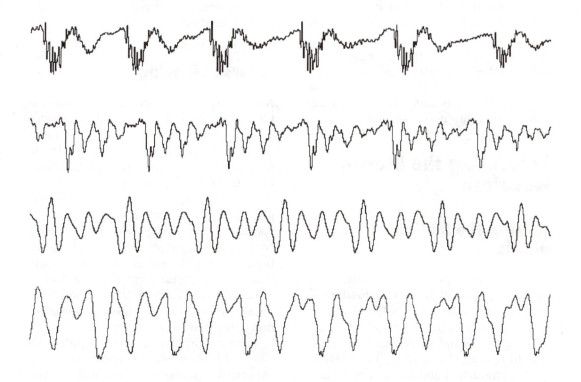

FIGURE 4–17. Speech waveforms of [i], [æ], [ɔ], and [u] (top to bottom channels). In each waveform, one can see five to six fundamental periods.

simplification is to ask the human operator for an estimate. If the program knows that the right answer lies in the vicinity of 100 Hz, it can rule out peaks which are much too close or too far apart.

The analysis then proceeds to identify candidate peaks, zero crossings, or valleys. Because this process is by no means fool-proof, there are various elaborations. Ideally, these methods find the period (and thereby the frequency) of *each* glottal period. That can be an advantage over autocorrelation or frequency-domain analysis, which must deal with at least several periods. Even when this analysis succeeds, however, it is not doing what a human being does. We do not look for just peaks, valleys, and zero crossings; we recognize a similarity in overall shape from period to period.

The most reliable approaches to tracking fundamental frequency today are those which use more than one method and then select a median (central) or modal (most frequent) value. Of course, these multiple analyses require more computing, but they offset the weaknesses of one method with the strengths of another. Different methods tend to fail in different situations, so the right answer is likely to be prominent within a set computed in several ways.

Recovering the Glottal Waveform

Sensing the Motion of the Glottis

One way to improve the accuracy of almost any method of tracking fundamental frequency is to start with the waveform at the glottis rather than at the lips. Plotting the glottal waveform is of value also in testing the source-filter view of speech production and in studying abnormalities of the vocal folds and in voicing. Phoneticians have observed the glottal waveform directly by passing tiny micro-phones down toward their glottises. This technique is not only uncomfortable but dangerous; if the fine wires holding the microphone should break, it may drop all the way into the lungs. There are now ways to pick up the glottal waveform externally. One is the *electroglottograph* (EGG), which tracks the motion of the vocal folds by passing radio-frequency waves through the larynx and measuring changes in impedance caused by the opening and closing of the folds. Even a simple and inexpensive *accelerometer*, a small contact microphone in effect, can measure the motion of the surface of the throat as it is pushed in and out by the pressure above or below the glottis. Figure 4–19 shows the sound pressure waveform of a vowel [a] (top channel) and the simultaneous motion of the throat as transduced by an accelerometer taped to the front of the throat below the larynx (middle channel). Fundamental frequency can be observed and measured more reliably in the latter by most methods.

Inverse Filtering

Another approach is based on the source-filter view of speech presented in Chapter 3. Recall that in this view, the spectrum of sound at the glottis is filtered by the transfer function of the vocal tract and the lips. In other words, the speech signal that radiates from our lips has a spectrum which is just that transfer function applied to the spectrum produced at the glottis. If we could undo the effect of the transfer function, we would recover the glottal spectrum, where the fundamental frequency is quite obvious, because the action of the vocal folds is by far the greatest perturbation in the flow of air at that point.

From x-ray films we know quite a lot about the shape of the vocal tract and therefore its transfer function in the normal production of most speech sounds (in English and some other languages, at least). If we compute a transfer function appropriate to a given steady-state stretch of speech, take its inverse, apply that inverse to the spectrum of the radiated speech, and then compute the waveform corresponding to that spectrum, we do indeed get a waveform which corresponds closely to the pressure waveform at the glottis. The bottom channel in Figure 4–19 shows the underlying glottal waveform as estimated by inverse filtering of the vowel waveform in the top channel. Note that when the glottis closes (where this trace falls sharply), pressure *below* the glottis rises, as shown in the middle channel. Again, measuring fundamental frequency or computing its contour over time is relatively easy in the estimated glottal waveform, because the effects of the transfer function, the resonances, are gone.

As you might expect, inverse filtering is computationally demanding, and it is still being developed. It requires a signal with accurate reproduction of low frequencies. You cannot apply inverse filtering to tape recordings from ordinary microphones, let alone from telephones, for instance. However, inverse filtering can provide noninvasive evidence of glottal and laryngeal abnormalities as well as helping to track fundamental frequency.

Conclusion

In this chapter we have presented some of the current techniques for analyzing speech. These techniques are continuously changing; in both spectral and fundamental frequency analysis, new mathematical approaches and new ways of displaying the signal and its components have been appearing regularly. The excitement of speech science today is not only in new understanding of speech and new practical applications of that understanding, but also in new ways to gain understanding. Similarly, the motivation for all this development has at least three sources: the basic desire to understand a central human activity, the desire to develop better ther-

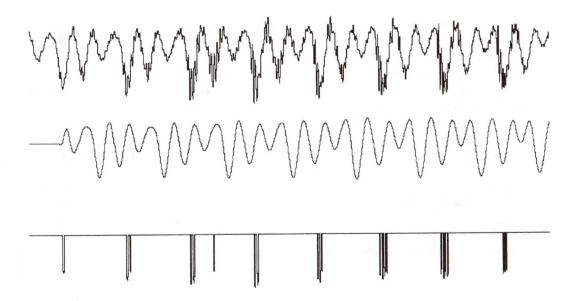

FIGURE 4–18. Top channel: speech waveform of the vowel [i]. Middle channel: the same waveform low-pass filtered at 850 Hz. Bottom channel: the same waveform amplitude-clipped, so that only negative peaks remain.

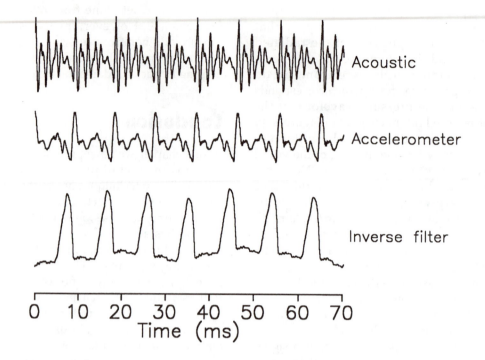

FIGURE 4–19. Top channel: speech waveform of the vowel [a]. Middle channel: output of accelerometer placed on the outside of the throat, just below the larynx. Lower channel: the waveform in the top channel after LPC analysis and inverse filtering to estimate the glottal airflow waveform.

apy for speech that has somehow gone wrong, and considerable commercial interest in speech synthesis and speech recognition. In particular, the difficulty of programming machines to recognize speech has forced us to recognize that what we thought we knew about speech even five years ago was incomplete.

One example can illustrate the unsolved problems: a child, a woman, and a man can each say the same sentence with the same intonation, and each can recognize that they have done so. Therefore, the three utterances must have something in common. Yet all of the techniques surveyed in this chapter

cannot define what that commonality is, at least not in such a general way that we can design a machine which can recognize words in context spoken by any normal talker. Notice that if we could do so, we would have a general transcriber, a hearing machine for the deaf, and other devices that respond to complex spoken commands. All of these practical goals and many others help to energize speech science today.

As a result of that energy, the ideas in this chapter, even more than those in some others, are subject to change. That is part of the excitement of speech analysis in the 1990s.

The Acoustic Characteristics of Vowels and Diphthongs

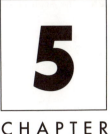

5

CHAPTER

Part 1: Vowels

General Issues in Vowel Production and Perception

In some respects, the vowels are the simplest sounds to analyze and describe acoustically. At least in the traditional understanding, vowels are associated with a steady-state articulatory configuration and a steady-state acoustic pattern. Supposedly, then, a vowel can be indefinitely prolonged as an articulatory or acoustic phenomenon. In this view, it is not necessary to consider the time dimension beyond choosing an instant that is taken as representative of the vowel production. In addition, vowels often have been characterized with a very simple set of acoustic descriptors, namely, the frequencies of the first three formants (vocal tract resonances), as shown in Figure 5–1. Assuming that a vowel is adequately represented by one time sample and by the frequencies of its first three formants,

about all that is needed to characterize the vowels in English is a three dimensional chart showing the formant-frequency values of each vowel. In fact, an even simpler representation often is used—the two dimensional vowel chart showing the frequencies of only the first two formants. The F1–F2 chart, like that shown in Figure 5–2, is perhaps the most widely used and best known acoustic description of a class of speech sounds. Almost every introductory textbook that touches on the acoustic properties of speech includes this chart in some form. In the following sections, we will consider the degree to which such a simple description suffices for the acoustic description of vowels.

Simple Target Model

This classic view of vowels and their perception may be termed the Simple Vowel Target Model. This model assumes that the vowel exists in a canonical form that is invariant across phonetic contexts and is sufficiently defined by a static vocal tract

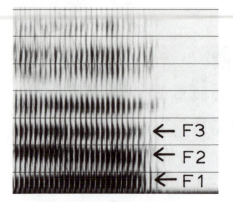

FIGURE 5–1. Spectrogram of the vowel /æ/, with arrows pointing to the first three formants F1, F2, and F3. The thin horizontal lines represent frequency intervals of 1kHz.

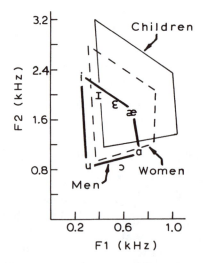

FIGURE 5–2. F1–F2 chart showing the vowel quadrilaterals for men (labeled with phonetic symbols), women, and children.

shape or by a point in the F1–F2 plane (or by a point in the F1–F2–F3 space). This model is implicitly assumed in many introductory (and some not-so-introductory) accounts of vowels. This model is not without limitations or difficulties. First, as becomes immediately evident in any F1–F2 chart that includes data for speakers who differ in age and sex, vowels that are heard to be phonetically equivalent by listeners very often have marked differences in their formant frequency values. A classical portrayal of the acoustic diversity for a given vowel is reproduced in Figure 5–3, which shows the F1 and F2 frequencies for several vowels produced by a sample of 76 speakers including men, women, and children (Peterson & Barney, 1952). As was explained previously, these differences are to be expected from acoustic theory, in that the resonance frequencies of a pipe are determined in part by the length of the pipe. The longer the pipe, the lower are the resonance frequencies. Obviously, a F1–F2 chart like that shown in Figure 5–3 does not give clear support for the Simple

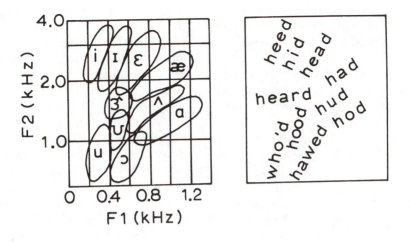

FIGURE 5–3. (Left) F1–F2 chart showing vowel ellipses that enclose the majority of the F1 and F2 frequencies reported by Peterson and Barney (1952) for vowels produced by men, women, and children. F2 frequency scale is logarithmic. (Right) Key words for vowels are positioned so as to correspond to the F1–F2 ellipses at the left.

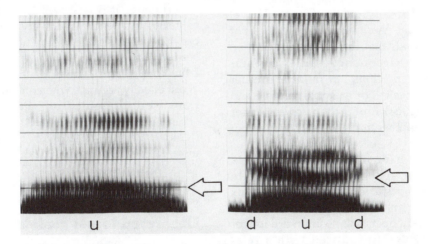

FIGURE 5–4. Spectrographic illustration of vowel undershoot. A sustained, isolated production of vowel /u/ at the left is taken as a target pattern. The production of the same vowel in the syllable /dud/ at the right shows a higher F2 frequency for /u/ than occurs in the target pattern. This difference is called *undershoot* and reflects the effects of phonetic context.

Vowel Target Model. This model can work only if some form of speaker normalization is applied. *Speaker normalization* for vowels refers to a process which eliminates, or corrects for, interspeaker differences in vowel formant frequencies. Normalization is not a trivial problem, and continuing efforts are being made to iden-

tify a reliable solution. (Miller, 1989, summarizes an evaluation of several alternative normalization strategies.)

Another limitation of the Simple Vowel Target Model is its inability to account for the phenomenon of *target undershoot* (Lindblom, 1963). This phenomenon is illustrated in Figure 5–4, which shows the formant patterns for a vowel produced in isolation and the "same" vowel produced in a CVC syllable. Note that the F2 frequency achieved in the CVC syllable does not reach the "target" value determined from the isolated vowel. It appears that the vowel in the CVC syllable undershoots the target. In fact, X-ray data on vowel articulation and acoustic data for vowels confirm that such undershoot effects are abundant in speech. Therefore, the F1–F2 points for a speaker's productions of the same vowel in different contexts will display a range of values. The Simple Vowel Target Model must account for this variation. One possible solution is to propose that listeners compensate for the acoustic undershoot by a perceptual overshoot that essentially corrects for the acoustic discrepancy.

Temporal or dynamic variations are another difficulty for the Simple Vowel Target Model. A close acoustic analysis of vowels reveals that they differ not only in the formant frequency values of their steady-state portions but in several other respects as well. For example, Lehiste and Peterson (1961) found that vowels differ from one another in the following ways:

1. Vowels have inherent differences in duration. Long or tense vowels have greater durations than short or lax vowels, and vowels produced with a relatively open jaw position are longer than vowels produced with a relatively close jaw position.

2. When vowels are produced in context with other sounds, they differ in their formant trajectories. For example, tense vowels tend to have proportionately short offglides (vowel to consonant transitions) and long steady states. Lax vowels, on the other hand, tend to have proportionately long offglides and short steady states.

Work by DiBenedetto (1989a, 1989b) also casts doubt on the simple vowel target model. She reported that a target defined by the time at which F1 reaches its maximum frequency is not an invariant attribute of the vowel. Rather, the temporal pattern of F1 had to be taken into account to determine an invariant correlate of vowel articulation. Her research showed that lower vowels are associated with higher F1 onset frequencies and F1 maxima near the onset of the vocalic portion of a syllable. These results indicate that a single F1 property, such as F1 maximum frequency, is not sufficient to make distinctions of vowel height.

These temporal or dynamic differences are not addressed by the Simple Vowel Target Model. Several experiments have demonstrated the relevance of such differences to vowels (Fox, 1989; Strange, Edman, & Jenkins, 1979; Strange, Verbrugge, Shankweiler, & Edman, 1976). In several experiments, it was shown that vowels in context could be identified very well even if only their transitional segments were presented (the steady-state segments were edited out). In fact, vowel identification was about equally accurate when only the transitions were presented or when only the steady state segments were presented (Jenkins, Strange, & Edman, 1983). For a more extensive critique of the Simple Vowel Target Model, see Jenkins (1987).

Elaborated Target Models

In recognition of these limitations of the Simple Vowel Target Model, some writers have proposed other models that can be called Elaborated Target Models. Most of these account primarily for the problem of speaker normalization. A usual solution is to transform the acoustic measurements of vowel formants to a perceptual or psychophysical space. Such a space may have dimensions scaled in the Bark transform (this transformation is defined in Appendix C). These efforts are designed to model the normalization of acoustic data performed by the auditory system. Therefore, a transform similar to that applied by the auditory system may solve the normalization problem.

Dynamic Specification Model

Strange (1987) believed that neither the Simple Vowel Target Model nor the Elaborated Target Model could adequately account for vowel perception. She proposed instead a Dynamic Specification Model in which temporal or dynamic information is used to identify vowels. Included in this information is the nature of the formant transitions into and out of a vowel steady state and the duration of the steady state. Obviously, a simple F1–F2 chart cannot adequately represent a vowel sound according to this theory. What is needed is a representation that includes temporally defined spectral information.

Some studies have not confirmed the experimental results on which the Dynamic Specification Model was based. These studies reported that isolated vowels were identified as accurately as vowels in context (Assman, Nearey, & Hogan, 1982; Diehl, McCusker, & Chapman, 1981; Macchi, 1980). But Fox (1989) observed that no investigation has demonstrated better identification for isolated vowels than for vowels in consonantal context. A conservative conclusion on the matter is that dynamic information of the kind carried in consonant-vowel and vowel-consonant transitions at least supplements the information carried by steady-state cues (Fox, 1983).

Vowel Identification: Templates vs. Constructed Patterns

The foregoing discussion introduced the problem of vowel normalization and three general theories of vowels that pertain to this problem. We can phrase the question quite simply: If speakers differ in the acoustic properties of their vowels, then how is it that a listener knows which vowel a given speaker is trying to produce?

One idea, introduced by Joos (1948), is that a listener actively constructs idiosyncratic vowel patterns for each speaker. These patterns, or reference frames, can be developed on the basis of a small number of utterances from that person. According to the reference frame hypothesis, the general acoustic context of a vowel provides the essential information from which the listener can construct a referential vowel space for a given speaker. Then, vowels produced by that speaker are interpreted within the vowel space. A variant of this idea is that listeners construct the referential vowel space on the basis of a speaker's vowel [i] (as in *he*). This vowel has special distinctive properties that make it a good "calibration" vowel (Matthei & Roeper, 1983). A weakness of this concept is that listeners cannot always wait for a speaker to produce vowel [i]. The warning, "Look out for that car," as it might be yelled by a passerby who notices a recklessly driven car, does not contain the handy calibration vowel. But the listener who waits for vowel [i] may well wait into eternity.

An alternative idea is that listeners acquire vowel templates based on their long-term experiences with the speech of various persons. These templates are like acoustic averages determined for men, women, and children (Bergem, Pols, & Koopmans-van Beinum, 1988). When listeners try to identify a vowel, they match the unknown vowel with an appropriate template vowel that is an average for men, women, or children. The appropriate template is selected on the basis of the pitch and timbre of the unknown vowel. Bergem et al. (1988) argue that the template theory is supported by the fact that listeners can identify with considerable accuracy even single vowels (without context) produced by any speaker (men, women, or children).

Nearey (1989) summarized the problem of speaker dependent overlap in the F1–F2 plane with respect to intrinsic and extrinsic factors. A purely intrinsic specification assumes that a vowel can be identified from the information contained within the vowel itself. Proponents of this view usually assume that the answer to the problem is to identify the appropiate parametric representation of vowel spectral properties. Nonlinear frequency transformations often are proposed as the solution. (Syrdal, 1984, used a Bark transform of formant frequencies; Miller, 1989, recommended using logarithms of the frequency ratios of formant frequencies.) A pure extrinsic specification holds that the necessary frame of reference lies in information distributed across vowels produced by a given talker. Examples of this approach are described in Gerstman (1968), Nordstrom and Lindblom (1975), and Nearey (1978).

Acoustic Description of Vowels

With the previous information as a backdrop, we will now consider the acoustic specification of vowels. The candidate parameters for the acoustic description are: formant pattern, spectrum, duration, and fundamental frequency.

Vowel Formant Pattern

Much of the experience with synthetic speech lends support to formant pattern as a primary cue for vowel perception. When vowels have been synthesized using the formant frequencies estimated from natural speech, the results have been generally satisfactory (Fry, Abramson, Eimas, & Liberman, 1962). Indeed, the bulk of current work on speech synthesis relies on a formant specification of vowels. Formant frequencies derived from analyses of natural speech are used to specify the formant pattern of synthetic vowels. The overall success of this approach certainly must be weighed as favoring formant descriptions, though not necessarily a description based only on static assumptions.

A *rough* rule of thumb in relating the vowel formant frequencies to vowel articulation is that F1 varies mostly with tongue height and F2 varies mostly with tongue advancement (that is, with variation in the antero-posterior position of the tongue). Caution should be followed in the use of this rule, because there are exceptions. However, multidimensional scaling experiments confirm the general accuracy of the rule (Fox, 1983; Rakerd & Verbrugge, 1985). Rakerd and Verbrugge (1985) reported the following significant correlations between perceptual dimensions and acoustic parameters of vowels: Dimension D1 (interpreted as advancement) with F2 and F3 frequency; Dimension D2 (interpreted as height) with F1 frequency; and Dimension D3 (interpreted as tenseness) with duration. In general, low vowels have a high F1 frequency and high vowels have a low F1 frequency. Back vowels have a low F2 and typically a small F2–F1 difference, whereas front vowels have a relatively higher F2 frequency and a large F2–F1 difference It appears, then, that a vowel's formant pattern can be used to identify a vowel and even to establish relationships between acoustic and perceptual parameters. From a review of several studies, Fox (1983) concluded that the most common dimensions in perceptual scaling studies of vowels correspond to front/back (advancement) and high/low (height) distinctions.

However, some experiments using synthesized vowels cast doubt on the role of formants. Of particular interest are experiments that have studied two-formant models of vowels. These studies have explored listener's identifications of various combinations of F1 and F2 patterns. Carlson, Fant, and Granstrom (1975) reported a study in which F1 was held at values appropriate for natural speech but F2 was varied experimentally. Sometimes the experimental F2' (the prime is used to distinguish this formant from a formant in real speech) varied over a range of values, including frequency values beyond those expected for F2 in natural speech. A graphic summary of the results is given in

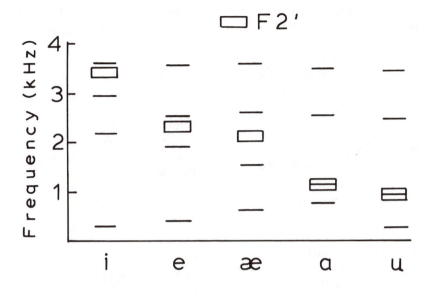

FIGURE 5–5. Stylized spectrograms to show effective second formant frequencies (F2') compared to natural second formant frequencies for five vowels. See text for explanation. Redrawn with permission from R. Carlson, G. Fant, and B. Granstrom (1975). "Two-formant models, pitch and vowel perception," in G. Fant and M.A.A. Tatham (Eds.), *Auditory Analysis and Perception of Speech* (pp. 55–82). London: Academic Press. Copyright 1975.

Figure 5–5. The open rectangular bar shows the frequency value of F2' that gave the most satisfactory acoustic result for each vowel. For the back vowels, F2' approximates the value for F2 in natural speech. However, for the front vowels, a very different result can be seen. F2' for vowels [e] and [æ] falls about midway between the natural F2 and F3. For vowel [i], F2' falls close to the natural F4.

These results are hard to reconcile with a simple formant model of vowel perception. Different approaches have been taken to predict F2' from acoustic measures of vowel formants (Bladon, 1983; Bladon & Fant, 1978; Paliwal, Lindsay, & Ainsworth, 1983). Bladon (1983) concluded from an evaluation of these approaches that the best explanation may rest in an auditory spectral integration of vowel formant energy within a broad bandwidth of about 3.5 Bark. As vowel formant energy moves into and out of this integrating bandwidth, nonlinearities in perceived vowel quality would result. The

3.5 Bark integration also has been indicated in other experiments on the perception of vowels and vowel-like sounds (Chistovich & Lublinskaja, 1979; Chistovich, Sheikin, & Lublinskaja, 1979). If nothing else, these experiments and attempted explanations tell us that the phonetic quality of a given vowel can be associated with more than one specific formant pattern.

Related work has attempted to determine the relationship between vowel formant frequencies and the optimal octaves in vowel perception. If a certain number of vowel formants, say the first three, are the principal determinant of vowel quality, then filtering experiments should show that the optimal octaves for vowel perception are located so as to contain these energy regions. (Octaves are a convenient way of breaking the frequency range into energy bands associated with perceptual effects.) The results of these filtering experiments are a little more complicated than that. Miner and Danhauer (1977) reported the following optimal octaves for the three vowels /i/, /u/, and /a/.

/i/: 1250-2500 Hz; 2500-5000 Hz; 5000-10,000 Hz (all of which approached the identification levels of the control (unfiltered) vowel.

/u/: 80-160 Hz and 160-315 Hz (which closely approximated the identification levels of the control vowel.

/a/: 630-1250 Hz and 1250-2500 Hz (the first of which was more effective than the second).

The Miner and Danhauer data indicate that the optimal octaves for vowel perception are not necessarily in the vicinity of the vowel second formant. In fact, only vowel /a/ conforms to the prediction that F2 is critical for vowel identification. Interestingly, for vowel /i/, three nonoverlapping bands were about equally effective for vowel identification (though not equal in listeners' judgments of distortion).

Although questions remain about the choice of formant pattern as the best acoustic description of vowels, many applications have satisfactorily used this approach. As will be discussed in more detail in Chapter 8, modern speech synthesis (speech production by machine) often relies on formant frequency specifications of sounds to produce machine-generated speech (so-called formant synthesizers). One advantage of the description of vowels by formant pattern is economy. In most cases, it is necessary to specify only the first three formants to achieve a good result. In addition, the formant patterns of vowels frequently are continuous with the formant patterns of neighboring consonants. Another advantage of formant description is that the formants typically are easily observed in acoustic analyses of speech. Indeed, in one approach to speech synthesis, salient acoustic properties such as formant patterns are traced from displays of natural speech and used as input specifications for synthesis. The synthesized pattern is thus a facsimile of the original natural speech.

Table 5–1 lists the values of the first three formant frequencies for several vowels produced by three groups of speakers: men, women, and children. These values should not be taken prescriptively, but rather as averages around which considerable variation may occur.

Vowel Spectrum

Vowels also can be described with respect to their spectra, and some investigators have proposed that spectrum is better than formant pattern in distinguishing vowels. Of course, the formant pattern is reflected in the spectrum of a vowel, but vowel spectra contain information in addition to formants. A graphical summary of the effects of selected spectral variations on vowel identification is presented in Figure 5–6. In spectral tilt the spectrum is rotated along a mid-frequency value to change the relative amplitudes of the low- and high-frequency portions. The effects of such spectral changes are usually slight. A spectral variation in which the depth of the spectral valleys is altered also results in relatively little effect on vowel identification. Logarithmic shifts in the intensity of the spectrum usually have little perceptual effect, except on loudness. Shifts in the relative position of spectral peaks frequently have pronounced effects on vowel perception. A spectral change in which the slope (rate of change in spectrum) changes near a spectral peak has large effects on vowel identification. A general conclusion to be drawn is that any spectral variation that affects the location of a peak can seriously affect the phonetic interpretation of the vowel spectrum.

Vowel Duration

The third parameter is vowel duration. Although duration is neglected in the traditional F1-F2 chart, it is almost always available as a cue in the physical signal of speech. Moreover, vowels can differ substantially in their durations, as illustrated

TABLE 5-1
Formant frequencies (in Hz) of the first three formants (F1, F2, F3) of ten vowels produced by 76 speakers including men, women, and children. Based on data reported by Peterson and Barney (1952). Values for F2 and F3 have been rounded to 50s. The vowel means may be taken to define the approximate formant frequencies of a neutral vowel for each group. Mean F2/F1 and F3/F2 ratios are shown at the bottom of the table.

Vowel	Men			Women			Children		
	F1	F2	F3	F1	F2	F3	F1	F2	F3
[i]	270	2300	3000	300	2800	3300	370	3200	3700
[ɪ]	400	2000	2550	430	2500	3100	530	2750	3600
[ɛ]	530	1850	2500	600	2350	3000	700	2600	3550
[æ]	660	1700	2400	860	2050	2850	1000	2300	3300
[ɑ]	730	1100	2450	850	1200	2800	1030	1350	3200
[ɔ]	570	850	2400	590	900	2700	680	1050	3200
[ʊ]	440	1000	2250	470	1150	2700	560	1400	3300
[u]	300	850	2250	370	950	2650	430	1150	3250
[ʌ]	640	1200	2400	760	1400	2800	850	1600	3350
[ɝ]	490	1350	1700	500	1650	1950	560	1650	2150
Mean	500	1420	2400	575	1700	2800	670	1900	3250
F2/F1	2.84			2.96			2.84		
F3/F2		1.69			1.65			1.71	

in Figure 5–7. Among the factors that influence vowel duration are: tense-lax (long-short) feature of the vowel, vowel height, syllable stress, speaking rate, voicing of a preceding or following consonant, place of articulation of a preceding or following consonant, and various syntactic or semantic factors such as utterance position or word familiarity. (For a good review, see Klatt, 1976.) Experiments indicate that although duration is not sufficient in itself to enable identification of any individual vowel, it does help the listener to distinguish spectrally similar vowels, such as [ae] versus [e] or to place vowels in large categories such as tense versus lax.

Vowel Fundamental Frequency

Vowels also vary in the fundamental frequency of phonation. These differences often are obscured by the many other fac-
tors that govern phonation, such as linguistic stress, speaker emotion, and intonation. But when these factors are controlled, reliable differences in inherent fundamental frequency can be observed. The general rule is that fundamental frequency varies with vowel height. That is, high vowels have a somewhat higher fundamental frequency on the average than low vowels. Figure 5–8 gives a graphical summary of two studies (Lehiste & Peterson, 1961; Peterson & Barney, 1952). It is doubtful if these fundamental frequency differences play a major role in vowel recognition, but they may be secondary cues.

Formant Bandwidth and Amplitude

The conventional F1–F2 chart specifies only the formant frequencies of vowels.

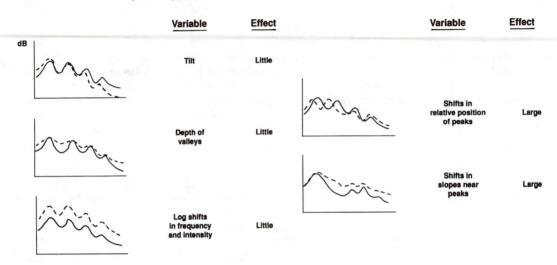

Variable	Effect		Variable	Effect
Tilt	Little		Shifts in relative position of peaks	Large
Depth of valleys	Little		Shifts in slopes near peaks	Large
Log shifts in frequency and intensity	Little			

FIGURE 5-6. Effects of various spectral changes on vowel identification. Spectral change variable is illustrated at the left and effect on identification is summarized at the right. Redrawn from J.D. Miller (1984), "Auditory processing of the acoustic patterns of speech," Archives of Otolaryngology, *110*, 154–159. (Reprinted with permission of the Archives of Otolaryngology.) Copyright 1984.

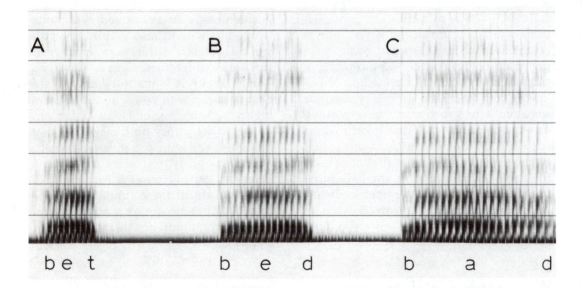

FIGURE 5-7. Spectrographic illustration of variations in vowel duration. Spectrograms are shown for (A) bet /bɛt/, (B) bed /bɛd/, and (C) bad /bæd/.

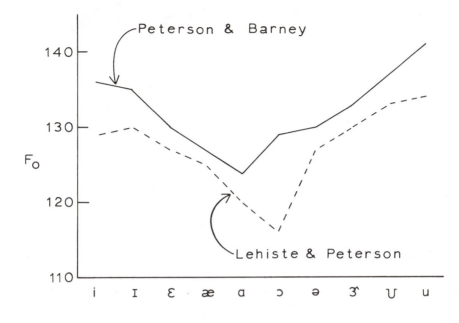

FIGURE 5–8. Mean fundamental frequency for different vowels as reported in two studies (Lehiste and Peterson, 1961; Peterson and Barney, 1952). Note that high vowels are associated with higher fundamental frequencies.

But each formant also can be described by two additional and interacting features, bandwidth and amplitude. In general, any resonance can be described by two numbers, its resonance frequency and bandwidth. Amplitude usually reflects the amount of energy available to the resonator. In describing vowels, it is useful to think of each formant as being described by three numbers: formant frequency, bandwidth, and amplitude. Because the last two typically interact, they need not always be specified individually. However, particularly for some applications in speech synthesis, independent control of bandwidth and amplitude is possible.

Bandwidth is related to damping, which is the rate of absorption of sound energy. The greater the damping, the greater the bandwidth of the sound. Sounds that are greatly damped tend to die out quickly; their energy is quickly dissipated. Sounds that are associated with very little damping tend to be sustained. A

practical application of this concept occurs with the acoustic treatment of concert or lecture halls. Frequently, halls that are enclosed with hard, flat walls are not acceptable acoustically. Sounds produced in these halls tend to echo or reverberate. The hard walls reflect the sound energy, so that the energy of a newly produced sound often competes with the reverberant energy of a previous sound. To reduce this unwanted reverberation, acoustic engineers often use draperies or acoustic tiles that absorb sound energy. The greater the absorption of sound, the less the problem with reverberation.

Each formant of the vocal tract during vowel production has a bandwidth. The usual convention in bandwidth measurement is to measure the width of the formant (or any resonance) between two points that are 3 dB below the peak on either side of it (Figure 5–9). The figure of 3 dB corresponds to the "half-power point," or the point corresponding to half of the acoustic power of the sound as

a - narrow bandwidth
b - moderate bandwidth
c - large bandwidth

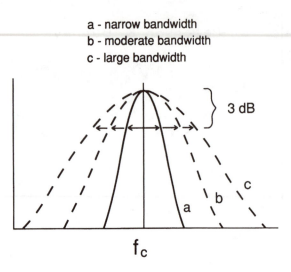

f_c

FIGURE 5–9. Variations in bandwidth for a fixed center frequency, f. Bandwidth is conventionally measured 3 dB down from the energy peak.

TABLE 5–2
Bandwidths of the vowel formants as estimated in five studies.

Bandwidth (Hz)	A	B	C	D	E
Formant 1	54	55	39	130	110
Formant 2	65	66	51	150	190
Formant 3	70	89	80	185	260

A – House and Stevens (1958), closed glottis condition.
B – van den Berg (1955)
C – Lewis (1936)
D – Bogert (1953)
E – Tarnoczy (1948)

determined by the peak. The effect of increasing formant bandwidth is illustrated in Figure 5–9 by the superimposed curves, each of which represents a resonance with a different bandwidth. If the human vocal tract were a hard-walled tube, like a metal horn, its damping would be considerably less than it is. Because the vocal tract is composed largely of soft, moist tissues, an appreciable amount of the sound produced in speech is absorbed by these tissues. Formant bandwidths determined by empirical measurement are summarized in Table 5–2. Formant bandwidth increases with formant number, so that the higher formants have larger bandwidths than does F1.

Experiments have shown that changing the bandwidth of formants has very little effect on vowel perception. In fact, it appears that the ear is not very sensitive to such changes. But even when the effect of bandwidth reduction is perceptually obvious, as when the bandwidth approaches zero, listeners can still identify vowel sounds. It is possible to synthesize a recognizable vowel by generating three simultaneous sinusoids having the frequencies of the first three formants of a vowel (Figure 5–10). The primary perceptual effect of formant bandwidth is on the naturalness of the vowel sound. Vowels that have unusually narrow bandwidths sound artificial even though listeners usually can identify these vowels. One can extend this idea to entire sentences. Remez and colleagues (Remez, Rubin, & Pisoni, 1985; Remez, Rubin, Pisoni, & Carrell, 1981) produced a type of synthetic speech that consisted only of three simultaneous sinusoids, adjusted to vary in frequency according to the formant frequency patterns of human speech. Sentences produced by this "sinusoidal synthesis" were generally intelligible if the listeners were told to expect speech sounds. (Interestingly, if the listeners were told to expect "science-fiction" sounds, they usually did not hear speech at all.) At the other extreme, increasing formant bandwidth eventually can reduce the distinctiveness of vowels, because the energy of the different formants begins to overlap. In such an instance, the vowel spectrum

loses the sharpness of its peaks and valleys (Figure 5–11). Nasalization of vowels has this effect, and it is interesting that nasalized vowels are less distinctive than their nonnasal counterparts (Lindblom, Lubker, & Pauli, 1977; Lubker, 1979).

Formant amplitude is related to formant bandwidth insofar as increases in bandwidth often lead to reductions in overall amplitude. That is, so long as the source energy (that is, the acoustic energy from the larynx) remains constant, increases in formant bandwidth are accompanied by reductions in formant amplitude. The relative amplitudes of the formants in a vowel are determined by the formant frequencies of the formants, the bandwidths of the formants, and the energy available from the source. The last of these probably is quite obvious, given that a resonator cannot create energy but rather depends on the energy from a source such as the vibrating vocal folds. As noted earlier in this paragraph, bandwidth can affect formant amplitude by determing the peak value of the formant. But why does formant frequency pattern affect formant amplitudes? The reason is

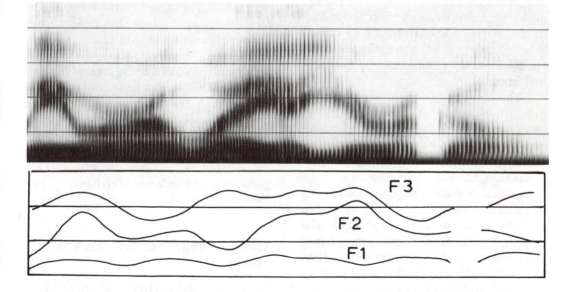

FIGURE 5–10. (Top) Spectrogram of the sentence, "We were away a year ago," and (bottom) sinusoids that vary in frequency according to the F1, F2, and F3 frequencies in the spectrogram at the top.

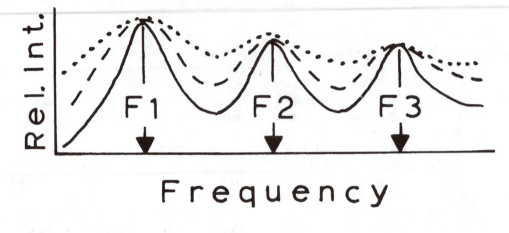

FIGURE 5-11.   Effects of increasing formant bandwidth on the spectrum of a vowel sound.   Bandwidth increases from the solid to the dashed to the dotted lines.

that in vowel production the formants interact. This interaction can be understood graphically as the algebraic addition of the overlapping formant curves at specific frequencies (see Chapter 2). When two formants are drawn closely together, they reinforce one another and both of their amplitudes increase. When these two formants move apart, their interaction is reduced and both of their amplitudes decrease. When F1 moves up in frequency, the higher formants are in effect boosted by the high-frequency tail of the F1 curve. When F1 moves down, the higher formants are not as strongly influenced by the high-frequency tail.

The amplitude envelope of a vowel determines judgments relating to vowel onset, such as hard (abrupt) or soft (gradual) attack. When the envelope of the vowel waveform reaches its maximum rapidly, listeners are apt to judge the vowel as having a hard attack. But when the envelope reaches its maximum value slowly, listeners tend to judge the vowel as having a soft attack. The perceived abruptness of vowel onset seems to be related to the logarithm of the time over which the amplitude envelope rises from 10% to 90% of its maximum value (Peters, Boves, & van Dielen, 1986). This feature does not necessarily affect vowel identification, but it can determine the likeli-

hood with which listeners will hear a glottal stop at vowel initiation. The faster the rise in the amplitude envelope, the more likely is a judgment of glottal stop occurrence.

Summary of the Acoustic Features of Vowels

A full account of the acoustic cues for vowel perception would seem to require consideration of each of these factors—formant pattern, spectrum, duration, fundamental frequency, formant bandwidth, and formant amplitude. Moreover, particularly when vowels are produced in the context of other speech sounds, it may be necessary to consider various dynamic aspects of the acoustic signal associated with the vowel in its phonetic context. These dynamic aspects primarily involve the formant trajectories of the syllable nucleus but also may include variations in fundamental frequency and formant amplitudes.

Formant Synthesizers and Vowel Sounds

As mentioned earlier, one of the best sources of support for the formant pattern as the chief acoustic representation for vowel perception is the success of the so-called *formant synthesizers*. Formant synthesis is a means of synthesizing speech by controlling circuits that generate formant-like energy patterns. This topic will be discussed in more detail in chapter 8, but this is a convenient juncture to illustrate how the acoustic characteristics of vowels can be realized by a machine.

Typically, each formant in a formant synthesizer is generated by a single resonant circuit. The center frequency of the formant is varied by changing the resonance frequency. There are two principal ways in which the component circuits are linked together to produce synthetic speech. One is a *parallel* configuration and the other is a *series* configuration. The parallel configuration (Figure 5–12a) splits the energy from a source to activate the resonant circuits individually. The outputs of the circuits are then summed to produce the output speech signal. With this config-

uration, the frequency, bandwidth, and amplitude of each formant can be independently controlled (although some bandwidth-amplitude interaction can occur). The series configuration (Figure 5–12b) is also called a cascade connection. In this case, the resonant circuits are arranged so that the output of one is the input to the following circuit. In some respects, the series connection models formant relationships that occur in natural speech. For example, in human speech and in the series configuration, the formant amplitudes are not independent; rather, the amplitudes of the formants depend on the formant frequencies. Therefore, the dependency of formant amplitudes on formant frequencies in a series configuration is more like the acoustic behavior of natural speech. However, this feature is not always advantageous. Particularly for experimental work involving independent

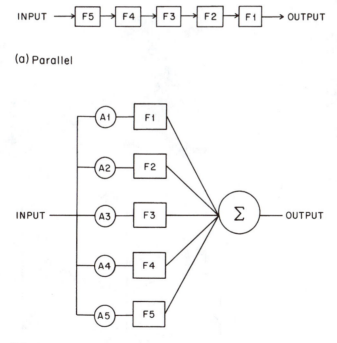

(a) Parallel

(b) Cascade

FIGURE 5–12. Two configurations of speech synthesis based on formants.

changes of formant amplitude and formant frequency, the parallel system is preferable. Notice that in both types of formant synthesis, a source-filter model is incorporated.

Whichever configuration of resonators is used, the formant synthesizer has become a popular choice. Such systems often produce synthetic speech of good to very good quality with modest demands on computer memory and processing. The success of formant synthesizers in producing highly satisfactory tokens of isolated vowels demonstrates that the formant specification of vowels has at least a face validity.

The first two or three formants (F1, F2, and F3) are the most important for vowel identification. Many English vowels can be satisfactorily distinguished from the first two formants alone. However, formant synthesizers often generate formants up through F4 or F5 to enhance the naturalness of the speech sounds. In most of

these synthesizers, F4 and F5 are fixed (no frequency variations are made with changes in vowel identity).

Part 2: Diphthongs

Vowels are also called monophthongs, meaning single (*mono-*) voiced sound (*phthong*). Another class of sounds, related to vowels, is the diphthongs. Diphthongs are like vowels in that they are produced with a relatively open vocal tract and a well-defined formant structure. Diphthongs are unlike vowels in that they cannot be adequately characterized by a single vocal tract shape or a single formant pattern. Diphthongs are dynamic sounds in which the articulatory shape (and hence formant pattern) slowly changes during the sound's production. Figure 5–13 shows

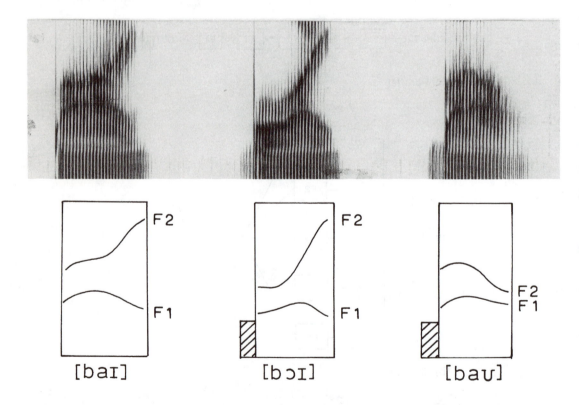

FIGURE 5–13. Spectrograms and extracted F1–F2 patterns for the words *bye*, *boy*, and *bough*. Note distinctive F1–F2 pattern for each diphthong.

spectrograms for three English diphthongs in the words *bye, boy*, and *bough*.

Most phonetic descriptions specify the starting (or *onglide*) and final (or *offglide*) positions of the diphthong. Some phoneticians use the term *nucleus* to refer to the onglide portion. The symbols in the International Phonetic Alphabet reflect this description. For example, the diphthong in the word *I* (or *eye*) is represented by a digraph such as /aɪ/, where the first symbol /a/ represents the onglide and the second symbol /ɪ/ represents the offglide. A similar approach can be taken to describe the diphthongs acoustically. As shown in Figure 5–14, each diphthong can be represented in the F1-F2 chart by a trajectory that begins with the formant frequencies of the onglide and ends with the formant frequencies of the offglide. Comparisons of the formant frequencies of diphthongs with those of simple vowels have been reported by Holbrook and Fairbanks (1962), and Lehiste and Peterson (1961). Limited data have been published for other languages, for example, Chinese (Ren, 1986); Dutch (Collier, Bell-Berti, & Raphael, 1982; Peturrson, 1972); Estonian (Piir, 1983); and Spanish (Manrique, 1979).

Particularly when diphthongs are produced in context or at fast speaking rates, considerable variation can occur in both the onglide and offglide formant values. Accordingly, these trajectory descriptions should be regarded more as suggested than as prescribed values. At least for some dialects, the rate of formant frequency change may be a characteristic feature of diphthong production. Gay (1968) reported that the rate of frequency change was essentially invariant despite variations in the onglide and offglide values. Possibly, then, the rate of formant frequency change is a perceptually important feature for the identification of English diphthongs.

Fox (1983) concluded from a perceptual scaling study of monophthongs and diphthongs in English that similar perceptual features were used for both types of vocalic elements. He also concluded that the perceptual structure of the monophthongs and diphthongs could be satisfactorily modeled in terms of four perceptual dimensions: front/back, high/low, low-back onset, and mid/nonmid. Interestingly, no dimensions were found that related to dynamic acoustic information

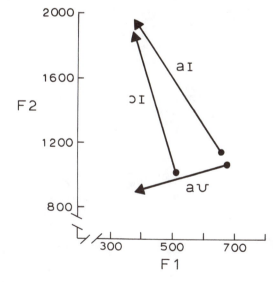

FIGURE 5–14. F1–F2 trajectories for the three diphthongs /aɪ/, /ɔɪ/ and /aʊ/. Arrowhead indicates direction of frequency change.

such as direction or magnitude of formant frequency change.

Summary

Vowels and diphthongs are associated with well-defined formant patterns, and formant frequencies have provided the dominant approach to acoustic characterization of these sounds. This is not to say that formant structure is all that needs to be considered, or that formant structure is the best way to characterize vowels. As noted earlier in this chapter, there are different views of the most accurate and economical acoustic description of vowels and diphthongs. However, formant pattern clearly has dominated the acoustic study of vocalic sounds. Much of the recent work emphasizes that linear frequency representations are not the best way to characterize vowel formants. Instead, proposals have been made for nonlinear frequency transformations such as the Bark transform or logarithms of formant–frequency ratios.

The Acoustic Characteristics of Consonants

6

CHAPTER

The acoustic characteristics of consonants are more complicated than those of vowels. All vowels can be described with essentially the same acoustic characteristics, such as duration or formant pattern, or some other spectral information. However, consonants differ significantly among themselves in their acoustic properties, and it is therefore difficult to describe all of them with any single set of measures. Some consonants involve significant noise generation, whereas others have virtually no noise components. Some consonants are produced with a period of complete obstruction of the vocal tract, whereas others are produced with only a narrowing of the vocal tract. Some consonants are strictly oral in their sound transmission, whereas others involve a nasal transmission of acoustic energy. Because of these differences, the consonants are discussed in groups that are distinctive in their acoustic properties: stops, fricatives, affricates, nasals, glides, and liquids.

In English, the stops are the phonemes /p b t d k g/ (also known phonetically as plosives and stop-plosives). The fricatives are /f v θ ʒ s z ʃ ʒ h/. The nasal consonants are /m n ŋ/. The glides are /w j/ (also called semivowels and approximants). The liquids are the lateral /l/ and the rhotic /r/. A great deal of acoustic information has been collected on consonant sounds. Because this background is important, a selective review of the literature is incorporated in this chapter. Therefore, literature citations will be much more frequent here than in most of the other chapters.

Stop Consonants

The essential articulatory feature of a stop consonant is a momentary blockage of the vocal tract. The blockage is formed by an articulatory occlusion, which for English, has one of three sites: bilabial, alveolar, or velar (there is also a glottal stop, but this will be discussed separately in another section). The term *stop plosive* is used by some writers to refer to the consonants /p t k b d g/, but the more general term *stop* is favored in this book. Not all stops involve the pressure release denoted by the word *plosive*, but all stops necessarily require an articulatory blockage, or stopping.

The articulatory and acoustic classification of stop consonants is diagrammed in Figure 6–1. The upper part of the diagram applies to word-initial, prevocalic stops, such as those produced in CV syllables. Prevocalic stops have both a closure phase and a release phase. (Accordingly, they may be called stop plosives.) The articulatory blockage has a variable duration, usually between 50–100 ms and is subsequently released with a burst of air as the air pressure impounded behind the obstruction escapes. Acoustically, the closure phase is associated with a minimum of radiated energy. Because the vocal tract is obstructed, little or no acoustic energy is produced. But upon the release, a burst of energy is created as the impounded air escapes. This burst is sometimes called a *transient* in recognition of its brevity. Typically, the burst is no longer than 5–40 ms in duration. It is one of the shortest, if not *the* shortest, acoustic events that is commonly analyzed in speech.

Stop releases are classified further as *aspirated* or *unaspirated*. *Aspiration* is a breathy noise generated as air passes through the partially closed vocal folds and into the pharynx. This noise is essentially that of the glottal fricative [h], as in the word *hat*. Naturally enough, the IPA represents aspiration with a superscript **h**. For example, [tʰ] denotes an aspirated voiceless stop. The aspiration closely follows the release burst and is distinguished from it mainly by the spectrum of noise

STOP CLASSIFICATIONS

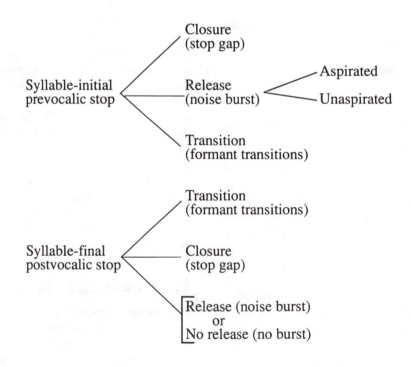

FIGURE 6–1.   Phonetic classification of stop consonants.

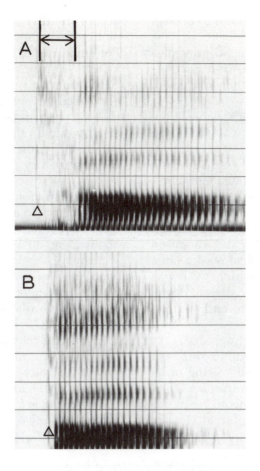

FIGURE 6–2. Spectrograms of (A) aspirated and (B) unaspirated stops. The double arrow in A indicates the interval of aspiration.

energy. In English, the voiceless stop plosives have aspirated releases except when they follow /s/. For example, the words *pie*, *too*, and *core* are produced with aspirated stops whereas the words *spy*, *stew*, and *score* are produced with unaspirated stops. Both aspirated and unaspirated stops will have bursts but only the former will have the [h]-like noise following the burst. Figure 6–2 presents spectrograms of aspirated and unaspirated stops. Note that the aspiration appears in a brief interval between the stop burst and the onset of vocal fold vibrations (voicing) for the following vowel. Voiceless stops in prevocalic position are characterized by a delay

in voicing relative to the release of the stop. This delay is on the order of 25–100 ms, depending on various factors to be considered later.

The voiced stops in English are normally unaspirated. Because the onset of vocal fold vibration begins close to the burst (with voicing just before, simultaneously with, or just after voicing onset), there is little opportunity for an interval of aspiration to occur. The vocal folds must be adducted for effective voicing, and the generation of turbulence noise requires some degree of glottal opening.

Aspiration of stops is phonemic in some languages, but not in English. The information given here pertains to English and will not directly apply to all languages. However, the general principles can be extended to stops in other languages (Fant, 1960a; Fischer-Jorgensen, 1954).

The voicing feature for syllable-initial stops can be specified quite well by a single number that gives the interval between the articulatory release of the stop and the onset of vocal fold vibrations. This time interval is called the *voice onset time* (VOT). The cross-linguistic application of the measure of VOT was described in a classic paper by Lisker and Abramson (1964). This article foreshadowed a large number of studies in which VOT was measured in normal adult speech, developing speech in children, and various speech disorders.

For voiced stops in English, VOTs assume a small range around zero. At VOT = 0, stop release and voicing onset are simultaneous. For example, a VOT of zero for the stop [b] in the word *bye* means that the release of the bilabial closure occurs simultaneously with the onset of voicing for a following diphthong sound. For small negative values of VOT (e.g., VOT = –10 ms), voicing onset briefly precedes the stop release. This situation is also called *prevoicing* or *voicing lead*, given that voicing precedes the release. For small positive values of VOT (e.g., VOT = +10 ms), the onset of voicing slightly lags the articulatory release. The term *short voicing lag* is used to refer to these VOT values. VOTs for voiced stops range from about –20 ms to about +20 ms. Voiceless stops have VOTs that range upward from about 25 ms to as much as 100 ms. The word *range* should be emphasized: There is no single value of VOT that will be used by all speakers or across all phonetic contexts. Generally, voiced and voiceless stops have VOTs in the ranges indicated—the 5-ms gray interval (from 20 to 25 ms) is a kind of boundary region. The VOT ranges for voiced and voiceless stops are illustrated in Figure 6–3. More will be said about voicing in a later section. Voicing is a great deal more complicated than might be

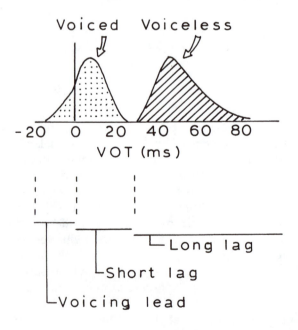

FIGURE 6–3. Distribution of voice onset time (VOT) values for voiced and voiceless stops, showing approximate VOT ranges for voicing lead, short voicing lag, and long voicing lag.

expected given the usual description of voicing as a binary opposition of voiced-voiceless. In fact, the voicing contrast is associated with a number of acoustic cues (Abramson, 1977; Port & Dalby, 1982).

For stops in syllable-initial position, the stop release entails a change in vocal tract shape from stop occlusion to vowel configuration. The articulatory transition from stop to vowel is associated with an acoustic transition in the form of shifting formants. We will call these formant shifts in CV sequences *CV formant transitions*. Much more is said about these transitions in a following section. For the moment, it is sufficient to emphasize that the formant shifts reflect changes in vocal tract shaping during the stop to vowel transition. The formant transitions are a very important acoustic cue for speech perception and have been the focus of numerous research efforts.

The lower part of Figure 6–1 shows the classification of stops in word-final, postvocalic position. These stops can be either released or unreleased. Their only

common feature, then, is a period of articulatory closure. When word-final stops are released, the acoustic evidence of the release is a short burst. The optional nature of the stop release is indicated in Figure 6–1. When the stop is not released (that is, when the closure is maintained until well after the utterance is completed and the oral pressure has dissipated), no burst appears. Obviously, then, the burst is not a reliable acoustic cue for word-final stops, but speakers can make a special effort to articulate the stop distinctly by producing a release burst. Stops in syllable-final position can be voiced or voiceless and, interestingly, an important acoustic cue for this contrast is often carried in the preceding vowel rather than in the consonant segment itself. Vowels are lengthened before voiced stops, so that vowel duration cues the voicing contrast for a postvocalic stop.

When the word-final stop is preceded by a vowel, as in Figure 6–4, an interval of formant transition joins the vowel and consonant segments. The VC formant transi-

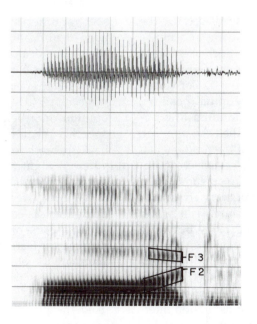

FIGURE 6–4. Waveform and spectrogram of the word *odd*. Notice convergence of F2 and F3 during the vowel-to-consonant transition near the end of the utterance.

tion can be regarded as the reverse of the CV formant transition discussed earlier. For CV sequences, the transition is from stop to vowel, whereas for VC sequences, the transition is from vowel to stop.

As the preceding, rather lengthy, discussion demonstrates, the articulatory and acoustic characteristics of stops are somewhat complex. But with the foregoing information as a foundation, we are prepared to examine in detail the acoustic properties of stop consonants. These properties are considered under the headings of stop gap (closure), burst, formant transition, and voicing. These four elements constitute the basic temporal sequence of stop production.

Stop Gap

The stop gap is the acoustic interval corresponding to the articulatory occlusion. As already noted, this interval is an energy minimum in the acoustic signal because little or no sound is radiated from the obstructed vocal tract. For voiceless stops, the stop gap is virtually silent because the vocal folds are not vibrating and hence voicing energy is absent. Such silent gaps are illustrated in the spectrogram and waveform shown in Figure 6–5. For voiced stops in other than word-initial position, the stop gaps usually contain a low-frequency band of energy called the *voice bar*. This band is the energy of the fundamental frequency of phonation. A spectrogram and oscillogram of voiced stop gaps can be seen in Figure 6–6. The primary criteria for identification of stop gaps are: (1) a region of reduced energy, typically between 50–150 ms in duration, and (2) other evidence of stop articulation preceding or following (or both) the stop gap. This other evidence may take the form of formant transitions, stop bursts, or aspiration intervals. Of course, not every silent interval in speech is a stop gap. Silent segments also are associated with pauses.

Release Burst

The transient that is produced on release of the occlusion is no more than 40 ms in duration and is usually much briefer. As noted earlier, the stop burst is one of the shortest acoustic events in speech. Accordingly, adequate determination of bursts can be made only if the analysis technique has a suitable temporal resolution. In other words, the method of analysis must be able to resolve intervals as brief as 10 ms if stop bursts are to be identified.

It has long been recognized that the spectrum of a stop burst varies with the place of articulation. The spectral variation is attributable to the fact that the short noise burst is shaped by the resonance properties defined by a particular articulatory configuration. To a certain degree, the spectral differences are visible even in spectrograms. As Figure 6–7 shows, labials tend to have a low-frequency dominance, alveolars are associated with high-frequency energy, and velars are characterized by a mid-frequency burst. A major research question has been whether these spectral differences are sufficient for phonetic identification.

A classical early experiment on this question was conducted with a pioneering approach to speech synthesis called *pattern playback*. With this technique, patterns painted on a belt provide a facsimile of speech. When these patterns are played back through an optical-to-acoustic conversion, identifiable speech sounds are produced. Although this technique is crude compared to modern methods of computer speech synthesis, it provided one of the first opportunities to manipulate the acoustic features of speech. This was a landmark development in acoustic phonetics and speech perception.

Liberman, Delattre, and Cooper (1952) used the pattern playback technique to generate the stylized speech stimuli depicted in Figure 6–8. The stop burst is represented acoustically as a short vertical

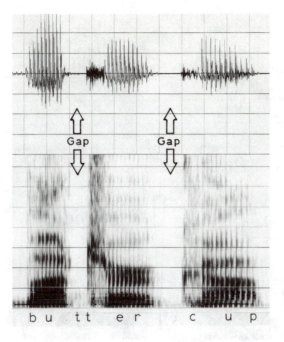

FIGURE 6-5. Waveform and spectrogram of the word *buttercup*. The arrows labeled "gap" point to the voiceless interval associated with the voiceless stops.

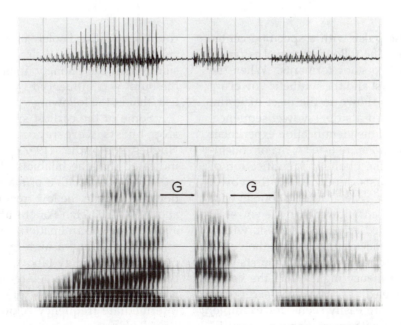

FIGURE 6-6. Waveform and spectrogram of the word *raggedy*. The intervals labeled "G" identify the voiced stop gaps.

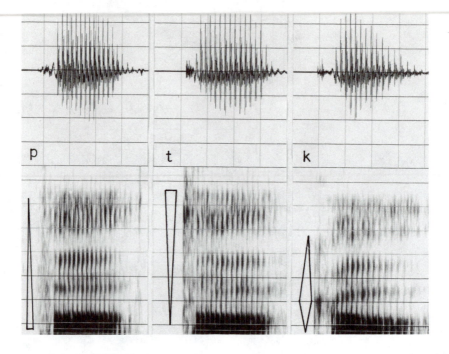

FIGURE 6–7. Waveforms and spectrograms of the syllables /p ɑ/, /t ɑ/ and /k ɑ/. Line drawings near the onset of each syllable suggest the spectral envelope of each burst—low frequency dominance for /p/, high frequency dominance for /t/, and mid-frequency dominance for /k/.

tic or noise pulse with a specified center frequency. The following vowel is represented by two static formants. When the synthetic burst and the synthetic vowel are combined as shown in the inset diagram, listeners heard a stop + vowel sequence. The results of the identification experiment are shown in Figure 6–9. A major conclusion is that the phonetic identification of the noise bursts depended on the vowel context. As a general rule, (1) bursts with a center frequency lower than the vowel F2 were identified as /p/, (2) bursts with a center frequency approximating the vowel F2 were heard as /k/, and (3) bursts with a center frequency higher than the vowel F2 were labeled /t/. However, exceptions to this rule are easily seen—for example, some bursts with energy above vowel F2 were heard as /p/ when the vowels were /o/ and /u/. This experiment established one important result, namely that stops

could be identified solely on the basis of a simplified burst cue. It also raised the possibility that the phonetic interpretation of the burst was influenced by acoustic context, that is, the following vowel.

Some of the earliest spectral data on stop bursts were reported by Halle, Hughes, and Radley (1957). Their results indicated that the bilabials /b/ and /p/ were associated with a primary concentration of energy in the low frequencies, from about 500-1500 Hz. For the alveolars /d/ and /t/, the spectral pattern either was relatively flat or had a high-frequency concentration of energy (above 4 kHz). The burst spectra for the velars /g/ and /k/ had strong concentrations of energy in the intermediate frequency regions of about 1.5–4.0 kHz.

Several more recent studies have determined the acoustic properties of bursts. In a series of studies on this issue,

Stevens and Blumstein (1978) and Blumstein and Stevens (1979) explored the possibility that a spectral template could be associated with each place of stop articulation. The original idea of these templates is illustrated in Figure 6–10: bilabial: a flat or falling spectrum; alveolar: a rising spectrum; and velar: a compact (mid-fre-quency) spectrum. Using these templates to classify naturally produced stops, Blumstein and Stevens (1979) were able to classify stops correctly in 85% of 1,800 stimuli produced by six talkers.

Published studies of stop recognition from bursts present a mixed pattern of results. The rates of correct stop identifica-

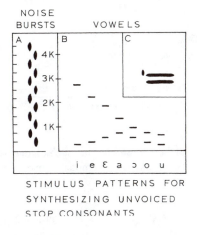

FIGURE 6–8.   Representation of synthesized stimuli used in a study of the phonetic classification of various noise bursts. Each noise burst in A was paired with each of the vowel formant patterns in B to yield stimuli such as that shown in C. Redrawn from A.M. Liberman, P.C. Delattre, and F.S. Cooper, "The role of selected stimulus variables in the perception of unvoiced stop consonants," *American Journal of Psychology, 65*, 1952, 497-516 (redrawn with permission). Copyright 1952.

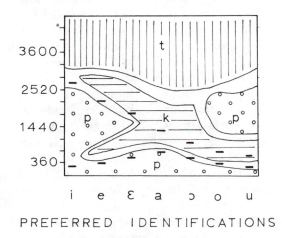

FIGURE 6–9.   Results of identification experiment for the stimuli represented in Fig. 6-8. Regions of /p/, /t/ and /k/ responses are shown. Redrawn from A.M. Liberman, P.C. Delattre, and F.S. Cooper, "The role of selected stimulus variables in the perception of unvoiced stop consonants," *American Journal of Psychology, 65*, 1952, 497-516 (redrawn with permission). Copyright 1952.

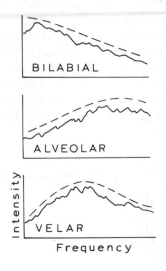

FIGURE 6–10. Spectral patterns of the release burst for bilabial, alveolar, and velar stops. Bilabial: flat falling pattern; alveolar: flat rising pattern; and velar: compact or mid-frequency peak.

tion in six studies were: 58% (Winitz, Scheib, & Reeds, 1972), 100% (Cole & Scott, 1974), 97% (Ohde & Sharf, 1977), 0–69% (Dorman, Studdert-Kennedy, & Raphael, 1977), 88% (Kewley-Port, 1983a), and 92–94% (Forrest, Weismer, Milenkovic, & Dougall, 1988). The large differences in the results of these studies are due in part to differences in procedures. What can be concluded is that at least under certain conditions, stops can be identified reliably from bursts alone.

Kewley-Port's (1983a) study indicated that effective classification of bursts should take temporal factors into account. Her classification matrix for stops is reproduced in Table 6–1. In this dynamic classification, the burst spectrum is categorized as falling, rising, or indeterminate; the onset of voicing is categorized as late, early, or indeterminate; and the presence of mid-frequency peaks (1-3 kHz) for at least 15 ms is noted. The bilabial vs alveolar distinction is based almost entirely on spectral tilt (the shape of the spectrum), whereas velars are identified by late voicing onset and the presence of mid-frequency peaks.

The relatively late voicing onset for velars indicates that VOT varies with place of stop articulation: The general rule is that bilabials have the shortest VOTs (including frequent prevoicing), alveolars have intermediate VOTs, and velars have the longest VOTs.

Other burst characteristics that have been suggested for stop identification are burst amplitude (Jongman & Blumstein, 1985; Ohde & Stevens, 1983) and relative spectral change from burst onset to voicing onset (Lahiri, Gewirth, & Blumstein, 1984). Jongman and Blumstein determined that burst amplitude could serve as one cue to distinguish alveolar and dental stops, with the former having a larger burst amplitude. Lahiri et al. tried to classify stops in Malayalam, French, and English. They discovered that static spectral features could not distinguish labial and dental stops, both of which have a diffuse-flat spectrum. (That is, they had a spectrum with widely and uniformly distributed energy.) But these stops could be identified with a dynamic cue based on a comparison of the ratio of change in the high frequencies (3500 Hz) to the ratio of

TABLE 6–1
Acoustic cues for classification of voiced stop consonants by their noise bursts alone. From Kewley-Port, 1983a.

Stop	Tilt of burst	Feature Late onset	Mid-frequency peaks
b	falling	no	no
d	rising	?	no
g	?	yes	yes

TABLE 6–2
Relationship between place of articulation for stops and the acoustic properties of burst spectrum, voice onset spectrum, and VOT.

Place	Burst onset spectrum	Feature Voice onset spectrum	VOT
Bilabial	Diffuse flat/falling	Low freq. dominance	Early
Dental	Diffuse flat/falling	High freq. dominance	Early
Alveolar	Diffuse rising	Diffuse rising	—
Palatal	Compact	High freq. dominance	?
Velar	Compact	Low freq. dominance	Late

change in the low frequencies (1500 Hz) over the time interval from stop release to voice onset. With this criterion, over 90% of the labial and dental stops were correctly classified. Essentially, this dynamic criterion describes a temporal change in spectral tilt. Similarly, Blumstein (1986) used a spectral tilt feature to distinguish palatal and velar stops in Hungarian. Because both of these stops have a compact spectrum at burst onset, a static spectral feature is not sufficient for their classification.

In summary, stops can be identified from their bursts if several features are examined over an interval of up to 40 msec extending from the onset of the burst to the onset of voicing. A fairly high rate of correct identification should be possible with the following information: spectrum at burst onset, spectrum at voice onset, and time of voice onset relative to burst onset (VOT). Places of stop articulation are

related to these acoustic properties in Table 6–2.

A statistical approach to the acoustic classification of word-initial obstruents was taken by Forrest et al. (1988). In their analysis, FFTs were treated as random probability distributions for which the first four moments (mean, variance, skewness, and kurtosis) were computed. Roughly, the moments can be interpreted as follows: first moment—mean or center of gravity of the spectrum; second moment—distribution of energy around the mean; third moment—spectral tilt; and fourth moment—degree of peakedness of the spectrum. A dynamic analysis based on moments from the first 40 ms of voiceless stop bursts yielded a correct classification rate of 92%. Moreover, the model constructed from the results for male speakers was able to classify the voiceless stops of female speakers at a rate of about 94%, indicating the generality of the analysis across speaker sex.

Formant Transition

In general, changes in vocal tract shape during speech are signaled acoustically by changes in the vocal tract resonances. The acoustic changes have approximately the same duration as the underlying articulatory changes. Thus, if the articulatory transition from stop occlusion to vowel configuration takes 50 ms, the acoustic transition also has a duration of about 50 ms. One fairly reliable temporal constant of stop articulation is that the transition from stop to vowel or from vowel to stop is about 50 ms in duration. Within this 50 ms interval, all formant frequencies shift from their values for the stop to their values for the vowel. Examples of formant transitions are shown in spectrograms and stylized formant trajectories in Figure 6–11. This figure illustrates that all visible formants accomplish their frequency shifts within an interval of about 50 ms. This relatively short transition time relates to the fact that stops are made with rapid articulatory movements.

The three syllables shown in Figure 6–11 are a good starting point for a discussion of formant transitions because they represent three different stops produced with the same vowel. In each syllable, the F1 frequency increases from stop to vowel. This change is fairly easily explained from acoustic theory because the F1 frequency during a stop occlusion is theoretically close to zero. Therefore, the F1 frequency will always increase during a stop to vowel transition (and will decrease during a vowel to stop transition). A very low F1 frequency usually means that the vocal tract is constricted to some degree for a consonant sound. The ultimate constriction is stop closure and it is for stops that the F1 frequency reaches its minimum, which would theoretically be zero for a hard-walled tube, but since the vocal tract is not really hard-walled, F1 only approaches zero during stop closure.

The formant frequency changes are not as simple for F2 and F3 as they were for F1. The F2 frequency increases slightly during the transition from [b] to [ɑ], but it decreases slightly for the [g] to [ɑ] transition and decreases markedly for the [d] to [ɑ] transition. This result holds the promise that the F2 transition may be sensitive to place of stop articulation. A similar suggestion is prompted by the results for F3. That is, the F1 transition appears to be a cue to *manner of production* (degree of constriction), and the F2 and F3 transitions

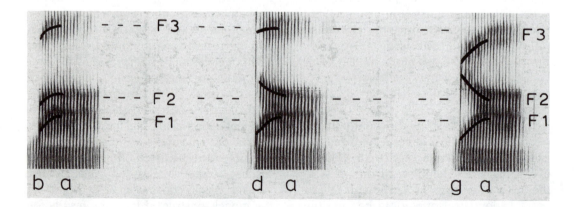

FIGURE 6–11. Spectrograms with highlighted formant transitions for the syllables /bɑ/, /dɑ/, and /gɑ/. Note distinctiveness of F2 and F3 transitions, but the uniformity of the F1 transition.

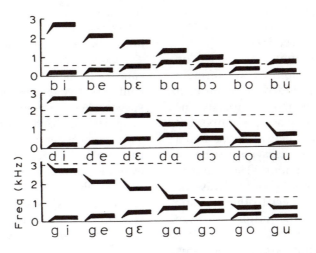

FIGURE 6–12. Stylized spectrograms (F1 and F2 patterns) for CV syllables composed of the stops /b/, /d/, and /g/ and each of seven vowels. The broken line in each CV series is an estimate of the F2 locus for that place of articulation. For example, the F2 locus for the bilabial /b/ is approximately 600 Hz. Adapted from Delattre, Liberman, and Cooper (1955).

may be cues to *place of production*. To evaluate this idea, we will revisit a significant part of the history of speech research.

Although formant transitions are evident in natural speech, they can be difficult to measure because of variability in their durations, rate of change, and terminal points. Because of these difficulties in the analysis of natural speech, it was easier to study formant transitions in synthetic speech. Early studies were performed with the pattern playback which allowed investigators to determine the perceptual qualities of various formant transitions. This work securely demonstrated that variations in the F2 transition between consonant and vowel were sufficient to produce stimuli identified as different stops. The problem that remained was to explain how stop identification related to the form of the transitions. It was immediately clear that a given consonant was associated with a variety of transitions, depending on the vowel context. Figure 6–12 shows the variety of stylized spectrographic patterns that applied to the three voiced stops /b d g/ in seven vowel contexts. Note in particular that /d/ could

have a rising transition, a flat transition, or a falling transition, depending on the vowel that followed it. Obviously, the direction of F2 shift was not in itself a sufficient cue to determine stop identity.

From examination of patterns like those in Figure 6–12, it was recognized that a unifying feature of the various F2 transitions might be the starting frequency. For example, all of the F2 transitions for /b/ were consistent with the hypothesis that the F2 starting frequency was very low, somewhere in the region of 600–800 Hz. For /d/, the F2 starting frequency appears to be about 1800 Hz. The results are not as simple for /g/, but it must be remembered that velar stops are not produced with a single site of contact but rather with a substantial antero-posterior (front-back) range associated with the vowel context. In the case of bilabials and alveolars, for which a definite point of occlusion is maintained across vowel contexts, the evidence for the hypothesized constant starting frequency of F2 is fairly strong. This starting frequency came to be known as the *locus*. The F2 locus for bilabials was estimated to be about 800 Hz and the F2 locus for alveolars, about 1800 Hz. At least two F2 loci were needed for /g/—one at about 3000 Hz and one at about 1300 Hz.

These locus values were based on experiments with simplified two-formant stimuli. When F3 is added to the formant pattern, a clearer picture emerges. For one thing, the F2–F3 relationship is important for velars, for which the transitions into a following vowel are characterized by an increasing F3–F2 separation. The results of perceptual experiments should always be interpreted with respect to the acoustic stimuli from which the judgments were obtained.

As a further illustration of the locus concept, Figure 6–13 shows several different F2 transitions for the stop /d/ produced with different following vowels. Despite the considerable divergence of the patterns, the starting point is essentially the same. Similar ideas can be applied to the F3 transition, and current understanding of formant transitions emphasizes the combined frequency shifts of F1 (a cue for manner of articulation) and F2 and F3 (cues for place of articulation). It also should be emphasized that the formant loci are consistent with the resonance frequencies calculated from acoustic theory

for each place of consonant articulation (Stevens & House, 1956). That is, the loci are grounded in acoustic theory.

Confirmation of the perceptual significance of formant transitions has come from contemporary experiments with synthetic speech. When the formant transitions are properly specified, listeners can identify stops even when bursts are omitted from the synthetic stimuli. Spectrographic examples of computer-synthesized stop + vowel syllables are shown in Figure 6–14. As compelling as some of the synthesis experiments have been, analyses of natural speech still do not provide strong support for the locus concept. Kewley-Port (1983b) concluded that none of the individual F1, F2, or F3 transitions were distinctive correlates of place of articulation when they were analyzed with respect to onset frequency and duration. In addition, the formant loci for F2 and F3 were so variable across vowel contexts that determination of a single locus frequency for each stop was tenuous (although the results for /d/ did converge on the expected value of 1800 Hz). A summary of Kewley-Port's F2 and F3 loci is given in Table 6-3.

A distinctive property of the F2 and F3 transitions for the velar stop is that both

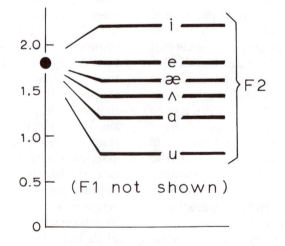

FIGURE 6–13. Composite illustration of the F2 patterns for syllables composed of an alveolar stop /d/ and six different vowels. F2 locus for /d/ is indicated by filled circle on frequency axis.

appear to emerge from the mid-frequency noise burst. This pattern is illustrated in Figure 6–15. Notice that F2 and F3 diverge from a common frequency region that is continuous with the burst. The pattern is similar to one that Stevens and Blumstein (1975) described as having a leading edge that is "wedge-shaped." The mirror-image pattern occurs for the VC transition, shown in Figure 6–15. The F2-F3 divergence or convergence is a useful cue for the velars and is a more reliable criterion than any single locus value.

Klatt (1979, 1987) suggested a modified-locus approach in which the starting frequency of the F2 transition is plotted against the F2 frequency of the following vowel. This approach yields a graph in which each point carries both consonant and vowel information. Klatt proposed that the frequency coordinates thus determined should be grouped into vowel subsets, such as front vowel, rounded vowel, back vowel, and unrounded vowel. Evidence for a locus theory is obtained if the data points for a given vowel subset fall on a straight line. A linear relationship indicates that the onset frequency of F2 for a given consonant can be predicted from the vowel target frequency. Sussman (1989) examined this possibility for two male speakers and presented locus equations for F2 and F3 of /b/, /d/, and /g/. He reported distinctive slopes for the linear locus equations. For example, for one speaker, the F2 slope value was 0.91 for bilabial place, 0.46 for alveolar place, and 0.67 for velar place.

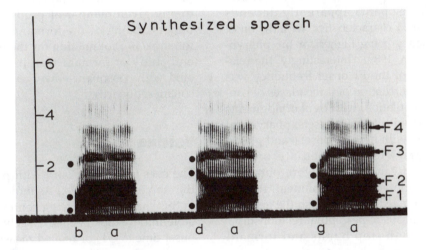

FIGURE 6–14. Spectrograms of synthesized CV syllables. The small filled circles near the onset of each syllable indicate the starting frequencies of F1, F2, and F3.

TABLE 6–3
F1, F2, and F3 loci for three places of stop articulation.
After Kewley-Port, 1983b.

	F1	Locus Estimate F2	F3
Bilabial	near 0	1100–1500	2200–2400
Alveolar	near 0	1800	2500–2700
Velar	near 0	1500–2500	2200–3000

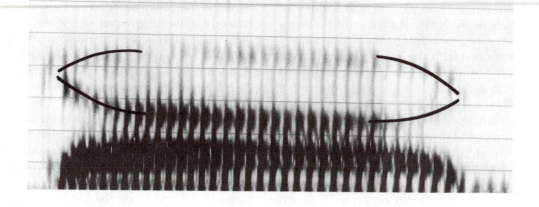

FIGURE 6–15. Spectrograms of the syllable /gæg/ with highlighted F2 and F3 transitions. Note wedge-shaped F2-F3 patterns.

Discrimination of pharyngeal and uvular consonants apparently depends largely on F1 characteristics, with the onset F1 frequency being higher for the pharyngeal (Alwan, 1989). Interestingly, the relative value of the F1 onset frequency was related to perception of three places of consonant articulation, with uvular judgments associated with low F1 onsets, pharyngeal judgments with high F1 onsets, and glottal judgments with intermediate onsets. Because Alwan's results were obtained with a single vowel environment, further studies are needed to establish the generality of this acoustic-perceptual relationship.

Although stop bursts and formant transitions have been considered separately, both are often available in speech perception. Therefore, they are complementary cues and their integration probably leads to a stronger phonetic percept than would be formed with either one alone. One additional important point is that the formant transition cue applies to consonants generally. For instance, we will discover in a following section that the nasal consonants produced like the stops with bilabial, alveolar, and velar articulations, have similar formant transitions. This result is not surprising if we remember that the formant transitions are a cue to

place of articulation and are not restricted to any given manner of production. An understanding of the formant transitions for stops is a foundation for the more general study of formant transitions associated with consonant-vowel or vowel-consonant sequences.

Voicing

The cues for voicing vary with position of the stop in the syllable. As indicated early in this chapter, the voicing contrast for syllable-initial stops is cued largely by voice onset time (VOT) or related measures such as aspiration. The cross-language significance of VOT was described by Lisker and Abramson (1964). VOT has been one of the most frequently measured phenomena in speech research. Baken (1987) gives a useful summary of VOT data for speakers of either sex and various ages. Klatt (1975) is a good source for data on the relationships among the temporal measures of VOT, frication, and aspiration in word-initial consonants and consonant clusters. Still another term encountered in discussions of syllable-initial voicing contrasts is "F1 cutback." The effect of F1 cutback is that the onset of F1 energy is delayed relative to higher formant energy for voiceless stops. The relative delay of F1 energy seems to be a useful cue for the voicing contrast. Fundamental frequency also can help to cue the voicing distinction: vowels following voiceless stops are associated with a higher onset of f0 than are vowels following voiced stops (Haggard, Ambler, & Callow, 1970). Apparently, several cues can contribute to the perception of voicing of syllable-initial stops.

As mentioned previously, vowel duration often is an important cue for the voicing of syllable-final stops. Vowels are lengthened before voiced stops (Chen, 1970; House & Fairbanks, 1953; Raphael, 1972). Chen reported that for English, the average ratio of vowel duration for vowels before voiceless as opposed to voiced consonants is 0.61. This is a rather large durational difference and one that should be readily perceived. Speakers can signal the voicing contrast in syllable-final position with other cues as well, including presence/absence of voicing during closure, duration of stop gap (with a longer duration for voiceless stops), strength of release burst or presence of aspiration (with a stronger burst or aspiration for voiceless stops), and perhaps even fundamental frequency (Hogan & Rozsypal, 1980; Wolf, 1978). There may be a hierarchy of acoustic cues for voicing, with timing information used only when other cues are unavailable or ambiguous (Barry, 1979; Hogan & Rozsypal, 1980; Port & Dalby, 1982; Wardrip-Fruin, 1982).

The voicing contrast for intervocalic stops, such as those for the word pair *rapid* vs *rabid* can have several acoustic cues, including duration of stop gap, strength of burst, fundamental frequency, duration of preceding vowel, formant transitions, and others (Abramson, 1977; Lisker, 1978). Although multiple cues are available, some are probably more commonly used than others. But it is important to recognize that several cues are available to signal voicing contrast in the intervocalic position.

Many of these same acoustic cues serve to signal the voicing contrast for other obstruents—the fricatives and affricates. Therefore, we will not repeat this information for each consonant class. Because the voicing cues are especially complicated for stops, the discussion of voicing for these sounds readily prepares the way to understand voicing for other consonants. Despite the multiplicity of acoustic cues for voicing, it is possible that all of them can be unified in terms of relatively simple underlying concepts. For examples of this attempt, see Lisker and Abramson (1971), Slis and Cohen (1969), and Stevens and Blumstein (1981).

Fricative Consonants

As discussed in Chapter 2, the essential articulatory feature of a fricative is a narrow constriction maintained somewhere in the vocal tract. When air passes through the constriction at a suitable rate of flow, a condition called *turbulence* results. Turbulence means that the particle motion in the air stream becomes highly complex, forming small eddies in the region just beyond the constricted segment. The aerodynamic condition of turbulence is associated with the generation of turbulence noise in the acoustic signal. Thus, fricatives are identified (1) by the formation of a narrow constriction somewhere in the vocal tract, (2) by the development of turbulent air flow, and (3) by the generation of turbulence noise.

Fricatives are not the only class of sounds involving noise generation. However, compared to stops and affricates, fricatives have relatively long durations of noise, and it is this lengthy interval of aperiodic energy that distinguishes fricatives as a sound class. It is risky to assign a particular duration to fricative noise segments, because the duration is influenced by numerous contextual factors. Klatt (1974, 1976) reported that the duration of fricative /s/ can range from 50 ms in consonant clusters to 200 ms in phrase-final position. You (1979) found that the duration of noise for a fricative varies with place of articulation, with average duration increasing in the following order: dentals, labials, alveolars, and palatals. It also appears that fricatives vary greatly in the stimulus duration that is needed for identification. Jongman (1989) studied fricative identification in edited consonant-vowel syllables (such as [si] and [fu]). The identification of /ʃ z/ was accomplished with only about 30 ms of frication, whereas /f s v/ needed about 50 ms for an equivalent rate of identification. The fricatives /θ ð / were identified reasonably well only when the entire frication interval was available.

One thing that can be safely said is that when stops, affricates, and fricatives are compared in an equivalent context, the fricatives will tend to have the longest noise segments. In a study of the noise segment durations for stops, affricates, and fricatives in the languages of Mandarin, Czech, and German, Shinn (1984) identified the following durational boundaries: 62–78 ms for the stop-affricate boundary, and 132–133 ms for the affricate-fricative boundary. That is, for his stimuli (isolated meaningful CV syllables), noise segments were likely to be labeled stops if they were less than about 75 ms, affricates if they were in the range of 75–130 ms, and fricatives if they were longer than 130 ms.

Fricatives in English are produced at five places in the vocal tract: labiodental—/f v/, linguadental—/θ ð/, lingua-alveolar—/s z/, linguapalatal—/ʃ ʒ/, and glottal—/h/. These nine fricatives may be classified into *stridents* /s z ʃ ʒ/ and *non-stridents* / f v θ ð h/. Some phonetics books use the term *sibilants* (and nonsibilants) rather than stridents (and nonstridents). Strident fricatives have a much greater noise energy than nonstridents, and the difference in amplitude often has been considered to be an important perceptual factor. But a perceptual experiment reported by Behrens and Blumstein (1988) cast some doubt on the phonetic sig-

nificance of the amplitude of the fricative noise. Behrens and Blumstein manipulated the amplitude of noise energy of the stridents /s ʃ/ and the nonstridents /f θ /. Listeners were asked to identify the amplitude-altered stimuli. Although decreases in noise amplitude for /s ʃ/ resulted in a substantial increase in the number of /f θ/ responses, increases in the noise amplitude for /f θ/ did not produce a corresponding increase in the number of /s ʃ/ responses. Although acoustic measurements consistently show differences in noise amplitude between the stridents and nonstridents, the perceptual significance of these differences is somewhat in doubt. Amplitudes of frication noise for voiceless fricatives produced by two speakers in three vowel contexts were reported to have the following ranges: /ʃ/ — 59–65 dB; /s/ — 57–68 dB; /f/ — 47–52 dB; /θ/ — 42–52 dB (Behrens & Blumstein, 1988). Another set of measures of frication amplitude were reported by Jongman (1989): /z/ — 70 dB; /v/ and /ð/ — 66 dB; /s/ — 65 dB; /ʃ/ — 64 dB; /θ/ — 54 dB; and /f/ — 53 dB. A proper interpretation of these values requires recognition of another property of fricatives, voicing.

Fricatives also are classified with respect to voicing as voiced or voiceless. The voiced fricatives /v ð z ʒ/ are produced with two sources of energy, the quasiperiodic energy of vocal fold vibration and the aperiodic energy of turbulence noise. The voiceless fricatives have only the latter source of energy. As the information in the preceding paragraph shows, voiced fricatives have a greater amplitude of the frication interval than their voiceless counterparts. In Jongman's (1989) study, frication amplitude for /z/ exceeded that for /s/ by 6 dB, and the amplitude for /v/ exceeded that for /f/ by 13 dB. Voiced fricatives tend to have shorter noise segment durations than voiceless fricatives (Baum & Blumstein, 1987; Crystal & House, 1988). However, there is considerable overlap in the durations of noise segments of voiced and voiceless fricatives

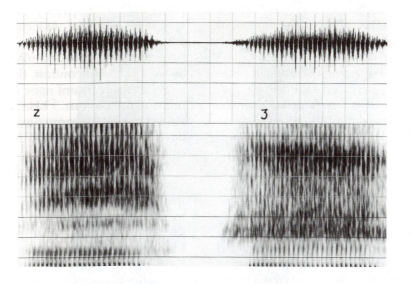

6-17. Waveforms and spectrograms for isolated productions of the fricatives /z/ and /ʒ/.

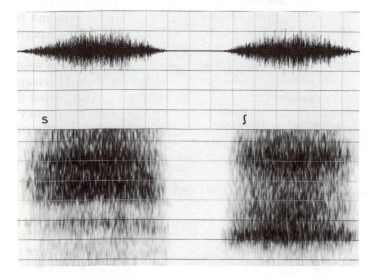

6-18. Waveforms and spectrograms for isolated productions of the fricatives /s/ and /ʃ/.

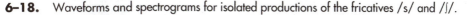

ed the resulting noise as /ʃ/ when er frequency of the pole was below kHz and as /s/ when the center ncy was between about 4-8 kHz. ue and Massone (1981) determined tive importance of different noise to fricative identification by filter- sounds with various low- and

high-pass circuits. Identification of /s/ appeared to depend on energy peaks at about 5 and 8 kHz, whereas identification of /ʃ/ was related to a peak at about 2.5 kHz. The results of this filtering study are consistent with the synthesis study of Heinz and Stevens (1961) in demonstrating the importance of a low-frequency noise when large numbers of these sounds are compared together. That is, the durational differences in noise segments are statistical, rather than categorical.

These classifications of English fricatives are summarized in Figure 6–16, which will serve as the framework for the following discussion of the acoustic properties of these sounds.

Stridents

The strident fricatives possess intense noise energy and are distinguished among themselves with respect to voicing and noise spectrum. The turbulence noise of voiced fricatives is modulated by the laryngeal vibrations. This quasiperiodic modulation is illustrated in Figure 6–17 with both a waveform and a spectrogram for [z] and [ʒ]. The spectrogram reveals how the turbulence noise is pulsed by the voicing source. The voiceless cognates [s ʃ] are shown in Figure 6–18. For these fricatives, continuous noise energy is evident in the waveform and the spectrogram.

It is clear from comparing the spectrograms in Figures 6–17 and 6–18 that the spectra for alveolar fricatives contain rela-

tively higher fre
spectra for palata
adult male talke
noise energy for
above 4 kHz. In
tives have signific
ing down to abo
values are only a
have to be scaled
children.

Spectrograms
nation of the deta
fricatives. For this
to use spectra de
such as FFT or LP(
LPC spectra for th
contained in Figure
lier with spectrogr
tive has more energ
compared to the pa
palatal fricatives h
maxima and mini
Apparently, these
are of relatively slig
perception of these
with synthesized f
Stevens (1961) mode
a single low-freque
nance) and a singl
applied to a white n

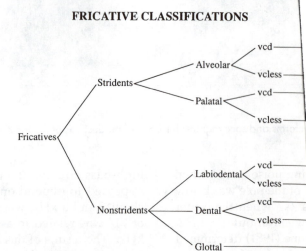

FRICATIVE CLASSIFICATIONS

FIGURE 6–16. Phonetic classification of fricative consonants.

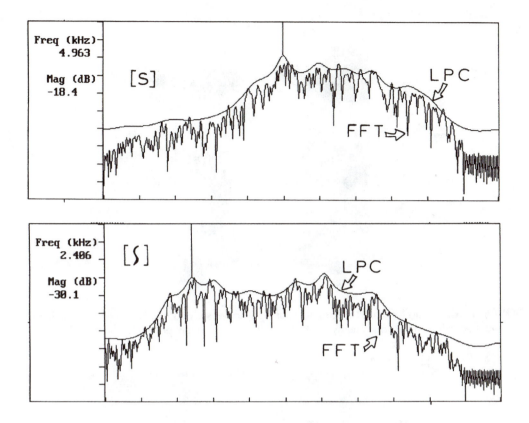

FIGURE 6–19.   FFT and LPC spectra for the fricatives /s/ and /ʃ/. Values shown at left pertain to vertical line on spectra.

region for /ʃ/ and a high-frequency noise region for /s/. Forrest et al. (in press) attempted to classify voiceless fricatives from the first four moments (mean, variance, skewness, and kurtosis) computed from FFTs of the frication noise. Among these statistical measures, skewness was found to be effective in distinguishing /s/ and /ʃ/, especially when a Bark transform was applied to the acoustic data. However, the statistical classification did not fare well with the nonstridents /f/ and /θ/. Nearly half of the /θ/ tokens was misclassified as /f/.

Another guideline for the spectral distinction between alveolar and palatal fricatives is based on a comparison of the major noise region of the fricative with the formant pattern of a vowel produced by the same talker. As shown in Figure 6–20, the lower frequency limit of the primary noise energy for [s] is close to the frequency of F4 for the vowel. For the palatal fricatives, the lower frequency limit of the major noise region is closer to the frequency of F3 for the vowel. As a test of this criterion, you might try to classify each labeled noise segment in Figure 6–21 as either [s] or [ʃ]. Each fricative occurs close to a vowel, making it convenient to compare the noise region of the fricative with the formant pattern of the vowel.

As described earlier for stops, consonants are joined to preceding or following vowels by an interval of formant transitions. Fricatives are no exception. The formant transition probably is secondary to the noise spectrum as a cue for the percep-

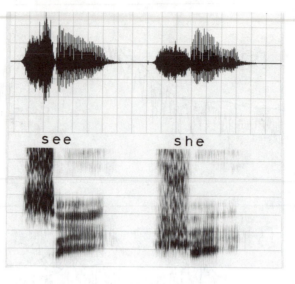

FIGURE 6–20. Waveforms and spectrograms of the syllables *see* and *she*. Notice relationship between the lower-frequency limit of noise energy for the fricative and the formant pattern for the following vowel.

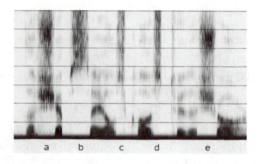

FIGURE 6–21. Spectrogram of the sentence, "The ship sails close to the shore." Try to classify the frication intervals as either alveolar or palatal.

tion of stridents. The spectrum is primary because the noise energy for stridents is intense and phonetically distinctive. Experimental demonstrations of this point were provided by Harris (1958) and LaRiviere, Winitz, and Herriman (1975a). Harris used a splicing technique in which the noise segment of one fricative was combined with the transition segment of another fricative. The identification of the strident fricatives from their noise segments was unaffected by this procedure, indicating that the noise spectrum was

highly distinctive. LaRiviere et al. studied fricative identification for edited stimuli in which different cues were available. Their results were like those of Harris in demonstrating that the stridents were well identified from the noise segment alone. However, it also was discovered that the transition interval could aid the identification of the stridents and that the relative value of the noise or transition interval varied with vowel context. For example, the noise segment for [s] was not as effective a cue in the [i] context as it was in the

[a] or [u] contexts. It may be concluded that although stridents can be identified fairly well from their noise segments alone, formant transitions can play a secondary role in improving fricative recognition.

Nonstridents

For these fricatives, we can consider the same major acoustic features discussed for stridents. The voiced nonstridents /v ð/ are shown as waveforms and spectrograms in Figure 6–22. The overall noise energy of the nonstridents is obviously less than that for the stridents. Quasiperiodic modulation of the noise by glottal pulses is evident for the voiced nonstridents in Figure 6–22 but is lacking for the voiceless nonstridents in Figure 6–23.

As a group, the nonstridents are weak in overall energy and possess fairly flat or

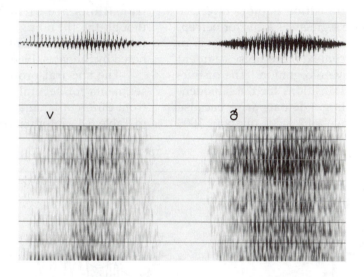

FIGURE 6–22. Waveforms and spectrograms for isolated productions of the fricatives /v/ and /ð/.

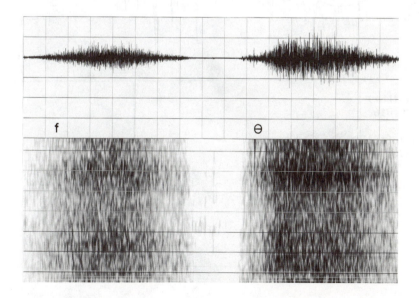

FIGURE 6–23. Waveforms and spectrograms for isolated productions of the fricatives /f/ and /θ/.

diffuse spectra. The spectral flatness is illustrated by FFT and LPC spectra in Figure 6–24. The pronounced difference in energy between stridents and nonstridents makes it unlikely that a strident would be confused for a nonstrident, or vice versa. When confusions occur, they are more likely to be among the stridents or among the nonstridents.

The experiments by Harris and LaRiviere et al. cited earlier indicated that the formant transition is more effective than the noise segment as a cue for perception of the nonstridents. However, in some vowel contexts, the noise segment can aid fricative recognition. The distinctive formant transitions for the labiodentals and the linguadentals arise because the former have a F2 locus of about 1000 Hz compared to a F2 locus of about 1400 Hz for the latter (assuming an adult male talker). The fricative /h/ typically is not associated with formant transitions. Not only is /h/ produced at the glottis and pharynx, but it can be almost completely coarticulated with a following vowel's vocal tract shape. For instance, in the word *he* [hi], the vocal tract configuration for the vowel [i] is assumed during the fricative production. Therefore, formant transitions are virtually absent even though the [h] noise segment often has a fairly marked formant-like structure (as noted by Strevens, 1960).

The spectral properties of the noise segments for several voiceless fricatives from different languages are summarized in Table 6-4. Information is given on rela-

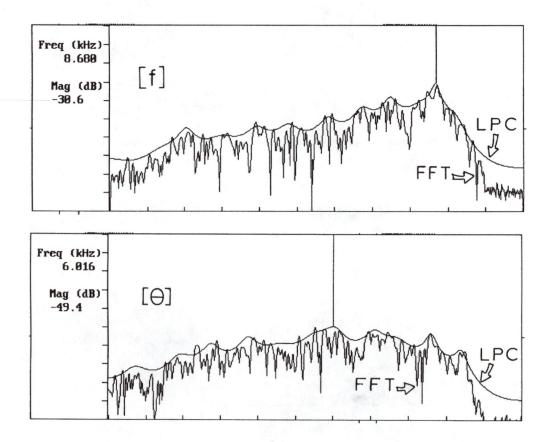

FIGURE 6–24. FFT and LPC spectra for the fricatives /f/ and /θ/.

TABLE 6–4
Spectral properties of voiceless fricatives.

IPA	Place	Frequency of Occurrence (rank)[a]	Relative Intensity[b]	Effective Spectrum Length[c]	Spectral Peaks (kHz)[d]	Spectral Peaks (kHz)[e]
Φ	Bilabial	–	Low	Long	–	–
f	Labiodental	3	Low	Long	1.5, 8.5	(0.5-0.6), 1.0-2.7
θ	Dental	6	Low	Long	–	(0.5-0.6), 1.5-2.3
s	Alveolar	1	High	Short	5.0, 8.0	1.0-2.7, 4.4-9.5
ʃ	Palatoalveolar	2	High	Short	2.5, 5.0	1.0-2.0, 2.3-5.3
ç	Palatal	7	High	Short	–	0.9-1.3, 2.7-4.4
x	Velar	4	Medium	Medium	–	1.0-1.7, 3.7-4.4
χ	Uvular	5	Medium	Medium	–	0.9-1.7, 3.1-3.7
h	Glottal	–	Medium	Medium	–	–

a   Based on frequencies of occurrence in 317 languages reported by Nartey (1982).
b, c   From Strevens (1960).
d   From Manrique and Massone (1981).
e   Interpreted from tables in Nartey (1982). Values indicate ranges over which prominent peaks occur. Parenthesized values indicate peaks present in some languages or contexts but not others.

Sources:

Manrique, A.M.B., and Massone, M.I. (1981). Acoustic analysis and perception of Spanish fricative consonants. *Journal of the Acoustical Society of America, 69,* 1145–1153.

Nartey, J.N.A. (1982). On fricative phones and phonemes: Measuring the phonetic differences within and between languages. UCLA Working Papers in Phonetics, No. 55, Department of Linguistics, University of California at Los Angeles.

Strevens, P. (1960). Spectra of fricative noise in human speech. *Language and Speech, 3,* 32–49.

tive intensity, effective spectrum length, and location of prominent spectral peaks. In addition, the rank frequency of occurrence as determined in a sample of 317 languages is noted. Although one should not make too much of the frequency of occurrence data, it is interesting that the most frequently occurring fricatives among these languages were the stridents /s/ and /ʃ/. Perhaps languages tend to select high-energy fricatives with prominent spectral differences.

The acoustic description of fricatives has considerable room for improvement. It has been difficult to identify measures that are economical, valid, and reliable. Measures such as effective spectrum length and location of prominent peaks are not always highly repeatable within or across observers. Anyone who intends to make spectral measurements for fricatives is well-advised to read the literature carefully and evaluate the reliability of any measures selected for use.

Affricate Consonants

There are only two affricates in English, /dʒ/ and /tʃ/. These are usually described as having a palatal place of articulation and to differ only in voicing. Some believe that the place of articulation is not truly palatal, at least not in comparison with the palatal fricatives /ʒ/ and /ʃ/. The affricate is a complex sound, involving a sequence of stop and fricative articulations. Like stops, the affricates are produced with a period of complete obstruction of the vocal tract. Like fricatives, the affricates are associated with a period of frication. The frication interval for affricates tends to be shorter than that for fricatives. Basically, then, acoustic description of the affricates entails a description of the stop portion and a description of the noise portion.

For the syllable-initial position, the primary acoustic cues that distinguish affricates from stops appear to be the rise-time of the noise energy and the duration of frication (Howell & Rosen, 1983). Rise time is particularly potent. Rise time is a measure of the time over which the amplitude envelope reaches its maximum or near-maximum value. For affricates, the mean rise time measured by Howell and Rosen was 33 ms, contrasted with a mean rise time of 76 ms for the fricatives. Thus, the affricates are characterized by a rapid build-up of acoustic noise energy, though not quite as rapid as that for stop consonants. The difference in rise time between affricates and fricatives is evident in Figure 6–25.

In the postvocalic position, the acoustic cues for the affricate-fricative distinction include the rise time and duration of the noise segment, the presence or absence of a release burst, the duration of the stop gap and the temporal and/or spectral characteristics of the preceding vowel (Dorman, Raphael, & Eisenberg, 1980).

Nasal Consonants

The nasal consonants, [m n ŋ] in English, are produced with closure of the oral cavity and radiation of the sound through the nasal cavity. As explained in the earlier chapter on acoustic theory, the obstructed oral cavity acts as a shunt or side-branch resonator. That is, even though the oral cavity is closed at some point, it nevertheless contributes to the resonant qualities of the nasal consonants. If it did not, then it would be impossible to distinguish the nasals in sustained, isolated productions. Although the nasal consonants are not always easily distinguished in such productions, they do not sound exactly alike.

The articulatory feature of velopharyngeal opening accompanied by oral cavity obstruction is linked to an acoustic feature of a *nasal murmur*. The murmur is the acoustic segment associated with an exclusively nasal radiation of sound energy. Although nasalization has effects beyond this interval, the murmur is a good place to begin our inquiry into nasal consonants.

As a first look at nasal murmur, Figures 6–26, 6–27, and 6–28 present spectrograms, waveform, and FFT spectra for sustained productions of the three nasal consonants of English. The spectrograms were prepared with an especially wide dynamic range to display the maxima and minima in the sound spectra. The spectral features of the nasal murmurs are also shown in the FFT spectra for the murmur portion of each nasal. Both the spectrograms and the FFT spectra illustrate that the nasal murmurs are associated with distinct regions of energy, similar to the formant patterns of sustained vowels (monophthongs). But the figures also show regions of greatly reduced energy. Unlike orally radiated vowels, which theoretically possess only formants in their transfer function, the nasals possess both formants and antiformants. As was discussed earlier, the antiformants can be thought of as interfering with, or preventing, the transmission of energy in the frequency range of the antiformant. Antiformants, like formants, can be described with two numbers, the center frequency and the bandwidth. It is important to recognize that the interaction of formants and anti-formants in the spectrum of a nasal sound is not a simple matter of assigning form-ants to spectral peaks and antiformants to spectral valleys. Although such a result may occur, other spectral consequences may occur as well. For example, if a formant and antiformant have exactly the same center frequency and bandwidth, the result of their interaction is a mutual cancellation. In fact, formants and antiformants often occur in pairs. When the mem-

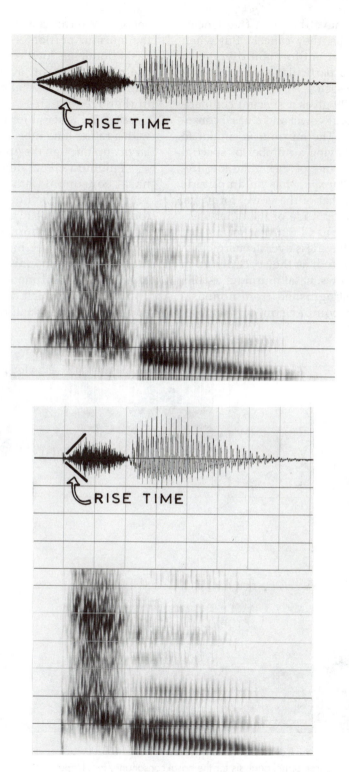

FIGURE 6–25.   Waveform and spectrogram for the word *shoe* and the word *chew* . Note gradual rise time of frication energy in the waveform for *shoe* (top) but a rapid rise of frication energy for *chew* (bottom).

bers of a pair have the same frequencies and bandwidths, they cancel. But when the formant and antiformant diverge in these values, a particular spectral consequence will be seen.

Figure 6–29 gives a spectral comparison of a nonnasal vowel and a nasal consonant murmur. The murmur is similar to the vowel in having a number of spectral peaks but only one of these, the low frequency *nasal formant*, has an amplitude comparable to that of the vowel formants. The reduced amplitude of the other spectral peaks in the nasal murmur means that the nasal will have less overall energy than the vowel. Indeed, as the spectrogram in Figure 6–30 shows, nasal murmurs usually are easily distinguished from nonnasal vowels by a comparison of the total

energy. We can conclude by stating that the murmur portion of a nasal consonant has a dominant low-frequency resonance, the nasal formant, accompanied by a number of much weaker resonances at higher frequencies. As explained in Chapter 2, the nasal formant is associated with a rather long tube extending from the larynx up through the opening of the nose.

Fujimura (1962) determined that the nasal consonants have three common properties. First, all of them have a first formant of about 300 Hz that is well separated from higher formants. Second, the formants tend to be highly damped (i.e., they have large bandwidths reflecting a rapid rate of absorption of sound energy). Third, there is a high density of formants and the existence of antiformants.

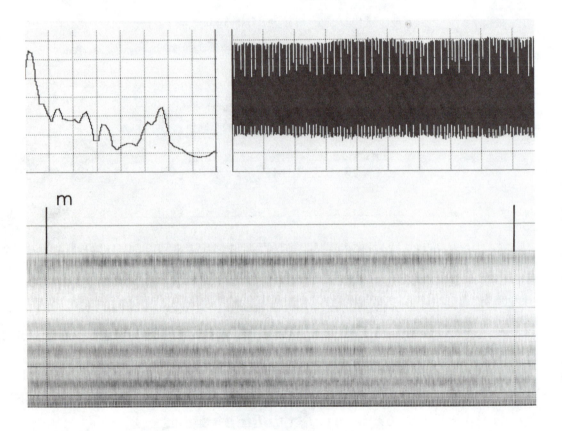

FIGURE 6–26. Three-panel analysis for the nasal consonant /m/. Upper left: long-term spectrum; upper right: waveform; lower half: spectrogram of sustained /m/. Long-term spectrum was calculated for the interval bounded by vertical lines in the spectrogram. This multiple display (and those in the following two figures) was produced with a Kay Elemetrics Corporation Model 5500 Sona-Graph.

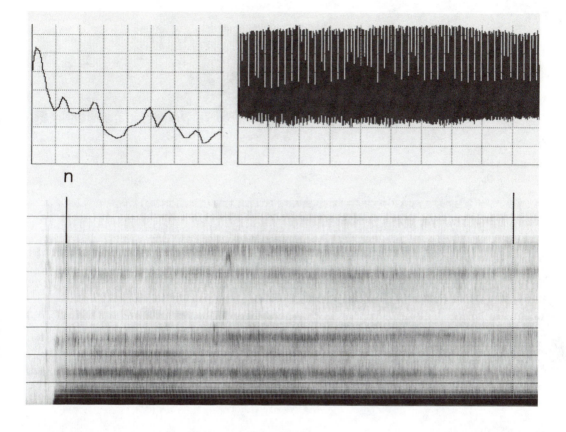

FIGURE 6–27.   Three-panel analysis for the nasal consonant /n/. Upper left: long-term spectrum; upper right: waveform; lower half: spectrogram of sustained /n/. Long-term spectrum was calculated for the interval bounded by vertical lines in the spectrogram.

A close examination of Figure 6–30 reveals that nasal consonants, like other consonants, are associated with formant transitions when they are produced in sequence with other sounds. In fact, the interpretation of the formant transitions associated with nasals is very much like that for the stops. The formant transitions can be interpreted according to place of articulation, so that similar patterns are observed for the stop-nasal pairs, /b/-/m/, /d/-/n/, and /g/-/ŋ/. This similarity is not surprising given that the F2 transition relates to the place of articulation and that the F1 transition relates to obstruction of the oral cavity. In many respects, the nasal consonants can be regarded as nasalized stops, that is, they share some fundamental properties with

the stop consonants (Ladefoged, 1975). The major differences between stops and nasals are explained by the effects of nasalization. A stylized representation of a stop-vowel and a nasal-vowel syllable is given in Figure 6–31. Because the stop /d/ and nasal /n/ are homorganic (having the same place of articulation), they differ only in the articulatory feature of nasality. The acoustic properties of the stop-vowel syllable include the release burst (b), transition (t), and the vowel steady state (ss). The properties for the nasal-vowel syllable are the murmur (m), transition (t), and vowel steady state (ss). The formant transition segment is highly similar for the two syllables.

Perceptual experiments by Kurowski and Blumstein (1984) demonstrated that

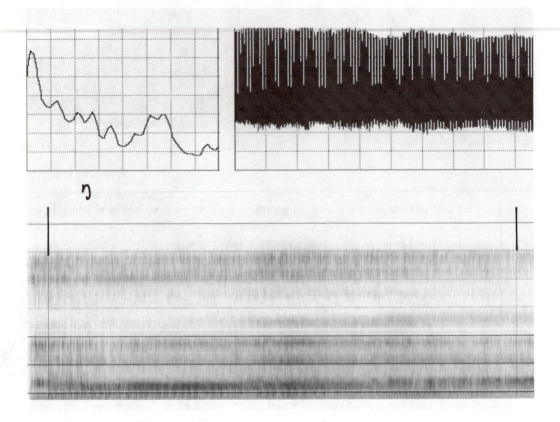

ŋ

FIGURE 6–28. Three-panel analysis for the nasal consonant /ŋ/. Upper left: long-term spectrum; upper right: waveform; lower half: spectrogram of sustained /ŋ/. Long-term spectrum was calculated for the interval bounded by vertical lines in the spectrogram.

the nasal murmur and the transitions are roughly equal in providing information on place of articulation. Their results also indicated that neither the murmur nor the transition is sufficient for perception of place of articulation. When the murmur alone or the transition alone was presented to listeners, the percentage-correct score for consonant identification was about 80%. Apparently, listeners rely on both cues, integrating them to form a single phonetic decision. Kurowski and Blumstein's conclusion stands in contrast to earlier work by Liberman, Delattre, Cooper, and Gerstman (1954) and by Malecot (1956) which indicated that place of articulation for the nasal consonants is cued primarily by the transition segment and not by the murmur. Repp and Svastikula

(1988) reported results for nasals in VC syllables that were in substantial agreement with those of Kurowski and Blumstein. Repp and Svastikula concluded that the vocalic formant transitions by themselves conveyed about as much information on place of articulation for /m/ and /n/ as did the nasal murmurs alone. However, full VC syllables containing [m] or [n] were not identified as well as full CV syllables with the same consonants. A possible reason for the poorer identification of nasals in VC syllables was the "relative absence of a salient spectral change between the vowel and the murmur in VC syllables" (p. 237).

In English, only the nasal consonants /m/ and /n/ occur in word-initial position (/ŋ/ cannot occur word initially), but

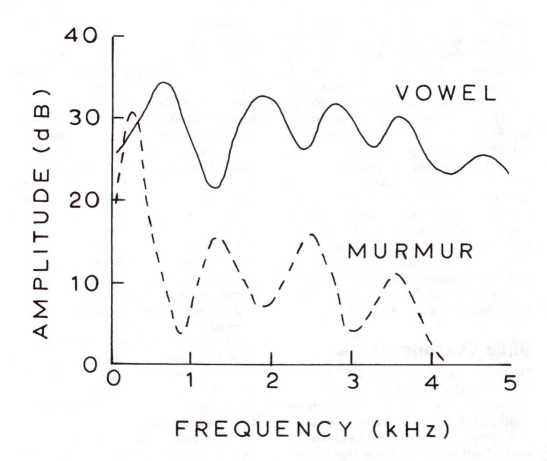

FIGURE 6–29.   Spectra of a nonnasal vowel and the murmur portion of a nasal consonant.

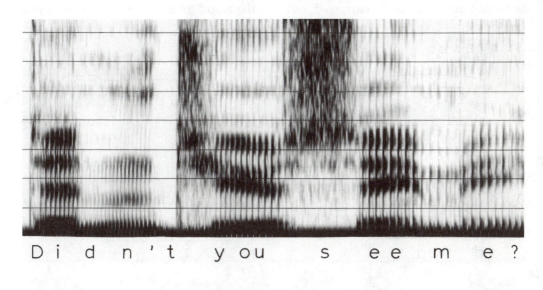

FIGURE 6–30.   Spectrogram of the sentence "Didn't you see me?" Compare nonnasal vowels, such as the /ɪ/ in *didn't*, with the nasal consonants, such as the /n/ in the same word.

all three nasals occur word-medially or word-finally. Taken together, the three nasal consonants account for about 10% of the sounds in adult running speech (Mines, Hansen, & Shoup, 1978) and occur at an average rate of about two per second.

The nasalization of the acoustic signal applies not only to the nasal consonants but also to certain surrounding sounds, particularly vowels. In general, vowels preceding or following nasal consonants tend to be nasalized to some degree. Experiments have shown that listeners are sensitive to the vowel nasalization and use this information to make perceptual judgments about the neighboring consonants. In other words, the acoustic cues for nasalization often can be found beyond the nasal consonant segment.

Glide Consonants

The two glides of English are /w/ and /j/. Ladefoged (1975) used the term *approximants* for these sounds, and the term *semivowels* also is used. All three terms are descriptive: the term *glide* describes the gradual articulatory motions that characterize these sounds; the term approximant describes the articulatory feature in which the vocal tract is markedly narrowed, but

not closed, at some point; and the term *semivowel* describes the vowel-like nature of these sounds. The glides are necessarily prevocalic. (Some phoneticians recognize a postvocalic variant, but we will not do so here.) The glide articulation therefore can be understood as a relatively slow movement that proceeds from a vocal tract configuration with a marked narrowing to a vocal tract configuration suitable for the following vowel. For /w/, there are really two regions of narrowing: at the lips and between the lingual dorsum and the palate (or velum). For this reason, /w/ is characterized phonetically as a labial-velar glide, quite similar in vocal tract configuration to the high-back vowel /u/. The labial and lingual movements for this glide are carried out with a close coordination, beginning and ending together. The glide /j/ has a vocal tract narrowing highly similar to that for vowel /i/. The tongue assumes a high-front position, nearly contacting the prepalatal region. The articulatory motion for glides is slow compared to the motion for stops and nasals.

Perceptual experiments have shown that the glides occupy a kind of midway position between stops and vowel-vowel transitions. The glide /w/ stands between the stop /b/ and a transition from vowel

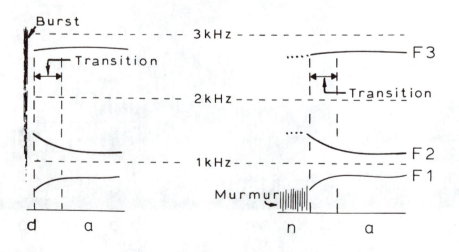

FIGURE 6–31. Stylized representation of stop + vowel and nasal + vowel syllables. Features include the stop burst, formant transitions, and nasal murmur.

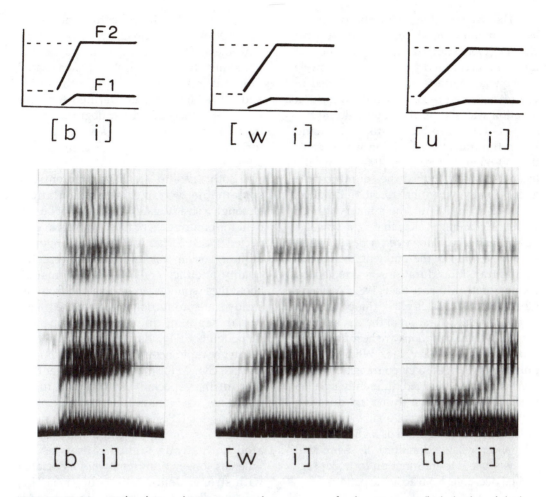

FIGURE 6–32.   Stylized F1 and F2 patterns and spectrograms for the utterances /bi/, /wi/, and /ui/. The frequency extent of transition is constant across the utterances but the duration of transition varies.

/u/ to another sound. Figure 6–32 shows spectrograms for three utterances that differ primarily in the duration of transition: syllable [bi] (as in the word *bee*), syllable [wi] (as in the word *we*), and the vowel + vowel utterance [ui] (which might be represented alphabetically as something like "oooeee"). The formant patterns for these three utterances are similar in their changes in frequency (e.g., the F2 transition extends over about the same frequency range), but they differ in the duration of transition. The transition duration is briefest for the stop [b], somewhat longer for the glide [w], and longest for the vowel + vowel utterance.

The glide [j] stands midway between the alveolar stop [d] and a transition from vowel [i] to another vowel. Diagrams illustrating this relationship are presented in Figure 6–33. The sample utterances are the syllable [du] (as in the word *do*), the syllable [ju] (as in the word *you*), and the vowel + vowel sequence [iu] ("eeeooo" as it might be rendered in a comic strip). As in the case of Figure 6–32, the formant patterns for the three utterances are similar in their frequency extent but different in the time taken to accomplish the shift in frequency. The transition is briefest for the stop [d], longer for the glide [j], and longer yet for the vowel + vowel utterance.

The perceptual experiments conducted by Liberman, Delattre, Gerstman, and Cooper (1956) showed that the duration of transition accounted for listener responses to phonetic contrasts like those depicted in Figures 6–32 and 6–33. When the transition duration was shorter than about 40–60 ms, listeners tended to hear a stop consonant. When the transition duration was greater than 40–60 ms but less than 100–150 ms, the listeners usually judged the sound to be a glide. Finally, when the transition duration exceeded about 100 ms, the listeners heard a vowel of changing color, that is, a vowel + vowel sequence. However, a qualification should be added: the phonetic interpretation of transition durations is affected by speaking rate (Miller & Baer, 1983; Miller & Liberman, 1979). This effect can be studied by changing the duration of the test syllable. Shorter syllable durations are heard as being produced with a faster rate. When syllable duration is changed, a given transition duration sometimes is judged differently by a listener. For example, a transition duration that is heard as a stop at a slow rate (long syllable duration) is heard as a glide at a fast rate (short syllable duration). It seems that listeners use rate information to make segmental decisions from acoustic patterns.

Liquid Consonants

The liquids /r/ and /l/ have some consonantal properties similar to stops and other properties similar to the glides. The similarity to stops is dynamic in nature: at least in some phonetic contexts, the articulatory movements for /r/ and /l/ are quite rapid. The similarity to glides is mainly in a shared sonorant (resonant) quality: both liquids and glides have a well-defined formant structure associated with a degree of vocal tract constriction that is less severe than that for the obstruents (stops, fricatives, and affricates).

Both /r/ and /l/ have a potentially sustainable characteristic articulation, although a steady state often may not be evident for occurrences of these sounds in connected speech. That is, a speaker can, upon request, sustain a sound with the essential quality of either /r/ or /l/. Information about these sounds can be obtained from the steady state production and from the transitional segment in connected speech. Although both liquids are associated with a relatively rapid acoustic change, it appears that the change for [l] tends to be faster than that for [r], especially with regard to F1. O'Connor, Gerstman, Liberman, Delattre, and Cooper (1957) reported that briefer durations of the F1 transition were associated with strong identifications of /l/ whereas longer durations were associated with strong identifications of /r/. This dynamic distinction between /l/ and /r/ is evident in other studies as well (Dalston, 1975; Fant, 1960a, b; Polka & Strange, 1985).

Probably the most distinctive spectral property of /r/ is a lowered F3 which is narrowly separated from F2 (Lehiste, 1964; McGovern, & Strange, 1977). Among

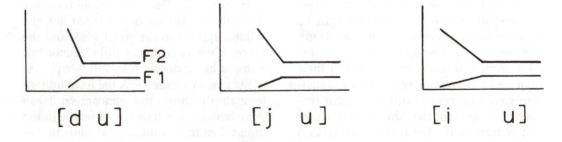

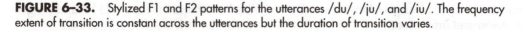

FIGURE 6–33. Stylized F1 and F2 patterns for the utterances /du/, /ju/, and /iu/. The frequency extent of transition is constant across the utterances but the duration of transition varies.

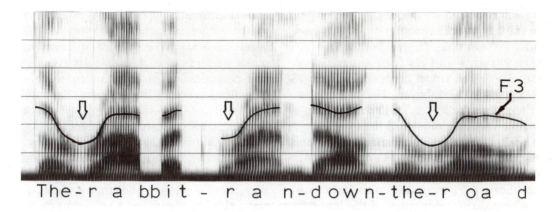

The-r a bbit - r a n-d own-the-r oa d

FIGURE 6–34. Spectrogram of the sentence, "The rabbit ran down the road," with the F3 trajectory highlighted. Arrows point to /r/ segments.

English sounds, /r/ has the lowest F3 frequency, and this feature alone often can be used to identify the occurrence of this liquid. This feature stands out clearly in Figure 6–34. As discussed in Chapter 5, a low F3 frequency also is a distinguishing feature for the rhotacized vowel /ɝ/. Generally, for English, [r]-coloring is associated with a low F3 that is close to F2. Nolan (1983) reported the following mean formant frequencies for /r/ produced in a list of words by fifteen 17-year-old males: F1—320 Hz; F2—1090 Hz, F3—1670 Hz. Dalston (1975) reports formant-frequency data for [r] produced by young adults and children. Data for children are particularly interesting because the /r/ is so frequently misarticulated in children's speech.

The /l/ is described phonetically as a *lateral* because the tongue tip makes a midline closure at or near the alveolar ridge, so that airflow escapes on either side (lateral release) of the occlusion. For /r/, there is a marked narrowing, without closure, of the vocal tract in the palatal region. Recall from Chapter 2 that a bifurcation of the vocal tract produces antiformants, and the lateral channels for /l/ constitute such a bifurcation. Antiformants arise during the time in which the lateral articulation is in effect. Thus, /l/ shares with the nasal consonants a steady state segment for which the transfer function

contains both formants and antiformants. Not surprisingly, then, the lateral and the nasals can be somewhat similar in their acoustic appearance. A spectrogram of syllable-initial [l] with a prolonged onset is shown in Figure 6–35. Mean formant frequencies for /l/ in three different studies were as follows: Nolan (1983): F1—360 Hz, F2—1350 Hz, F3-3050 Hz; Lehiste (1964): F1—295 Hz, F2—980 Hz, F3—2600 Hz; Al-Bamerni (1975): F1—365 Hz, F2—1305 Hz, F3—2780 Hz. The F1 and F2 values for [l] are similar to those for /r/, but the F3 value for /l/ is about 1 kHz higher than that for /r/.

Figure 6–36 depicts the differences in formant pattern between /r/ and /l/. This figure shows a schematic spectrographic representation in which three acoustic cues are manipulated to produce stimuli that vary from *rock* to *lock*. One is a temporal cue in which the steady state and transition durations of F1 are varied from an /r/ pattern (short steady state and long transition) to an /l/ pattern (long steady state and short transition). Another cue is the relative onset frequency for F2, which varies from a relatively low value for /r/ to a relatively higher value for /l/. The third cue is the relative onset frequency for F3, varying from a relatively low F3 for /r/ to a relatively high F3 for /l/.

Phonetics books frequently comment on the allophonic complexity of the liquids. For example, /l/ has both light and dark variants and its formant pattern varies with the vowel context (Tarnoczy, 1948; Lehiste, 1964, Nolan, 1983). Various writers describe for /r/ syllabic and non-syllabic variants, initial and final variants, as well as articulatory variants such as retroflex and bunched (Lehiste, 1964; Shriberg & Kent, 1982). These variants complicate the description of the articulatory or acoustic properties of the liquids, and this limitation should be kept in mind whenever generalizations are proposed. It seems necessary to recognize at least two major variants of each liquid: prevocalic and postvocalic. Justification for such a classification comes from Lehiste (1964) for /r/ and from Giles (1971) for /l/. Both of these studies indicate that prevocalic liquids differ from postvocalic liquids, and that these two categories may predominate over other allophonic distinctions. A further complication is that many phoneticians classify postvocalic /r/ as a vowel.

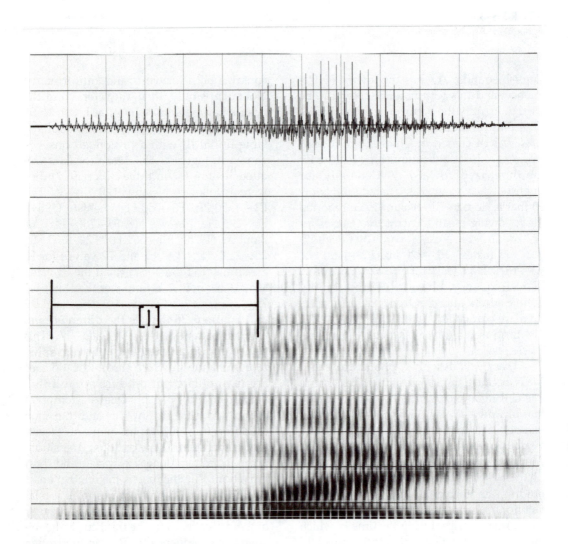

FIGURE 6–35. Waveform and spectrogram of the word *law* produced with a prolongation of the /l/ steady state (labeled on spectrogram).

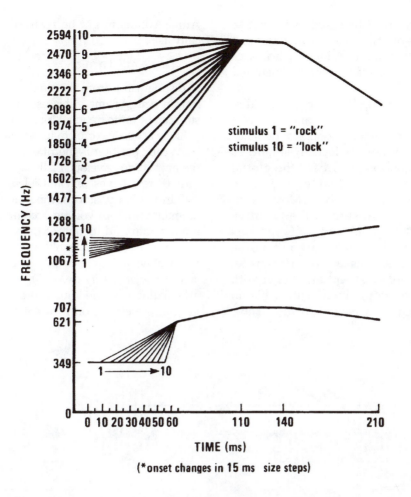

stimulus 1 = "rock"
stimulus 10 = "lock"

(*onset changes in 15 ms size steps)

FIGURE 6–36. F1, F2, and F3 patterns used in synthesizing a range of stimuli between *rock* and *lock*. Reprinted from L. Polka and W. Strange, "Perceptual evidence of acoustic cues that differentiate /r/ and /l/." *Journal of the Acoustical Society of America, 78,* 1985, 1187–1206. (Reprinted with permission of the American Institute of Physics.) Copyright 1985.

We will not attempt to resolve these issues here; suffice it to say that /l/ and /r/ can be acoustically described in terms of formant pattern.

The Allophones [ɾ] and [ʔ]

Several allophones have been mentioned in the preceding sections. For example, the released and unreleased allophones of the stop consonants were discussed as a part of the general section on stops. But because they have special properties, the two allophones [ɾ] and [ʔ] are given a separate section in this chapter. [ɾ] is described phonetically as a lingual flap (or, alternatively, as a one-tap trill). This sound is made as a very rapid tongue movement from one vocal tract configuration, typically for a vowel, to a brief contact with the alveolar ridge or the postdental region. The contact is followed by a rapid movement away from the constriction. The flap is an allophone of both /t/ and /d/ in words like *latter* vs *ladder*, and *writer* vs *rider*. In its spectrographic appearance, the flap is remarkable primarily for its brevity. Compared to distinctive productions of /t/ and /d/, the flap has a short overall duration and a very brief closure period. These features are illustrated in Figure 6–37.

The glottal stop [ʔ] also is used allophonically for the stops /t/ and /d/, and occasionally for other phonemes, depending on dialect and idiolect. It is hard to identify a good keyword for the glottal stop, because of its variable production among speakers and dialects. Most speakers use the glottal stop in the negative expression "unh unh," and many speakers use [ʔ] in the word *bottle*. In addition, the glottal stop serves a junctural role. Abutting words that end and begin with vowels often are produced with a glottal stop between the vowel elements. Thus,

Anna Adams might be realized phonetically as

[æ n ə ʔ æ d ə m z]

to distinguish it from the similar sound pattern in Ann Adams. This use of the glottal stop can be quite frequent for some speakers. A likely acoustic correlate for glottal stops in prevocalic position is the rate of increase in the amplitude envelope of the vowel waveform (Peters, Boves, & Van Dielen, 1986).

In medial positions, the glottal stop is an interruption of voicing accomplished by a momentary adduction of the vocal folds. The interruption can be observed on acoustic displays as a gap or period of reduced acoustic energy (Figure 6–38). Because the articulation is carried out at the level of the larynx, the effects on formant pattern are

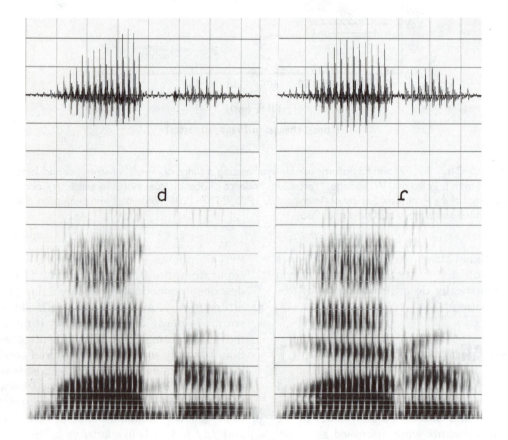

FIGURE 6–37. Waveforms and spectrograms for the word *ladder* produced with an intervocalic stop /d/ (left) and an intervocalic flap /ɾ/ (right).

subtle. In particular, the glottal stop usually is not associated with marked formant transitions typical of the oral stops. A glottal stop in word-initial position often is acoustically evident through the rapid rise of energy for the voiced sound. This short rise time resembles "hard glottal attack," or a forceful and abrupt onset of voicing energy. Upon release of the glottal stop in word-initial position, a brief burst of energy often can be seen in oscillograms or spectrograms. Usually, the spectral composition of the burst is continuous with that for the following vowel, as would be expected if the acoustic energy produced at the level of the vocal folds activated the formants appropriate for the following vowel sound. Although some phonetics books describe the glottal stop as voiceless, this classification should not be taken too literally. Given that the glottal stop is produced with a sustained closure of the vocal

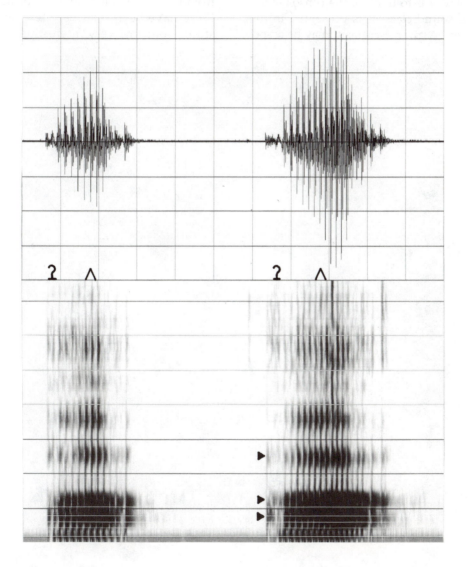

FIGURE 6–38. Waveform and spectrogram for the utterance [ʔ ʌ ʔ ʌ]. Note glottal stops in initial and medial positions. Small arrows point to F1, F2, and F3 frequencies, which are essentially continuous from glottal stop release into the following vowel.

folds, the laryngeal dynamics of the sound are rather like those for voiced stops.

Summary

Consonant sounds involve a variety of acoustic characteristics and therefore a variety of possible measures by which they can be characterized. One way of managing the complexity is to think of the consonants in major sound classes, as presented in this chapter. A given consonant may be associated with several cues, and it appears that consonant identification frequently involves an integration of separate cues, for example, burst and formant transition for stops, murmur and formant transition for nasals, noise interval and formant transition for fricatives, and formant steady state and transition for liquids. Many of these basic ideas apply to consonants in other languages as well. However, some languages have consonants that are quite different from those in English, and, unfortunately, there have been relatively few acoustic studies of some very interesting sounds.

Acoustic Effects of Context and Speaker

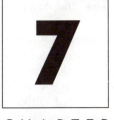

CHAPTER

Most of what has been said so far oversimplifies the problem of speech analysis in various applications. The simplification arises largely from the fact that important sources of variability in the acoustic properties of speech have been neglected. Some of the sources of variability have been briefly mentioned, but it is the task of this chapter to consider them in more detail. In particular, this chapter will consider the effects of phonetic context and speaker on the acoustic pattern of speech. Phonetic context refers to the phonetic environment in which a sound occurs, including neighboring sounds and prosodic characteristics such as speaking rate and stress pattern. Speaker age and sex are important because they determine vocal tract length and certain aspects of overall vocal tract geometry. Other speaker variables include dialect and disorder. This chapter discusses a number of issues that may arise in

applications of the acoustic analysis of speech. They are discussed under the headings of: coarticulation, speaking style (clarity and rate), speaker variables (age and sex), and speech disorders. These are not totally independent topics, and some recurring analysis problems will be encountered. However, it is convenient to discuss them under separate topics.

Coarticulation

The descriptions of speech sounds in the earlier chapters have largely ignored the effects of context, that is, the production of sounds in combinations to form syllables, words, and phrases. It is in fact rather artificial to describe a given sound in terms of its isolated, discrete production. Speech usually involves strings of sounds uttered in rapid succession. In such strings, the individual sounds can lose some of their distinctiveness. Frequently, the boundaries between sounds are blurred. To take one example, consider the simple word *am* [æm]. In the typical production of this word, the vowel [æ] is nasalized, that is, produced with some degree of nasal resonance because the velopharyngeal opening for the nasal consonant [m] is anticipated during the vowel. In effect, an articulatory (and acoustic) feature of the consonant is produced *in advance* during the preceding vowel. For another example, most speakers produce the word *stew* [stu] with lip rounding that begins during the [s]. The lip rounding is actually required for the rounded vowel [u] but begins well before the vowel itself is articulated. No such lip rounding is observed for the [s] in a word like *stay*, which does not involve a rounded vowel.

From these examples, we can see that the segments of speech interact, so that some of their features are coproduced or coarticulated. The term *coarticulation* refers to events in speech in which the vocal tract shows at any one instant adjustments that are appropriate for two or more sounds. The direction of a coarticulatory effect can be described as forward (anticipatory) or backward (retentive). In forward coarticulation, an articulatory feature for a phonetic segment is apparent during the production of an earlier segment. Consider the examples in the preceding paragraph. For the word *am*, the property of nasalization (open velopharyngeal port) occurs during the vowel that precedes the nasal consonant. Thus, this word shows evidence of the forward coarticulation of nasalization. In the second example, forward coarticulation of lip rounding is evident for the [s] in the word *stew*.

Coarticulation is reviewed in depth by Sharf and Ohde (1981), who consider the physiologic, acoustic, and perceptual aspects of this speech phenomenon. They also review models of speech production that attempt to account for the coarticulatory patterns of speech. A more recent review of speech production models is available in Kent, Adams, and Turner (in press). For the purposes of this text, coarticulation is mainly of interest in understanding the modifications of a given sound by the context in which it appears. The discussions of vowel and diphthong production in Chapter 5 and consonant production in Chapter 6 should be tempered with the knowledge that sounds in context often are mutually influenced. Some investigators of coarticulation described the process as one of "feature spreading," insofar as a feature of one sound is anticipated during an earlier sound in the string or retained by a later sound. Whether or not this characterization is theoretically correct, it does convey an essential property of many coarticulatory effects that can be observed in the acoustic signal. Recall that in the word [æm], the vowel [æ] is nasalized because of the influence of the following nasal consonant [m]. The nasalization is present as a modification of the vowel [æ] produced nonnasally. Specifically, antiformants may be present, along with the appearance of a low-frequency nasal formant and a broadening of formant bandwidths. These acoustic features of nasalization are in effect "spread over" to influence the production of the vowel segment.

Figure 7–1 shows several examples of coarticulation. Notice that in each case illustrated, there is a blending or shingling of articulatory features across neighboring speech sounds. Some features are particularly likely to have a large temporal range. Among these features are lip rounding and nasalization. Other features tend to affect only the immediately adjacent segments.

When sounds are produced in context, a number of temporal adjustments usually occur. Generally, a sound produced in context is shorter than the "same" sound produced in isolation. In addition, the duration of a segment tends to become shorter as more elements are added to the sound string. For example, when elements are added to a given consonant to produce two- and three-element consonant clusters (such as /p/, /sp/ and /spr/), the duration of the consonant decreases (Haggard, 1973; Schwartz, 1970; Umeda, 1977). A similar effect occurs for syllables. The duration of a monosyllabic base, such as *stick*, becomes progressively shorter in syllable-suffixing sequences like *stick, sticky, stickiness* (Lehiste, 1972). These durational effects occur even as the speaker tries to produce speech at a constant rate.

Suprasegmentals

A major consequence of coarticulation is that the articulatory and acoustic characteristics of phonetic elements are affected by the surrounding elements. Therefore, allowances should always be made for contextual effects. The acoustic descriptions offered in this chapter do not take account of all of the coarticulatory variations in speech, which are too numerous to

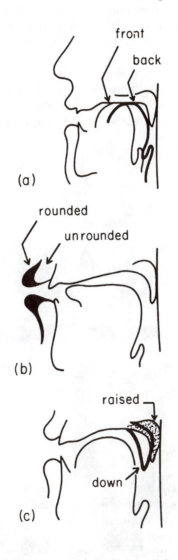

FIGURE 7–1. Examples of coarticulation: (a) variation in place of articulation of velar consonant, depending on vowel context; (b) variation in lip rounding for /s/, depending on following vowel; and (c) variation in velopharyngeal articulation during vowel, depending on following consonant.

summarize briefly. The acoustic properties for any given element will depend on a number of factors, including those associated with phonetic context, speaker, speaking style (e.g., casual vs. formal), speaking rate, dialect, and situation. A talker can adjust speech patterns in a number of ways and for a number of purposes. Few systematic investigations have been conducted to show the nature of these variations. Some very brief comments will be given here on some selected factors and their acoustic effects. The comments are arranged under the headings of clear speech, prosody (intonation), and speaking rate. These are *suprasegmental* properties of speech in the sense that they typically have effects that are expressed beyond segmental boundaries. Frequently, suprasegmental features are described in terms of units larger than segments, for example, syllables, phrases, or breath groups. This is not to say that suprasegmental properties are without effects at the segmental level.

Clear Speech

One factor is the difference between clear speech (speech produced in an effort to be highly intelligible) and conversational speech (in which clarity may be compromised). Figure 7–2 gives a spectrographic comparison of clear and conversational speech. Compared to conversational speech, clear speech is (1) slower (by virtue of longer pauses between words and

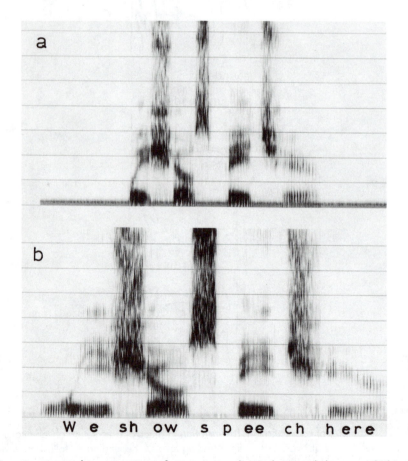

FIGURE 7–2. Spectrographic comparison of conversational speech (a) and clear speech (b). Both spectrograms are for the sentence, "We show speech here."

lengthening of some speech sounds), (2) more apt to avoid modified or reduced forms of consonant and vowel segments, and (3) characterized by a greater rms intensity of obstruent sounds, particularly stop consonants (Picheny, Durlach, & Braida, 1986). When talkers make an effort to be easily understood, they modify their articulation to make speech slower and more acoustically distinctive. In conversational speech, vowels often are modified or reduced, thus losing some of their acoustic distinctiveness. Similarly, stops occurring in word-final position in conversation frequently are not released, so that the burst cue is not available to listeners. But in clear speech, vowels are not likely to be modified or reduced, and stop consonants (and consonants in general) tend to be released.

Lindblom (1990) proposed that speakers vary their speech output along a continuum from *hypospeech* to *hyperspeech* (the H&H hypothesis). This hypothesis is based on the idea that speakers adapt to the various circumstances of communication, in effect tuning their production patterns to communicative and situational factors. Lindblom cites evidence that "clear speech" (hyperspeech in the H&H hypothesis) is not simply loud speech; it involves an articulatory reorganization (Moon & Lindblom, 1989). Adams (1990), however, concluded from an X-ray microbeam study of speech movements that changes in speech clarity did not reflect a reorganization of speech motor control. The changes that Adams did observe, such as increases in maximum displacement and peak velocity of articulatory movements, occurred so as to maintain a fixed velocity/displacement ratio.

Prosody, Especially Intonation

Imagine how many ways a speaker can produce the simple sentence, "I'll give it to you." It could be a declarative (a factual statement), a question ("I'll give it to you?"), or a checked form in which the speaker requests more information, as in, "I'll give it to you—PAUSE (on Monday? Tuesday?)." It could convey a wide range of emotion, from a graceful offering to a reassuring agreement to a grudging or even bitter concession, for instance. The sentence also can be produced with different stress patterns, by placing the emphasis on the capitalized words in the following versions: "I'LL give it to you." "I'll GIVE it to you." "I'll give it to YOU." Or it could be produced with different internal pausing, such as a pause after *it*, or a pause after *to*. All of these modifications fall in the category of *prosody*. For the purposes of this book, prosody will be defined as the suprasegmental features of speech that are conveyed by the parameters of fundamental frequency (perceived primarily as vocal pitch), intensity (perceived primarily as loudness), and duration (perceived primarily as length). The term suprasegmental indicates that the phenomena of interest are not confined to phonetic segments. In fact, they often are observed over much larger intervals—syllables, words, phrases, sentences, and even discourses.

The term prosody is not easily defined in a way that agrees with all that has been written about it. Definitions disagree in some respects, so the reader should be wary in applying any one definition to different writings on the subject. One major disagreement is with the pair of terms, prosody and intonation. Some writers regard them as synonyms, others mark an important distinction between them. We will follow Johns-Lewis (1986) in considering intonation as a part of prosody. Intonation is similar to prosody in that its parameters are vocal frequency, intensity, and duration. But intonation refers to a narrower range of phenomena, generally the patterns of pitch rises and falls and the patterns of stress in a given language. Prosody includes these effects but also embraces tempo (pause and lengthening), loudness, and other phenomena. Some writers include speaking rate as a part of tempo and therefore as a part of prosody.

The purpose here is not to provide a rigorous and comprehensive definition of prosody and related concepts. This is a matter of intense debate within linguistic theory and goes beyond the modest scope of this chapter. Rather, our purpose is to summarize the acoustic correlates of basic prosodic phenomena: vocal fundamental frequency, intensity, and duration. The measurement of all three parameters was discussed in Chapter 4. The ways in which these parameters are regulated will determine how the sentence "I'll give it to you" takes acoustic form and is perceived. These parameters influence each other in complicated ways; we will sketch a few basic prosodic effects without attempting to describe their interactions in detail.

One way to approach prosody is to consider its shape on several levels of linguistic or communication structure. At the level of the discourse, for instance, *new*, as opposed to *given*, information is highlighted prosodically. Behne (1989) showed that in a minidiscourse like:

"Someone painted the fence."
"Who painted the fence?"
"Pete painted the fence."

the new information ("Pete" in the above exchange) is made longer and higher in fundamental frequency. She also showed that the same cues are deployed somewhat differently in French. Prosodic cues vary across languages, just as segmental ones do.

Another discourse effect on prosody is *contrastive stress*, which can occur on almost any word, phrase, or clause which the speaker considers to contradict or contrast with one that was previously stated or implied in the discourse. For instance, one says, "I'll GIVE it to you" when one believes that some other verb (like "sell") was incorrectly assumed by the listener.

At the level of syntax, too, prosody plays essential roles. At this level, we encounter juncture and pause phenomena marking multiword units. One of the best-known and most important of these in

English is *phrase-final lengthening,* in which the last stressable syllable in a major syntactic phrase or clause is lengthened. For example, if we contrast the two sentences:

(a) Grapes, melons, and apples are my favorite fruits

(b) Apples, grapes, and melons are my favorite fruits

the first syllable of *apples* will be longer in (a) than (b) because in the first example this word is at the end of the subject noun phrase. (Although the word *apples* contains two syllables, only the first one can be stressed.) To an even greater degree, *fruits* will be longer in both sentences than it would be if it stood in the middle of a phrase. Klatt (1976) provides a classic survey of this and related phenomena that determine durations of speech elements. Read and Schreiber (1982) showed that listeners use phrase-final lengthening to recognize the structure of (i.e., to parse) spoken sentences. They argued that children rely more on this prosodic cue than adults do, and in fact that prosody provides the language-learner with an accessible starting point for learning the complex syntactic structures of language.

Also at the level of syntax, the fundamental frequency contour typically declines across clauses or comparable units. The origin, nature, and measurement of this fundamental-frequency tilt are the subjects of argument (Cohen, Collier, & t'Hart, 1982). One view is that declination is linear—fundamental frequency falls gradually and linearly throughout a sentence (Maeda, 1976; Sorensen & Cooper, 1980; Thorsen, 1985). This pattern often is described as a universal property of spoken language. Other writers have disputed the linear declination hypothesis, especially for spontaneous speech (Lieberman, Katz, Jongman, Zimmerman, & Miller, 1985). Lieberman (1967) proposed a *breath-group theory* in which variation is allowed in the nonterminal part of the fundamental-frequency contour. That is, if a declarative sentence is divided into nonterminal and terminal parts, the former can take various forms whereas the latter typically shows a rapid fall in fundamental frequency. Support for this proposal comes from studies showing that an important acoustic cue for syntactic structure is the fall in fundamental frequency and intensity at the end of the breath group (Landahl, 1980; Lieberman & Tseng, 1981; Lieberman et al., 1985). Also in support of this more flexible view of intonation, Umeda (1982) described declination as situation-dependent: the pattern of fundamental frequency becomes more complex as the complexity of contextual information increases.

At the level of the lexicon, too, prosody plays a role. English has many noun/verb pairs like 'import versus im'port, in which the stress pattern is the major spoken contrast. Another lexical effect is the stress pattern on compounds versus phrases. For example, the compound noun 'blackboard contrasts with the noun phrase black 'board (board that is black). Stress in English, whether contrastive or lexical, is not merely a matter of intensity but involves all three acoustic parameters—duration, intensity, and fundamental frequency—of which duration may be the most salient and reliable (Fry, 1955). Stress also affects segmental properties such as vowel and consonantal articulation (Kent & Netsell, 1971; de Jong, 1991). Segments in stressed syllables tend to have larger articulatory movements than syllables in unstressed syllables. In a sense, the movements in stressed syllables are more contrastive, and this contrastivity is also realized in the acoustic patterns of speech. Therefore, a vowel in a stressed syllable usually has a distinctive formant pattern, that is, one that resembles the presumed target pattern for the vowel as might be defined in an isolated production. Acoustic distinctiveness usually decreases in unstressed syllables.

Some linguistic accounts distinguish types of stress-like effects such as stress and accent (Lehiste, 1970), but a recent theory (Beckman, 1986; Beckman & Edwards, 1991) proposes a unified representation with four levels:

Level 1: syllables with reduced nuclei, such as the second syllable in *vita*.

Level 2: syllables similar to those above except that they have full vowels, e.g., *veto*.

Level 3: syllables may be selectively given more stress by assigning to them a pitch accent.

Level 4: syllables can receive a marking called *nuclear accent* (or *phrase accent*) in which the last accented item in a phonological grouping assumes the most prominent accent.

This proposal illustrates the complexity of stress, which may involve several different, interacting phenomena. Consider a speaker who wants to place pitch accent on the word *tuba*. The accent cannot be placed on the second syllable, which is a reduced nucleus. Rather, the accent must be placed on the stressed syllable. In this way, the various levels of the stress representation can interact without destroying essential phonological patterns.

To the prosodic effects at these levels of formal linguistic description, one could add sociolinguistic patterns, such as those of geographic and social dialects. For example, a British pronunciation of "Are you going?" may have level pitch on the first two words, with pitch accent on *go* while an American pronunciation may have rising pitch on the first three syllables, followed by a sharper rise on *-ing*. Like many such transatlantic differences, this one may covary with socal status, actual or desired.

Finally, affect (attitude, commitment, mood, emotion) can strongly influence prosody. One example is the occurrence of rising intonation on what is intended as a declarative utterance, a pattern of which may suggest a lack of certainty, a desire to elicit a response from the listener, or even a lower social status than one's listener.

When one contemplates the possible interactions of all these (and more) sources of prosodic variation, one cannot wonder that prosody is generally less well understood than segment structure. We can describe quite well (although not completely) the formant structure of the vowel [a], but we have scarcely begun to describe the prosodic differences between using that vowel as an exclamation of sudden discovery ("Ah!") and as listener's interjection, warning the speaker that something controversial or offensive is about to be said. Still less have we systematically compared the uses of prosody across languages.

What is clear, however, is that prosody is not merely the melodic and rhythmic decoration of language. It is true that arhythmic, monotone speech can be understood if other cues are intact, but it is equally true that segments can be obliterated without affecting intelligibility (Warren, 1970, 1976) and that "intact" words extracted from conversation can be unintelligible when presented in isolation (Craig & Kim, 1990; Kent, in press). These observations merely show that no one aspect of speech is essential, given the redundancy of the whole. More adequately, prosody might be regarded as the fabric of speech, within which segments are the individual stitches or fibers. Prosodic patterns span the linguistic levels, holding together the many influences that make up the rich tapestry of language in context. Prosody serves essential, if sometimes subtle, functions in communication, and its acoustic foundations are no less important in the speech signal than those which distinguish segments.

The next section addresses what many consider to be an aspect of prosody—speaking rate. Rate effects are summarized under a separate heading primarily for ease of writing and not to suggest that speaking rate is distinct from prosody.

Speech Rate

Obviously, when a person speaks faster, the overall duration of an utterance decreases. However, what is not clear is how the alteration affects the various components of an utterance, including vowels vs consonants, stressed vs unstressed syllables, and movement durations vs steady-state durations. Part of a speaker's competence is the ability to produce an utterance at various rates, ranging from very slow to moderate to very fast. Acoustic studies of rate changes reveal how speakers accomplish variations in rate, how these changes are signaled to listeners, and how these alterations affect various classes of speech sounds.

As speaking rate increases, the durations of the components of speech necessarily get smaller. What is not so obvious is the manner in which reductions of duration are distributed across the components. The reduction is not constant. Generally, pauses and steady-state segments for vowels and consonants tend to be sacrificed more than transitional or dynamic aspects of the speech signal. However, at very fast speaking rates, segments and even unstressed syllables may be deleted. Rapid rates also tend to be accompanied by *undershoot*, as described in Chapter 4. Particularly for vowels, it appears that the actual production can deviate from the spatial configuration that occurs for an isolated production of the sound.

Some examples of speaking rate variations are shown in Figure 7–3, which contains spectrograms for a slow and rapid rate of speech for the sentence, "It starts at six o'clock." The difference in overall duration is immediately evident from the spectrograms. The rapid-rate production takes only about half as long as the slow-rate production. Other differences can be detected by a careful examination of the spectrographic features.

Changes in speaking rate also can affect a number of phonetic characteristics of speech, including the actual deletion of

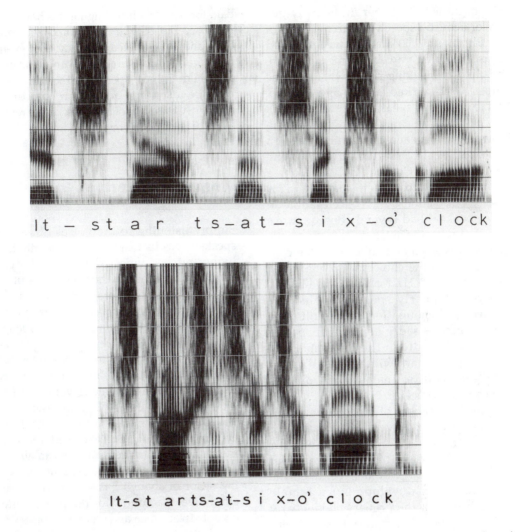

FIGURE 7–3. Spectrograms of the sentence "It starts at six o' clock" produced at two rates: moderate and rapid.

segments or even syllables (Dalby, 1986). Attempts to use acoustic measures to study the effect of speaking rate obviously must be used with recognition of changes in the phonetic structure of the speech signal.

Despite the complexity of speaking rate changes in natural speech, a relatively simple technique seems to work reasonably well in making rate changes in speech synthesis: make linear (proportionate) adjustments in the durations of all phonetic segments. This method is used in some commercial speech synthesizers.

Speaker Variables: Age and Sex

To a very large extent, the early work in acoustic phonetics focused on the adult male speaker. There were a number of reasons for this focus, including social and technical factors. Only rather recently has the study of acoustic phonetics been broadened to encompass significant research on populations other than men. This is not to say that children and women were neglected altogether in the early history of acoustic speech research. Peterson and Barney's (1952) classic study included acoustic data on vowels for men, women, and children, making it clear that acoustic values vary markedly with age and sex characteristics of speakers (see Chapter 5). However, the research effort given to the speech of women and children has been on a smaller scale than that given to the speech of men. Consequently, there is a continuing need to gather acoustic data for diverse populations. The concentration on male speakers had several consequences, not all of which facilitated research on the speech of women and children. One consequence was the choice of an analyzing bandwidth (300 Hz for the "wide-band" analysis) on early spectrographs that worked well enough for most adult male voices but was sadly deficient for many women and children. The unsuitability of the analyzing bandwidth probably discouraged acoustic analyses of women's and children's speech.

The implications of the male emphasis may have reached even to theory; Titze (1989) commented, "One wonders, for example, if the source-filter theory of speech production would have taken the same course of development if female voices had been the primary model early on" (p. 1699). Klatt and Klatt (1990) remarked on the same point: "informal observations hint at the possibility that vowel spectra obtained from women's voices do not conform as well to an all-pole model, due perhaps to tracheal coupling and source/tract interactions" (p. 820).

One might think that acoustic data for women and children could be extrapolated quite easily from data collected for men's speech. After all, acoustic theory (Chapter 3) tells us that the length of the vocal tract is one determinant of formant frequencies. Given that resonance frequencies change systematically as the length of a pipe is changed, one might expect that scaling factors could be determined to permit the derivation of acoustic data for women and children from the data for men. Such scaling factors have been proposed but they are calculated with difficulty and have limited accuracy. But even if accurate factors were determined, women and children have speech characteristics that must be taken into account in both theory and analysis. The following sections review some of these problems.

Women's Speech

Simply listening to the voices of various speakers tells us that women generally have higher-pitched voices than men. Indeed, women's voices are on the average about one octave, or about 1.7 times, higher than men's. This difference in fundamental frequency relates primarily to the membranous length of the vocal folds (Titze, 1989). Figure 7–4 illustrates the scaling of the glottis in terms of three variables that account for differences between men's and women's voices. A scaling factor (computed by Titze to be about 1.6) based on the membranous length L_m accounts almost entirely for differences in mean fundamental frequency, mean airflow, and aerodynamic power. An additional scaling factor of about 1.2 based on vibrational amplitude A accounts for the power differences between men and women's voices.

But women's voices may differ from men's in many ways. In particular, it has been suggested that women's voices have the following attributes (relative to men's):

A. breathy;

B. weak;

C. more glottal leakage (air escaping through the glottis even during its "closed" phase;

D. less abrupt flow termination;

E. larger open quotient (meaning that the vocal folds are open longer during each glottal cycle);

F. more symmetric vocal pulses (about the same time given to the opening and closing portions);

G. shorter pulses;

H. higher fundamental frequency;

I. different range of fundamental frequency;

J. lower Sound Pressure Level;

K. more dominant fundamental frequency (first harmonic);

L. steeper spectrum slope (i.e., a faster roll-off of harmonic energy with frequency);

M. more noise fill in interformant regions;

N. higher formant frequencies;

O. larger formant bandwidths;

P. different coupling, or interaction, between subglottal and supraglottal cavities;

Q. greater interaction between source and filter.

These various items are not necessarily independent of one another; for example, breathy voice, glottal leakage, more dominant first harmonic and noise fill may all be related. The list is simply a compilation of characteristics that may have to be taken into consideration for a full understanding of women's voice (see Klatt & Klatt, 1990 for additional discussion).

It was recognized early in attempts to produce women's speech from speech synthesis that a woman's voice is not simply a man's voice produced with higher fundmental and formant frequencies. Attempts to use this simple alteration met with limited success. The voice simply did not sound feminine. More recent work (Klatt & Klatt, 1990) showed that synthesis of

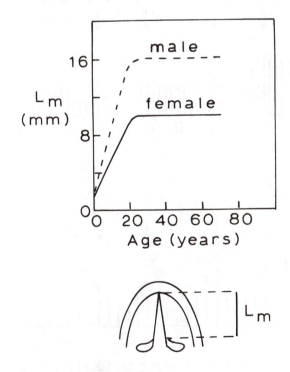

FIGURE 7–4. Variation in length of vocal fold, L_m, with age in males and females. Redrawn from I. Titze, "Physiologic and acoustic differences between male and female voices," *Journal of the Acoustical Society of America, 85,* 1989, 1699–1707. (Reproduced with permission from the American Institute of Physics.) Copyright 1989.

womens' voices should include provision for: (a) a voicing source model that offers flexible control of open quotient, spectral tilt, aspiration noise associated with breathiness, flutter timed to glottal pulses, and diplophonic double pulsing; (b) an extra pole-zero pair to simulate a tracheal resonance, and (c) pitch-synchronous adjustment of the first-formant bandwidth to simulate one component of source/tract interaction. Price (1989) noted that the glottal waveforms for female voices tended to have shorter closed quotients and less sharp excitation than the waveforms for male voices.

The higher fundamental frequency of women's voices can present occasional difficulties in acoustic analysis. As fundamental frequency increases, there is a corresponding increase in the interval between harmonics of the laryngeal source spectrum (Figure 7–5). At some harmonic spacings, it becomes difficult to discern the location of formants in the spectrum. The problem is essentially one of sampling: widely spaced harmonics do not reveal much detail about the spectral envelope. Early spectrographs were particularly limited in the analysis of high-pitched women's speech because they were equipped with a standard 300-Hz analyzing filter for wide-band analysis. This filter worked satisfactorily for most men's voices because it typically embraced at least two harmonics and therefore resolved formants rather than harmonics. But for many women's voices, this filter bandwidth corresponded to a harmonic interval. As a result, spectrograms had harmonic-formant interaction, as illustrated in Figure 7–6.

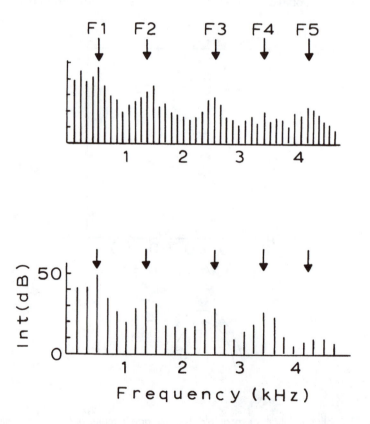

FIGURE 7–5. Effect of change in fundamental frequency on vowel spectrum. Top: spectrum for vowel produced with low fundamental frequency; bottom: spectrum for same vowel produced with high fundamental frequency. Approximate formant frequencies are shown by arrows.

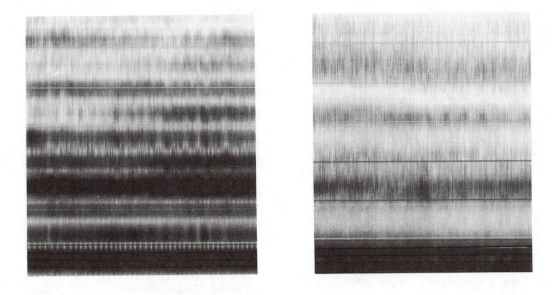

FIGURE 7-6. Spectrograms to illustrate formant-harmonic interaction. The spectrogram at the left was produced with a high fundamental frequency, so that the analyzing bandwidth resolves individual harmonics of the voice. The spectrogram at the right is the same vowel spoken by the same woman but with a lower fundamental frequency, so that the analyzing bandwidth resolves formants.

This occurrence made it difficult or impossible to tell when a band of energy on the spectrogram represented a formant or a harmonic.

One solution to this analysis problem is to increase the analyzing bandwidth. As a general rule of thumb, the bandwidth of the analyzing filter should be two to three times as large as the speaker's fundamental frequency. For example, the analyzing bandwidth for a woman who has a fundamental frequency of 300 Hz should be at least 600 Hz. There are upper limits to the size of the analyzing filter—making it too large defeats the purpose of acoustic analysis. For instance, a filter as wide as 1000 Hz would likely embrace not only harmonics but closely spaced formants as well. One approach taken to analyze women's and children's speech with the fixed-bandwidth analyzing filters on older spectrographs was to play back the speech signal at a slower speed than the speed used for recording. When the slowed signal was fed to the spectrograph, the

effective result was a change in analyzing filter bandwidth proportional to the difference in recording/play back speed.

Another issue in the acoustic analysis of women's speech is the overall frequency range of analysis. As a rule of thumb, the frequency value for a particular acoustic feature will be on the order of 20% higher for a woman than for a man. This upward shift of frequency values should be taken into account especially for sounds with high frequency components. Whereas a frequency range of 8 kHz may be quite satisfactory for the analysis of fricative energy for men, this range may not be adequate to represent the fricative energy for women speakers.

A number of studies point to the conclusion that women's voices differ from men's on dimensions other than fundamental frequency. These dimensions are pertinent to the optimal analysis of women's speech. A frequently reported characteristic of women's voices is that they are breathier than men's. Several acoustic correlates have been identified in the study of breathiness and related features in women's voices. Henton and Bladon (1985) determined that for speakers of RP (Received Pronunciation) British, the amplitude of the first harmonic, relative to the amplitude of the second harmonic, was about 6 dB stronger for women than for men. Klatt and Klatt (1990) reported a similar difference for male and female speakers of American English but noted that there was considerable variation within their male and female groups. Bless, Biever, and Shaikh (1986) concluded from stroboscopic observations of the larynx that women were four times as likely as men to have a posterior glottal chink during the closed period of the cycle. Using inverse-filtered, glottal-flow waveforms, Holmberg, Hillman, and Perkell (1988) found greater acoustic evidence of breathiness for women than for men. Similarly, Klatt and Klatt (1990) discovered a tendency for female voices to have a greater excitation of F3 by aspiration noise ("noise in F3") than male voices. Klatt and Klatt also concluded that the partial glottal opening in breathy voices causes an increase in the bandwidth of the first formant, "sometimes obliterating the spectral peak at F1 entirely" (p. 835). They commented that this effect, combined with the appearance of extra pole-zero pairs associated with tracheal coupling, can create problems for models that expect a formant-like representation of sounds across speakers who differ in age and sex.

In summary, there is much to consider in analyzing women's speech. The points mentioned should be weighed in the choice of analysis tools and parameters. For example, the all-pole model assumed in many LPC analysis routines may not be well-suited to breathy women's voices, which may be characterized by tracheal pole-zero pairs, wide F1 bandwidth, and significant noise excitation of the F3 frequency region.

Children's Speech

Because children have shorter vocal tracts and shorter vocal folds than adults, it is expected that children will have relatively higher fundamental and formant frequencies than adult speakers. This statement is generally true, but it should be recognized that children are a diverse population having a range of speech characteristics. To a first approximation, we may say that the speech of prepubescent children is characterized by higher formant and fundamental frequencies than observed for adult speech. After puberty, the situation changes markedly, particularly for males. The well-known "voice change" in adolescent males brings about a sizeable reduction in vocal fundamental frequency, which typically drops by about an octave.

This review begins with a consideration of infant vocalizations. Although a relatively small number of studies have been published on infant vocalizations, the available reports are sufficient to give an overall characterization of these early sounds. Compared with speakers of other ages, infants have the shortest vocal folds and the shortest vocal tracts. It is therefore not surprising that they have the highest fundamental and formant frequencies. Acoustic research summarized by Kent and Murray (1982) has shown that infants have the following approximate means for a mid-central vowel:

Fundamental frequency—400 Hz,

First formant frequency—1000 Hz,

Second formant frequency—3000 Hz, and

Third formant frequency—5000 Hz.

The formant frequencies are spaced at intervals of about 2000 Hz, compared to about 1000 Hz for adult males (for whom the first three formant frequencies of the mid-central vowel are about 500, 1500, and 2500 Hz). Using the formulas given in Chapter 2, we can calculate the length of the infant's vocal tract given these acoustic measures of formant frequency. The estimated length of about 8 cm agrees quite well with actual measurements made of an infant's vocal tract length.

The mean value of fundamental frequency of 400 Hz should not be taken too strictly. Infants have large ranges of fundamental frequency, with minimum values reaching down to the adult male range and maximum values extending to 1000 Hz or higher. This large range can make the measurement of fundamental frequencies of infants rather challenging, especially for analysis instruments that have a limited range of fundamental-frequency measurement. But range is not the only obstacle, as will be seen in the following.

Several other characteristics of infant vocalizations have been noted in acoustic studies. One of these is the relative frequency of occurrence of intonation contours. Kent and Bauer (1985) and Robb, Saxman, and Grant (1989) reported that Rise-Fall, Flat, and Fall contours were the most frequently occurring. For example, Kent and Bauer's data showed that Fall and Rise-Fall together accounted for about 77% of the intonation contours produced by five 1-year-olds. In the Robb et al., study, the three contours Rise-Fall, Flat, and Fall accounted for 67% of the contours in comfort-state vocalizations.

Infants also tend to produce a large variety of phonation types. Observations have been made of harmonic doubling (the abrupt appearance and often equally abrupt disappearance of a harmonic series at one-half the original fundamental frequency), fundamental frequency shift, biphonation (a double series of fundamental frequencies), vocal tremor (a periodic variation of fundamental frequency and/or voice amplitude), and noise components (Kent & Murray, 1982; Kent & Bauer, 1985). Robb and Saxman (1988) determined that 6% of 1,200 noncry vocalizations from 14 infants had instances of harmonic doubling, fundamental frequency shift, or biphonation. These variant phona-

tion types can present problems for vocal analysis, especially for unwary investigators. Figure 7–7 shows a narrow-band spectrogram of an infant vocalization in which several phonation types appear. Such rapid and extreme variations in phonatory characteristics are not uncommon.

The overall frequency range of analysis is an important consideration in the analysis of infants' vocalizations. The fundamental frequencies of infants and young children may exceed the nominal range of many pitch analysis systems. Also, the frequency values for some acoustic properties may be considerably higher for children than for adults. Bauer and Kent (1987) reported that the primary energy ranges for fricatives produced by infants sometimes fell above 8 kHz, the upper frequency limit of conventional spectrography. Examples of frication spectra obtained from infants are shown in Figure 7–8. Notice that significant regions of noise energy extend to 16 kHz. It is always wise to determine carefully the upper limits required for an analysis before setting analysis parameters, for example, sampling rate for A/D conversion.

As children grow, their vocal tracts lengthen and their formant frequencies decrease accordingly. In fact, formant frequencies continue to decrease across the age span for most people, because the facial structures grow gradually larger even into old age (Kent & Burkhard, 1981). There is, therefore, a kind of acoustic "lifeline" in which the formant frequencies for a particular sound gradually decrease over an individual's lifetime (Figure 7–9). The pattern of formant-frequency change as a function of age is not simple. Vocal tract growth is not a simple matter of overall lengthening. Particularly in males, the vocal tract has disproportionate growth in the pharyngeal region compared to the oral region. Figure 7–10 gives a comparison of a newborn's vocal tract with that of an adult male. Not only does the newborn have a shorter vocal tract, but there are differences in the relative size and shape of

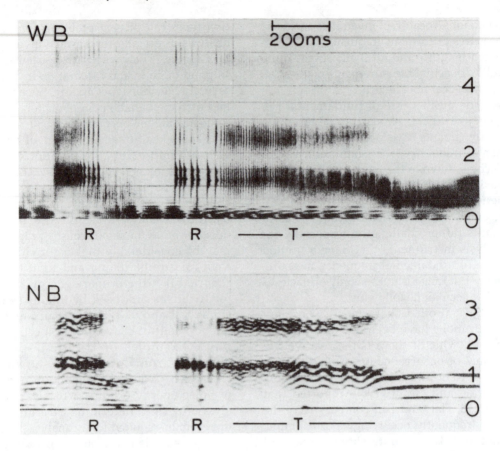

FIGURE 7–7. Wide-band (WB) and narrow-band (NB) spectrograms of an infant's vocalization. Note variation in phonatory pattern, including vocal roll or fry (R) and tremor (T).

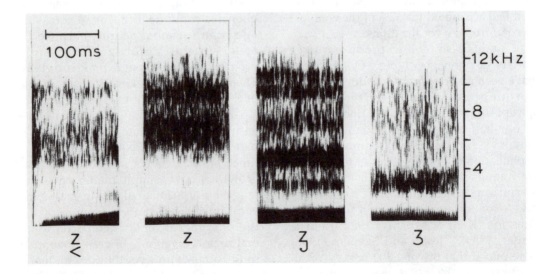

FIGURE 7–8. Spectrograms of fricatives produced by infants younger than one year. Phonetic symbols are shown at the bottom of each sample.

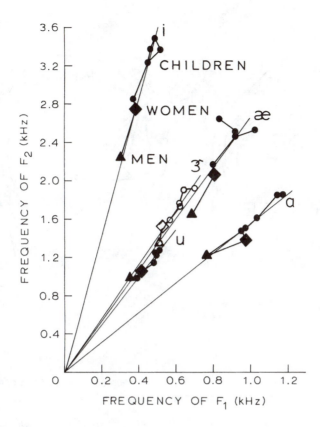

FIGURE 7–9.   Variation in F1 and F2 values for five American English vowels, as produced by groups of children, women, and men. The filled circles represent data for different age groups of children. The data are plotted to show "isovowel lines" or lines that connect the mean F1–F2 data for the various age-sex groups.

vocal tract structures. In particular, the newborn has a gradually sloping oropharyngeal channel compared to the nearly right-angle orientation between the oral and pharyngeal cavities in the adult. The larynx position in the neonate is relatively much higher—so high, in fact, that the epiglottis (a cartilage that closes over the laryngeal opening during swallowing to prevent food from entering it) nearly touches the soft palate. The infant also has a relatively shorter, broader oral cavity that is nearly filled by the tongue. A classic paper on normalization of formant-frequencies for speakers of different ages and sexes is Fant (1975); other papers on this subject were cited in Chapter 5.

Speech development is much more

than changes in vocal tract size and geometry. Oller (1986) described the acoustic properties of the *canonical syllable*, which is intended to represent the great majority of syllables in the world's languages. Presumably, the emergence of this syllable is a major accomplishment in vocal development. Oller proposed the following acoustic properties for the canonical syllable:

1. The power envelope has peaks and valleys that differ by at least 10 dB.

2. The peak-to-peak duration of the syllable is in the range of 100-500 ms.

3. The nucleus of the syllable is associated with a periodic source (i.e., voicing energy) and a relatively open vocal tract

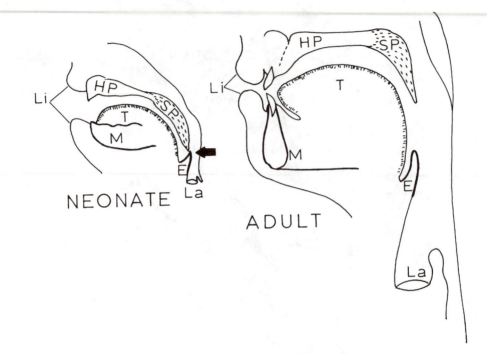

FIGURE 7-10. Drawings of the vocal tracts of a human neonate (newborn) and adult. T = tongue, HP = hard palate, M = mandible, Li = Lips, E = epiglottis, and La = larynx.

that affords full resonance (i.e., has a well-defined formant pattern).

4. The syllable possesses at least one margin of low resonance and relatively obstructed vocal tract. This margin has properties like those of obstruent consonants.

5. Smooth formant transitions occur between the margin(s) and nucleus, with a transition duration in the range of 25-120 ms.

6. The intensity range should be greater than about 30 dB.

7. The range of fundamental frequency should not exceed about one octave (doubling).

The canonical syllable may be an important unit for the integration of the perception and production of speech. The values just given should be regarded as hypothetical and subject to revision by research.

Following an interval of canonical babbling (babbling formed largely of canonical syllables), the infant usually begins to produce early words. The ages of these accomplishments vary considerably among children, but canonical babbling typically appears between 6–12 months of age, and the child's first words generally occur between 10–15 months. It seems reasonable to expect that experience in syllable babbling assists the child with the production of early words.

Compared to adults, children tend to have longer segment durations (slower speaking rates) and greater variability in repeated productions of an utterance (Kent & Forner, 1980). These effects are consistent with motor development generally. As children acquire a motor skill, their performance typically becomes faster and more reliable. Studies of temporal patterns in children's speech are helping to shape the understanding of speech development; the reader is referred to Allen and Hawkins (1980) for a good example of this effort. Spectrograms readily show the durational differences that often occur between children's and adults' productions of similar utterances. An example is given for the phrase "took a spoon" in Figure 7–11.

Acoustic methods are useful in studying phonetic and phonological variations in children's speech. Consider the child who deletes the /s/ fricative in words like *spoon*. Recall that voiceless stops following /s/ are unaspirated. If a child deletes the

/s/, is a following stop aspirated or unaspirated? The former would be predicted if the deleted fricative is not represented in the child's phonological representation, that is, the representation is something like /p u n/. But the unaspirated allophone would be predicted if the phonological representation includes the "missing" /s/, in which case the representation would be similar to the adult /s p u n/. Figure 7–12 shows two wideband spectrograms of the phrase *took a spoon* recorded from the same child within

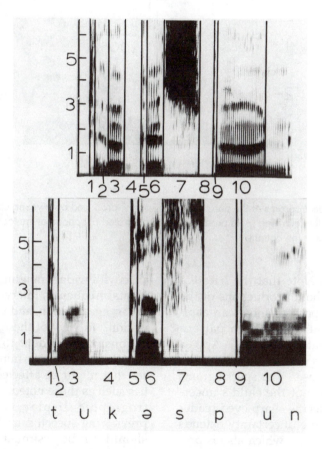

FIGURE 7–11. Spectrograms of the phrase "took a spoon" produced by an adult male (top) and a young child (bottom). The numbers identify the following acoustic segments: 1 – release burst of [t], 2 – aspiration interval, 3 – vowel [ʊ], 4 – stop gap for [k], 5 – release burst for [k], 6 – vowel [ə], 7 – frication for [s], 8 – stop gap for [p], 9 – burst for [p], and 10 – vowel [u]. Note generally longer segment durations and higher frequency energy for the child's production. Reprinted from R.D. Kent, "Sensorimotor aspects of speech development," In R.N. Aslin, J.R. Alberts, and M.R. Peterson (Eds.) *Development of Perception* (Vol. 1). (Reproduced with permission of Academic Press, New York). Copyright 1981.

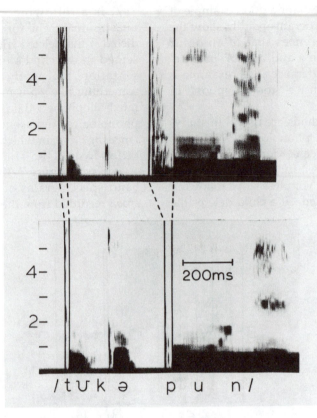

FIGURE 7-12. Spectrograms of the phrase "took a spoon" produced by a young child. The [s] in *spoon* is deleted and the following [p] is produced as an aspirated allophone at the top and as an unaspirated allophone at the bottom.

the same session. Note that the fricative /s/ is deleted in both productions of the phrase. The top pattern shows an aspirated stop /p/ but the bottom pattern shows an unaspirated stop /p/. Apparently, the child was uncertain about which stop allophone to use. The spectrograms give clear evidence of the child's uncertainty. Actually, as the sharp-eyed reader may have noted, the uncertainty extends even to the /t/ in *took*, which also is produced as unaspirated and aspirated variants.

Children's voices may present some of the same complications reviewed earlier in this chapter for women's voices. In addition, children often can be highly variable in their speech and voice characteristics; for example, producing an utter-ance with widely ranging values of funda-mental frequency, intervals of breathiness or laryngealization, and unexpected nasal-ization. In view of these possible compli-cations, it is prudent to preview speech samples before performing detailed analy-ses that might be affected by characteris-tics such as those noted. A real-time spec-trographic display is very useful in previewing speech samples. Above all, it should not be assumed that the default values of analysis parameters (usually determined from the speech of adult males) will be optimum for the analysis of children's speech. Generally, analysis parameter values for women's speech will be more suitable than values for men's speech when analyzing the speech pat-terns of children.

Speech Disorders

Speech disorders often present many challenges to acoustic analysis. One problem is that the acoustic properties predicted for normal speech may be missing or altered in speech disorders. It is not uncommon for an investigator to discover that acoustic measures easily applied to normal speech have to be modified to apply to some speakers with disorders. Some speech-disordered persons have highly variable phonatory and articulatory function, so that analysis parameters are not equally suitable over a stretch of speech. For example, a stutterer may have rapid and marked changes in fundamental frequency during a speech sample of interest. Therefore, an analyzing bandwidth that works well for one portion of the signal may not be appropriate for another portion. Similar rapid variations in phonatory and articulatory characteristics of speech can occur in speakers who are deaf or dysarthric.

A comprehensive account of the acoustic analysis of speech disorders would require several volumes. However, certain issues are encountered frequently enough that some preparation can be given in a few pages. What follows then, is a highly selective description of the application of acoustic analysis to speech disorders. Sample analyses will be described for individuals with cleft palate, deaf talkers, individuals with dysarthria (a condition in which the speech musculature is impaired because of neurological disease or damage), and individuals with verbal apraxia (a neurological disorder in which a major difficulty appears to be in the selection and regulation of segments and their associated movements).

A particularly troublesome feature of many speech disorders is unexpected nasalization, arising from velopharyngeal incompetence. Nasalization can severely compromise the acoustic analysis of a speech signal. In speakers with severe velopharyngeal incompetence, the entire signal can be influenced by a high degree of damping (therefore reduced signal energy and large formant bandwidths) and by antiformants (which can further reduce overall energy of the signal and can complicate the determination of formant locations). A severely nasalized speech signal usually has a greatly reduced acoustic contrast among its segmental components. An example of such reduction is given in Figure 7–13, which shows spectro-

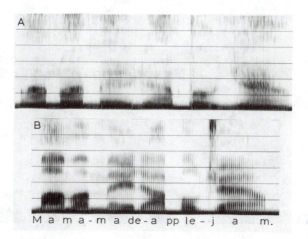

FIGURE 7–13. Spectrograms for the sentence, "Mama made apple jam," produced by a speaker with velopharyngeal incompetence (hypernasality) at the top (A) and by a speaker with normal nasality at the bottom (B). The pattern in A has a general loss of acoustic contrast among its component segments.

grams for a normal production of "Mama made apple jam," and a recitation of the same sentence by a speaker with severe velopharyngeal incompetence. When dealing with nasalized speech, it should be remembered that the acoustic correlates of nasalization are numerous and complex in their potential effects on the acoustic signal. Interpretation of acoustic records can therefore be difficult. For example, the following correlates of nasalization may appear in spectrograms of nasalized vowels (Kent, Liss, & Philips, 1989):

1. increase in formant bandwidth, so that formant energy appears broader;

2. decrease in the overall energy of the vowel (compared to non-nasalized vowels);

3. introduction of a low-frequency nasal formant with a center frequency of about 250-500 Hz for adult males;

4. a slight increase of the F1 frequency and a slight lowering of the F2 and F3 frequencies; and

5. the presence of one or more antiformants.

A general difficulty in acoustic analysis of speech disorders is that individuals with the same disorder may vary greatly from one another in their acoustic speech characteristics. Speakers with hearing impairment are notable for such interindividual variability. Some examples are shown in Figure 7–14 and Figure 7–15. Figure 7–14 contains several spectrograms of a portion of the simple phrase "took a spoon" produced by six deaf adolescents. The spectrograms shown focus on the production of the fricative [s] in the word "spoon." The following patterns can be seen: (a) This speaker produced a fairly normal fricative, as evidenced by the conspicuous noise energy at higher frequencies; (b) Here the speaker interrupts the frication segment so that its midsection is nearly silent, somewhat resembling a stop gap; (c) This attempt begins with a fairly good fricative but it is cut short and followed by a noticeable silent gap; (d) The production is characterized by a burst of diffuse noise energy closely preceding the onset of the vowel [u]; (e) The speaker represented here tended to laryngealize

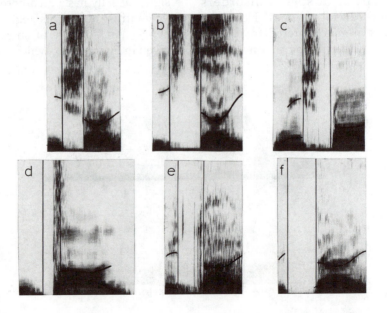

FIGURE 7–14. Spectrograms of the phrase "a spoon" (extracted from the sentence, "I took a spoon and a dish") produced by speakers with profound hearing loss or deafness. The individual patterns a–f are described in the text.

consonant segments, as indicated in this spectrogram by the continuation of voicing through the marked interval and the appearance of pronounced glottal pulses; and (f) In this case, there is no frication energy, but the location of the [s] is marked by a silent interval of approximately the right duration of the [s] energy in normal speech.

Figure 7–15 gives examples of phonatory, resonance, and prosodic variations in the speech of the deaf. All of the patterns shown are for the first three words of the sentence, "Buy Bobby a puppy." Spectrogram **a** shows the result for a speaker with a continuously breathy voice. Note that there is little evidence of periodic voicing energy and that the formants are excited by noise. In spectrogram **b**, the speaker tends to laryngealize consonants and word

boundaries, and to produce speech with little variation in fundamental frequency or F2. The fundamental frequency is superimposed as the broken line averaging a little less than 125 Hz, and the F2 frequency is drawn as a solid line on the spectrogram. Note the glottal roll (R) near the end of the pattern. Spectrogram **c** is the result for a speaker with a highly variable fundamental frequency (see the superimposed broken line representing the fundamental frequency contour) and a strong tendency to nasalize speech. The nasalization caused a virtual disappearance of F2 energy (see dotted line). Finally, spectrogram **d** shows the pattern for a speaker who produced nearly equally stressed, widely separated syllables in a kind of sing-song cadence. This speaker's speech is slow (compare the duration of **c** with that of the other three

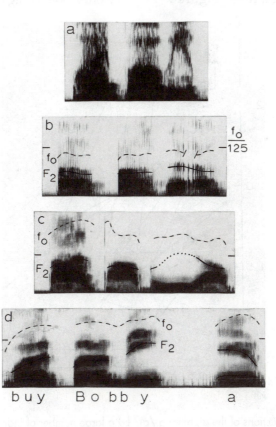

FIGURE 7–15. Spectrograms of the first three words of the sentence, "Buy Bobby a puppy," produced by individuals with profound hearing loss or deafness. The fundamental frequency (f0) contour is superimposed on the spectrograms in b, c, and d. See discussion in text.

patterns) and deliberate (note the distinct formant patterns).

The variability among deaf speakers is further illustrated in Figure 7–16, which shows the F1-F2 trajectories for the diphthong in *buy* produced by 23 deaf adolescent speakers. The trajectories are drawn as straight lines connecting the apparent onglide of the diphthong with its apparent offglide. The trajectories differ in onglide frequency, offglide frequency, and to a lesser extent even the direction of movement in the F1–F2 plane (e.g., some speakers have a downward rather than the expected upward frequency shift for F2).

Acoustic contrast among speech segments is reduced in a number of speech disorders. One in particular is Parkinson's disease, which is typically characterized by reduced articulatory movements and a rigid speech musculature. Figure 7–17

allows a comparison of a normal control speaker and a speaker with Parkinson's disease saying the phrase "strikes raindrops." Selected acoustic segments are numbered at the top of the production by the control speaker. Note that the acoustic contrastivity is much reduced in the production by the speaker with Parkinson's disease: vowel formants are obscure, stop gaps for /t/, /k/, /d/, and /p/ are missing (in fact, they are spirantized—filled with noise energy), and the oral-nasal resonance contrast is weakened (compare the /n/ in *raindrops* with its surrounding oral sounds). Some speakers with Parkinson's disease have a dysarthria in which words are uttered in short rushes or accelerated patterns. Figure 7–18 shows narrow-band (top) and wide-band (bottom) spectrograms for a short-rush production of the words "something beyond his reach." The

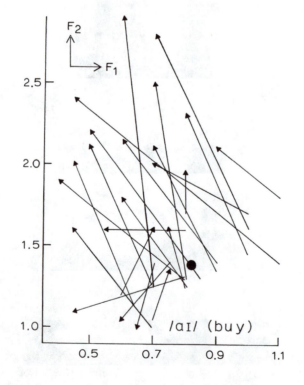

FIGURE 7–16. Productions of the diphthong /aɪ/ by a large number of individuals with profound hearing loss or deafness. The result for an individual speaker is represented in the F1-F2 plane as a line running from the onglide to the offglide (arrowhead). The mean F1 and F2 values for the onglide are indicated by the filled circle.

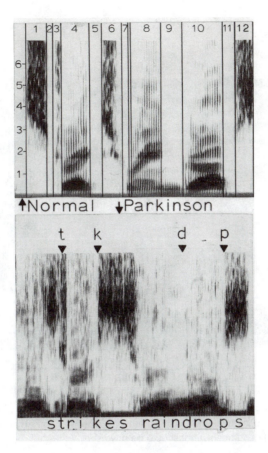

FIGURE 7–17.   Spectrograms of the phrase "strikes raindrops," produced (top) by a person with normal speech, and (bottom) an individual with Parkinson's disease and dysarthria. The arrowheads in the result for the speaker with Parkinson's disease indicate spirantized stop gaps (that is, stop gaps containing frication energy).

production is continuously voiced (notice the continuous voicing bar and the uninterrupted glottal-pulse vertical striations) and poorly articulated. The speaker accomplishes the rapid speaking rate by neglecting many phonatory and articulatory adjustments.

Acoustic analyses can be helpful in the study of speech disorders that disturb timing and sequencing. One such disorder is verbal apraxia (or apraxia of speech), which is a disorder of the sequencing or programming of speech movements. Dyspraxic speech tends to be slow, intermittent, and variable. The spectrograms in Figure 7–19 illustrate normal (a) and two

dyspraxic (b and c) productions of the word *please*. Differences in word duration are immediately evident, with the dyspraxic productions being more than twice the duration of the control. The second formant is labeled in each spectrogram. Note that the dyspraxic productions have slower F2 changes than the normal production. This analysis shows that the dyspraxic productions are longer and, moreover, have slower rates of acoustic (and, by inference, articulatory) change.

A general question about dyspraxic speech is whether the errors are phonemic (substitutions of one phoneme for another) or involve phonetic distortions (such as

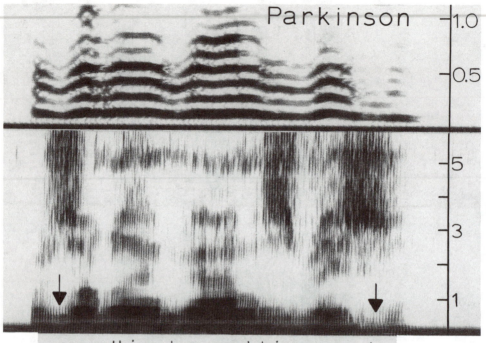

FIGURE 7–18. Narrow-band (top) and wide-band (bottom) spectrograms of the phrase "something beyond his reach," produced by a speaker with Parkinson's disease. The arrows point to intervals of continuous voicing (voicing of segments that should be unvoiced).

might result from incoordination). Figure 7–20 illustrates the use of a spectrogram to evaluate a particular error in dyspraxic speech. The word analyzed is the monosyllable *shush*. The illustration shows both wide-band (top) and narrow-band (bottom) spectrograms. The word was produced disfluently with a false start; note the initial frication segment followed by a production of the whole word. Fig 7–20 demonstrates how acoustic analysis can help to answer the question. Note that the initial fricative production of *shush* is not entirely voiceless: evidence that vocal fold vibrations begin during the fricative interval appears in both the wide-band spectrogram (note circled voice bar) and narrow-band spectrogram (note circled harmonic pattern). Apparently, this speaker commits errors in the coordination of voicing with oral articulatory function, such that the

resulting pattern is not a phonemic error but a phonetic or motoric lapse.

Variations in VOT for the prevocalic stop /d/ in *dad* are illustrated in Figure 7–21. Results are shown for four dyspraxic speakers, arranged in order of increasing duration of prevoicing. The VOT interval is highlighted with a vertical bar and attached arrow. The speaker represented in (d) has a particularly long interval of prevoicing. A similar pattern in cerebral-palsied speech was described by Farmer and Lencione (1977).

A related speech disorder in children is a controversial disorder often given the name, developmental verbal apraxia. Children with this disorder have considerable difficulty in producing speech with normal rate and phonetic accuracy. Figure 7–22 contains three spectrograms showing: (a) a normal speaker saying the

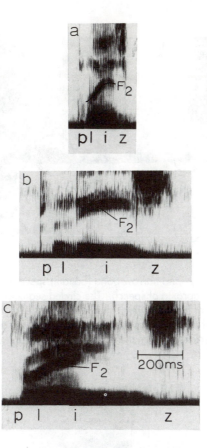

FIGURE 7–19.   Spectrograms of the word *please* produced by (a) a person with normal speech, and (b and c) persons with apraxia of speech. The apractic productions are greatly lengthened compared to the normal pattern. Reprinted from R.D. Kent and J.C. Rosenbek, "Acoustic patterns of apraxia of speech," *Journal of Speech and Hearing Research, 26,* 231–249. (Reproduced with permission from the American Speech-Language-Hearing Association, Rockville, MD.) Copyright 1987.

word *spaghetti*, (b) a verbally dyspraxic child saying the same word, and (c) a second attempt by the same child as in (b). The characteristics of slowness, intermittency, and variability are represented acoustically in patterns (b) and (c) by long overall duration and long segment durations (slow speaking rate); long pauses (intermittent, broken speech); and inconsistency between the two productions (variability). Similar characteristics have been observed in adult (or acquired) apraxia of speech (Kent & Rosenbek, 1983).

A promising role of acoustic methods in speech pathology is to monitor changes in speech production that may occur as the result of management or as the result of disease progression. Acoustic analysis permits a quantification of selected features of speech production. One example is the use of acoustics to study the change in speech in an individual with amyotrophic lateral sclerosis, a degenerative and fatal neurologic disease. Sample spectrograms of the word *sigh* from one speaker are shown in Figure 7–23 for two different times: (a) at about the time of the initial diagnosis, and (b) several months after diagnosis. One can see in the spectrograms that as the disease progresses there

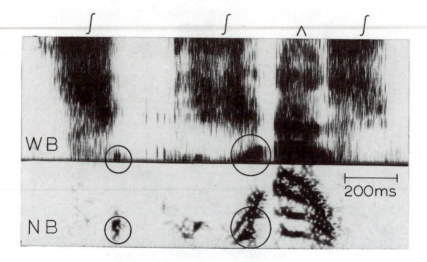

FIGURE 7–20. Wide-band (top) and narrow-band (bottom) spectrograms of a dysfluent production of the work *shush* by a person with apraxia of speech. The circled segments indicate brief voiced intervals during the production of the initial fricative (which should be voiceless). Reprinted from R. D. Kent and J.C. Rosenbeck, "Acoustic patterns of apraxia of speech," *Journal of Speech and Hearing Research, 26,* 231–246. (Reproduced with permission from the American Speech-Language-Hearing Association, Rockville, MD.) Copyright 1987.

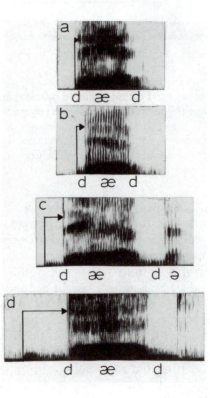

FIGURE 7–21. Spectrograms of the word *dad* produced by (a) a person with normal speech, and (b–d) persons with apraxia of speech. The interval marked by an arrow is the voice onset time (VOT) for the initial [d].

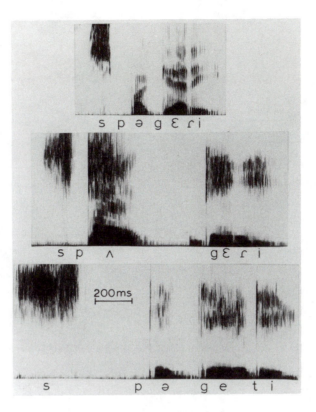

FIGURE 7–22. Spectrograms of the word *spaghetti* produced by a normal adult speaker (top) and (middle and bottom) a child with developmental apraxia of speech. The child's productions are characterized by lengthened segments and a highly variable pattern.

is a deterioration of the noise energy for /s/ and a flattening of the formant pattern for the diphthong. Acoustic methods can be used to detect subtler changes as well, possibly changes that cannot be reliably detected by the ear alone.

The spectrograph made possible an objective examination of speech disorders. However, one problem with the spectrograph is that it often leaves the user with a considerable analysis task. The spectrogram in itself is rarely sufficient; the user has to derive measures, often by a rather tedious process. Much faster analyses, resulting in quantitative measures, are being used today. For example, LPC formant tracking identifies formant patterns automatically, thus saving the effort and time that otherwise would be given to manual formant tracing from spectro-

grams. A sample of automatic quantitative analysis is given in Figure 7–24. The analysis pertains to the same dysarthric speaker's productions of the word *sigh* shown in Figure 7–23. The multiparameter analyis of Figure 7–24 shows: (a) LPC formant tracks for the first two formants, (b–e) the fourth, third, second, and first spectral moments, respectively, (f) the rms envelope, and (g) the fundamental frequency contour. Note that Figure 7–24 reflects the deterioration of /s/ frication as changes in the spectral moments, particularly the first moment, and the reduced formant movements of the diphthong as a flattening of the LPC formant tracks. This multiparameter analysis yields a great deal of information about the speech pattern, all of it obtained semiautomatically on a personal computer.

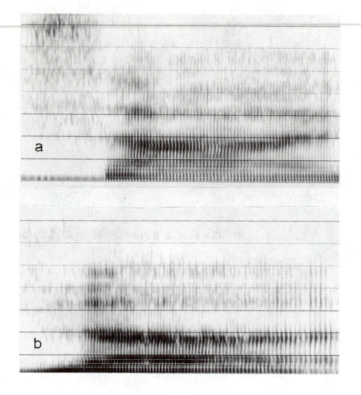

FIGURE 7–23. Spectrograms of the word *sigh* produced by a woman with amyotropyhic lateral sclerosis (Lou Gehrig's disease). The result in (a) was recorded at an early point in the disease and the result in (b) was recorded at a later point when the disease was highly advanced.

As one final illustration of acoustic analysis to speech disorders, consider the condition of *aglossia*, or absence of the tongue. In some cases of lingual cancer, it is necessary to remove the tongue. Interestingly, some speakers who have had such surgery manage to recover fairly intelligible speech. One individual who had essentially total removal of the tongue (plus part of the jaw) was nonetheless able to produce understandable sentences. Sample spectrograms of his productions of the words *four* and *five* are shown in Figure 7–25. Note that formants are present—the vocal tract continues to be a resonating system, even without the tongue—but the formants have conservative shifts in frequency.

For more detailed discussions of the acoustic characteristics of disordered speech, the reader is referred to an article on acoustic characteristics of dysarthria by Weismer (1984), a book on clinical measurement of speech and voice (Baken, 1987), and a collection of articles on spectrographic analysis edited by Baken and Daniloff (1990).

Other Applications and Issues

The application of acoustic analysis is rapidly expanding to a broad range of topics. These cannot be discussed in any detail in this book, but a general list of topics and selected references is provided below:

Vocal correlates of psychological stress: (Brenner & Shipp, 1987; Hollien, 1980). This topic addresses the questions: Is psychological stress evident in a speaker's

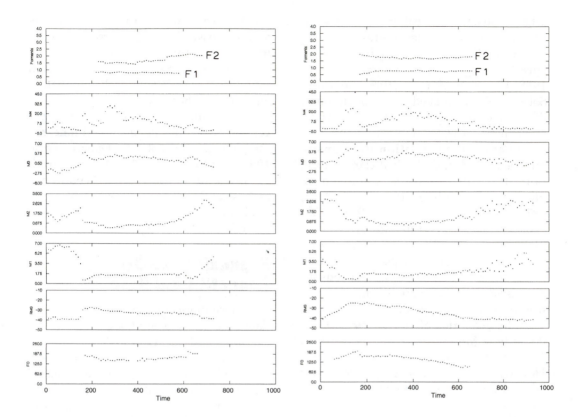

FIGURE 7–24. Multiparameter acoustic analysis of the utterances shown spectrographically in Figure 7–23. (left) Analysis of the production from an early point in the disease. (right) Analysis of the production from a late stage in the disease. See text for discussion.

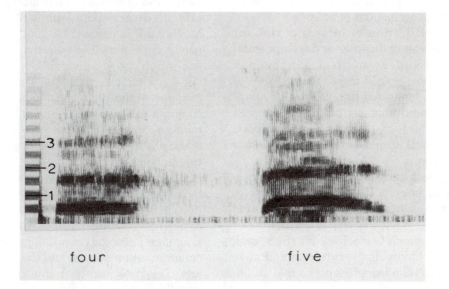

FIGURE 7–25. Spectrogram of the numbers *four* and *five* produced by a man with aglossia (absence of tongue, which was removed due to cancer).

articulation and voice patterns? If so, what are the acoustic correlates of stress?

Acoustic correlates of intoxicated speech: (Klingholz, Penning, & Liebhardt, 1988; Pisoni & Martin, 1989; Sobell & Sobell, 1982). Inebriated talkers often sound "under the influence." What are the acoustic-phonetic correlates of intoxication?

Speaker identification by acoustic methods: (Black et al., 1973; Bolt et al., 1970; Bolt et al., 1973; Endres, Bambach, & Flosser, 1971; Hollien, 1974, 1980; Poza, 1974; Reich, Moll, & Curtis, 1976). Can "voice prints" be used like finger prints to identify individuals in crimes associated with a recording of the suspect's voice, as in bomb threats, harrassing calls, and conspiracy cases? The cited papers bring the controversy into relief if not resolution.

The acoustics of the singing voice: (Schutte & Miller, 1983; Sundberg, 1977, 1987) and musical sounds (Sundberg, 1991). How does the trained singing voice differ from the untrained voice? What is the singer's formant and why is it important?

Acoustic diagnosis of voice disorders: (Davis, 1976; Kasuya, Ogawa, & Kikuchi, 1986). Can acoustic measures be used to identify and classify voice disorders? How well do acoustic measures correlate with perceptual evaluations of voice?

Identification of infants at risk for communication disorder or developmental disability: (Kent, in press; Lindblom & Zetterstrom, 1986; Murry & Murry, 1980). It has been suggested that certain developmental conditions can be identified even from the birth cry. What are the prospects for a clinical acoustic assessment of infant vocalizations?

Speech technology for the management of speech disorders: (Bernstein, Goldstein, & Mahshie, 1988; Kewley-Port et al., 1991). What are the implications of acoustic speech technology for the speech training of individuals with communicative disorders? Can machines play a role in clinical management?

Speech synthesis for the vocally disabled: (Edwards, 1990). Persons who are unable to communicate vocally often can use speech synthesizers as an assistive communication aid. What are the alternatives and how can they be used?

Determining the nature of speech perception difficulties in persons with hearing impairment: (Clement, 1991; Dubno,& Levitt, 1981; Gordon-Salant, 1987). Are certain acoustic features especially difficult to hear because of hearing loss? If so, what are the implications for the design of hearing aids or other devices to assist speech perception?

Expanding the Acoustic Phonetic Data Base

The preceding comments indicate that the data base of acoustic phonetics is expanding to include a much broader range of speakers, speaking conditions, and issues than studied in the past. Data are being collected on infants, children, women, speakers of various dialects and individuals with various speech and voice disorders. This broader research effort is important to make the acoustic analysis of speech, automatic speech recognition and speech synthesis, and other speech technologies applicable to diverse populations of speakers. Much work remains to be done, but, fortunately, current methods of acoustic analysis are much more adaptable to different speaker characteristics than was the spectrograph of the 1950s and 1960s. The spectrograph was a powerful tool in its day, but modern computer systems and digital spectrographs go far beyond the original spectrograph in speed, flexibility, and ease of use.

Speech acoustics stands today as a well-developed science with a variety of applications in engineering, computer science, education, psychology, linguistics, speech-language pathology, audiology, industry, communication science, and the performing arts. This book is only an introduction to a rapidly developing field.

Speech Synthesis

CHAPTER

Purposes

With a few billion people on the planet who can produce natural speech more or less fluently, why would anyone want to create *synthetic speech*? This question seems especially pertinent considering the poor quality of some synthetic speech today. However, synthetic speech has several good uses, some of which are actually quite important.

Toys

One of the first widely known uses for synthetic speech was in toys and games, such as the Texas Instruments *Speak & Spell*™, which (in one of its several modes) pronounces words for a child to spell on its keyboard. When it was introduced in 1978, this toy surprised many speech scientists as well as business competitors; few people were aware that synthetic speech of commercial quality could be produced by an integrated circuit (a "chip") so low in price that it could be at the heart of a toy. The potential for talking toys and games is now limited only by our imaginations.

Word Processing and Reading

A short step from a talking toy for young spellers is a word processor which reads back what one has written. Most primary school teachers today encourage children to write while, or even before, they learn to read. In the process, children frequently ask, "What did I write?" Upon command, a talking word processor attempts to speak what a child has written. This same feedback can be helpful to older writers, too — even to adults, and especially to the visually impaired. An extension of this idea is the reading machine, of which one notable example is the Kurzweil Personal Reader™, sold by Xerox Imaging Systems. A reading machine links a scanner which can recognize printed characters to a synthesizer which takes those characters as input and produces speech as output.

Prosthesis

Not everyone can speak fluently, or speak at all. Those who have not developed or have lost the capability may nonetheless be able to control a speech synthesizer, which enables them to interact with other people via spoken language, face-to-face or over the telephone. This replacement can be vital in a world in which most communication, including most urgent communication, is oral. For an up-to-date review of speech synthesis as an aid, see Edwards (1991), which gives particular attention to the interface, that is, the ways in which a person can control a synthesizer. Edwards includes several case studies of devices, as well as appendices listing equipment and manufacturers.

Manufacturing and Control

In many situations, workers' eyes and hands are fully occupied; examples are aircraft pilots during takeoffs and landings, as well as factory workers who are controlling a machine that demands their attention. In such cases, spoken messages from the aircraft or other machine, rather than more lights, gauges, and beeps, can be essential to getting a crucial message across. Such applications do not necessarily require *synthetic* speech; if the messages are relatively few and brief, they can be recorded digitally and played back on command. It is this approach which telephone companies use today to answer "directory assistance" requests or to provide error messages. The same technique is used in systems for telephone inquiries about bank balances, reports to the home office from sales representatives on the road, and course registration at universities. When the potential messages become extremely numerous or unpredictable (as

with word processing), recorded speech is no longer feasible and synthetic speech becomes necessary. As systems for information and control become more complex and the quality of synthetic speech improves, we may well find ourselves listening more often to machines that talk.

Speech Research

Despite this growing list of commercial applications, the use of synthetic speech that is most important to speech science is as the ultimate check on our analysis of speech. In fact, analysis and synthesis are often paired as complementary parts of an investigation. If we conclude from spectrographic analysis that a certain formant pattern is crucial to the production and comprehension of [æ], for instance, the real test of that hypothesis is to synthesize that pattern and see whether it sounds like [æ]. After the development of the sound spectrograph, one of the most important steps in modern speech research was the development of the "pattern playback" synthesizer at Haskins Laboratories in the 1950s. (See the discussion in Chapters 5 and 6.) This device was simply the inverse of a spectrograph: given a spectrogram as input, it produced the corresponding speech as output. That is, it scanned a spectrogram and produced sound at the indicated frequencies and intensities over time. What made the device so important was that the spectrographic pattern at the input could be hand-drawn instead of printed by a spectrograph. Thus researchers tested the hypothesis that the first two or three formants are crucial to the quality of vowels by drawing just those formants and listening to the corresponding synthetic speech. In this way re-searchers discovered the importance of formant transitions in conveying the place of articulation of stop consonants, for example. It would be difficult to test such ideas by analyzing natural speech because brief events like formant transitions cannot be manipulated separately from the vowels to which they are attached. When we listen to formant transitions by themselves, they sound like chirps, not stop consonants.

Synthesis is essential not only in studies of the speech signal and its production, but also in studies of how people perceive speech. For example, as we have seen, there are several acoustic differences between "voiced" and "voiceless" stops: in the occurrence of aspiration, the duration of the stop and of a preceding vowel, the fundamental frequency of a following vowel, and the occurrence of voicing during the closure, to name a few. Which of these most affects listeners' ability to hear this distinction? Is any one of them necessary? We could scarcely have studied such questions without synthetic speech, because we could not control these features individually by editing natural speech.

In modern synthesis, we can control almost any feature of speech which is thought to be important, including qualities of the voice source as well as of articulation and resonance. Given the rapidity with which change occurs in the speech signal, such control can be tedious, but it is the ultimate test of our understanding.

In the remainder of this chapter, we will describe three types of speech synthesis: formant synthesis, synthesis by rule, and synthesis based on linear predictive coding (LPC). These are all based on acoustic models of the speech signal and are most commonly used today. Each has been implemented on ordinary microcomputers; anyone with a personal computer with a little ancillary equipment can experiment with synthetic speech. This fact has certainly accelerated progress in the field.

An alternative to acoustic synthesis is articulatory synthesis, which creates speech from a model of the changing shape of the vocal tract during articulation. In starting from articulation, this approach is more thorough; it includes more of the speech process and enables us to test hypotheses about articulation directly.

However, it is correspondingly more intricate and demanding. Only recently has it become possible to create computer models of articulation which run relatively rapidly. If one's goal is to produce high-quality synthetic speech in a reasonable amount of time, the acoustic-based approaches are still preferable.

Formant Synthesis

The most basic acoustic synthesis is simply to recreate the changing formants of speech, each one being specified as a frequency and bandwidth, updated every 5 ms or so during an utterance. A few such formants (resonances) together with suitable inputs, namely periodic and noise sources to mimic voicing and frication respectively, have proven sufficient to produce recognizable speech. In essence, this was the approach of the pattern playback synthesizer, although it was primitive compared to modern devices; for example, its voice source did not vary in f0 or other parameters. Formant synthesis received a big boost in 1980 with Dennis Klatt's publication of a more elaborate model, complete with a computer program which synthesized speech on a laboratory computer (Klatt, 1980). Because speech synthesis had commercial value, this publication was a generous contribution on Klatt's part. Variants of this model are now available as working computer programs from several sources at little or no cost. Klatt updated the model, especially as to voice quality, in Klatt and Klatt (1990), and Sensimetrics Corporation offers a microcomputer program based on this second model.

The basis for Klatt's model is the source-filter theory, as discussed in Chapter 2. Figure 8–1 is Klatt's block diagram of his (1980) cascade/parallel formant synthesizer. There are two sound sources, one for voicing (labeled "voicing source") and one for frication (labeled "noise source"). These drive two resonating systems, a cas-

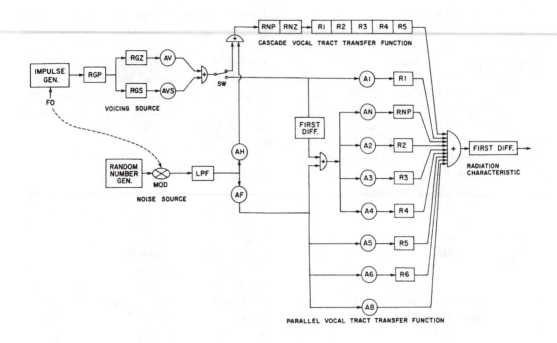

FIGURE 8-1. Block diagram of cascade/parallel formant synthesizer (Klatt, 1980).

cade (or serial) resonator for vowels and a parallel resonator for fricatives. In the cascade resonator, the output of the first formant resonator (R1) becomes the input to the second formant resonator (R2), and so on. Thus the formants influence each other: the relative amplitude of each depends partly on how close it is in frequency to other formants, as in the natural articulation of vowels. There is no need for a separate amplitude control for each formant as there is in the parallel resonator, in which each formant is developed independently. The cascade synthesizer models the production of speech sounds in which the excitation source is at the larynx and the entire vocal tract serves as a resonator, while the parallel synthesizer models the production of fricatives, in which the noise source is higher, usually in the oral cavity, and only that part of the vocal tract which is in front of the source serves as the resonator.

Let us trace the cascade system in Figure 8-1 from source to output. The voicing source generates a train of im-pulses like that produced by the vocal folds. The

boxes labelled RGP, RGZ, and RGS are essentially filters which smooth this simulated glottal waveform and shape its spectrum. AV controls the amplitude of voicing; it is set to zero during voiceless sounds. This source then enters the resonating system, in which RNP and RNZ represent nasal pole and nasal zero, respectively, and R1 to R5 represent formants 1 through 5. For each formant, the user specifies a frequency and bandwidth for every few milliseconds (ms) of speech.

Tracing the parallel system, we find a noise source which begins with a random number generator, since frication noise begins with turbulence that is quasirandom in frequency and amplitude. MOD provides for mixing the noise and voicing sources for voiced fricatives. LPF is a low-pass filter which shapes the source spectrum, and AH and AF control the amplitude of aspiration and of frication, respectively. Aspiration noise goes to the cascade resonator because aspiration generated at the larynx, like voicing, uses the entire vocal tract as a resonator. Aspiration can be mixed with the voice source to produce (among other things) a breathy voice quality, as in some female voices. The noise source for fricatives goes through the parallel resonators, each with its own amplitude control. The boxes labeled "First Diff" are high-pass filters; the one at the output simulates the emphasis given to higher frequencies as sound radiates from the lips.

Altogether, the 1980 Klatt model has 39 parameters (control values), of which 19 are fixed. The user must specify the other 20 for every 5 ms of speech to be produced. Thus for a syllable of, say, 250 ms, the 20 variable parameters must be set 50 times, for a total of 1000 specifications. Most of these values do not change constantly. For example, during a vowel, AF (amplitude of frication) and the amplitudes of all of the parallel formants can be set to zero and remain there. In principle, f0 and AV (amplitude of voicing) could be set to constant values during a syllable in which fundamental frequency does not change. However, even in such a syllable, more life-like speech will result if these two values vary a little, as they do in natural speech. In some implementations of the Klatt synthesizer, the user can set key parameters at points of major change, and the program will fill in the rest, using linear or other interpolations. Thus one would set the fundamental frequency at the beginning and end of the voiced portion of a syllable, and the program would fill in f0 at all points in between, creating a linear or nonlinear slope and perhaps introducing slight variation, known as jitter.

Table 8–1 lists suggested values for F1, F2, F3, and duration for most phonemes of English. These are "default" values, in the sense that they might be used as starting points in synthesis before one takes context and individual variation into account.

Figure 8–2 shows two spectrograms of utterances of "seep." The lower one is of

TABLE 8–1

Suggested values for synthesis of phonetic segments. Shown for each IPA phoneme are: CPA—computer phonetic alphabet, WORD—Keyword, F1—frequency of first formant, F2—frequency of second formant, F3—frequency of third formant, and DUR—inherent duration, and, optionally, OTHER—additional features that must be represented in synthesis. The terms listed under OTHER are described at the end of the table. For diphthongs, both the onglide and offglide formant frequencies are specified (a linear transition between brief steady states can be used in synthesizing the formant shifts). For consonants, the formant frequency values are characteristic values in the sense that they can be used to specify formant transitions between the consonant and a neighboring sound (especially a vowel). These values correspond to the idea of formant loci, or characteristic formant frequencies for the consonant.

IPA	CPA	Word	F1	F2	F3	DUR	Other
			VOWELS AND DIPHTHONGS				
[i]	IY	beet	300	2200	3000	160	
[ei]	EY	bait	550	1900	2650	190	
			400	2100	2700		
[oʊ]	OW	boat	575	900	2400	220	
			450	800	2350		
[æ]	Æ	bat	650	1750	2400	230	
[aʊ]	AO	bought	575	850	2400	240	

(continued)

TABLE 8-1 (continued)

IPA	CPA	Word	F1	F2	F3	DUR	Other
		VOWELS AND DIPHTHONGS (continued)					
[ɑ]	AA	Bob	750	1150	2400	240	
[ɑɪ]	AY	bite	750	1250	2500	250	
[ɔɪ]	OY	boy	550	850	2525	280	
[aʊ]	AW	bout	750	1325	2700	260	
			575	900	2250		
[ə]	AX	about	600	1300	2450	120	
[ɜ˞]	RR	bird	500	1350	1700	180	
[ɪ]	IH	bit	400	2000	2550	130	
[ɛ]	EH	bet	525	1850	2500	150	
[ʌ]	AH	but	650	1200	2400	140	
[ʊ]	UH	book	450	1050	2250	160	
		SONORANT CONSONANTS					
[w]	W	wet	300	600	2200	80	GLIDE
[r]	R	red	425	1300	1600	80	LIQUID
[l]	L	let	375	875	2575	80	LIQUID
[j]	Y	yet	300	2200	3050	80	GLIDE
[m]	M	met	275	900	2200	70	NASAL
[n]	N	net	275	1700	2600	65	NASAL
[ŋ]	NG	sing	275	2300	2750	80	NASAL
		FRICATIVE CONSONANTS					
[f]	F	fin	150	1100	2400	120	NOISE
[v]	V	van	150	1100	2400	60	NOISE
[θ]	TH	thin	200	1600	2200	110	NOISE
[ə]	DH	this	200	1600	2200	50	NOISE
[s]	S	sip	200	1800	2600	125	NOISE
[z]	Z	zip	200	1800	2600	75	NOISE
[ʃ]	SH	ship	200	1300	2400	125	NOISE
[ʒ]	ZH	azure	200	1300	2400	70	NOISE
[h]	H	hat	(set to match vowel)			80	NOISE
		AFFRICATE CONSONANTS					
For affricates, use values for a similar fricative, but include stop gap to represent the closure portion and shape the noise with a rapid rise time.							
		STOP CONSONANTS					
[p]	P	pat	150	800	1750	85	B, AF
[b]	B	bat	150	800	1750	80	B
[t]	T	tip	150	1800	2600	85	B, AF
[d]	D	dip	150	1800	2600	65	B
[k]	K	come	150	2350	2750	65	B, AF, V
[g]	G	gum	150	2350	2750	65	B, V
[ɾ]	DX	butter	150	1800	2600	20	FLAP

(continued)

TABLE 8-1 (continued)

TERMS LISTED UNDER OTHER:

AF — affrication is required unless stop follows [s]. Aspiration noise can be simulated with a flat-spectrum noise.

B — burst may be needed; burst is a brief noise segment (10–30 msec) shaped according to place of articulation. A simple rule for spectral shaping: bilabials—flat or gradually falling spectrum; alveolars—flat or gradually rising spectrum; velars—mid-frequency peak in spectrum.

FLAP — sound is a flap, which involves a very brief closure.

GLIDE — sound is a glide and is associated with gradual formant shifts (about 75–100 msec duration).

LIQUID — sound is a liquid; brief steady state and transition may be required. Transition tends to be faster for [l] than [r].

NASAL — sound is characterized by nasal murmur, which can be simulated with a strong low-frequency band of energy (nasal formant).

NOISE — sound requires a substantial interval of noise, shaped according to place of articulation. For labio-dentals /f v/ and linguadentals /θ ð/, use a low-energy, flat-spectrum noise. For alveolar /s z/ and palatals /ʃ ʒ tʃ dʒ/, use a more intense noise shaped by high-pass filtering. The noise energy should lie principally above 4 kHz for alveolars and above 3 kHz for palatals (these values are for adult males; scale upward for women and children). For glottal /h/, use aspiration noise as described for AF.

V — sound is a velar, which does not have a single set of characteristic formant frequencies. Formants have to be adjusted for vowel context. A basic rule is to give F2 and F3 a "wedge" shape into or out of a neighboring vowel; e.g., for /gi/, F2 and F3 should begin close together and quickly separate during CV transition.

---

natural speech, and the upper one of speech produced with the Klatt and Klatt (1990) synthesizer as implemented by Sensimetrics. Only moderate efforts were made to shape the synthetic speech. Note that it has little sound energy above 5 kHz, while in the natural speech the [s] has intense energy up to the 8 kHz range of the spectrogram. The synthetic speech has less variable amplitude, more abrupt transitions, more intense aspiration of the [p], and less noise in the higher frequencies than the natural speech.

Figure 8–3 shows an amplitude spectrum taken near the middle of the [i] in each utterance; the lighter trace is for the natural speech. Notice that the synthetic vowel has a wider bandwidth for F2, and a considerably higher F3. In fact, the tilt of the spectrum in the higher frequencies is wrong.

Figure 8–4 shows the waveforms and f0 contours of each utterance; counting from the top, channels 1 and 3 are the nat-

ural speech, which has more gradual change in both amplitude and f0. In principle, all of these differences could have been eliminated if we had tailored the relevant parameters in sufficient detail.

Table 8–2 lists the 60 parameters of this synthesizer, with a brief description of each. The default values are those for a "neutral" schwa–like vowel. Column 2, headed V/C, indicates whether that parameter is variable or constant; the "constant" ones can be changed, but are set only once for each utterance. For example, DU (duration) is a constant, in this sense. Among the variable parameters, those marked V have been altered, while those marked v do not vary over the course of the utterance and have not been changed from their default values.

Table 8–3 lists the 15 parameters that have been varied, that is, those marked V. Roughly, from 0–245 ms are the values for [s], from 250–495 are the values for [i], from 500–585 are the values for the closure

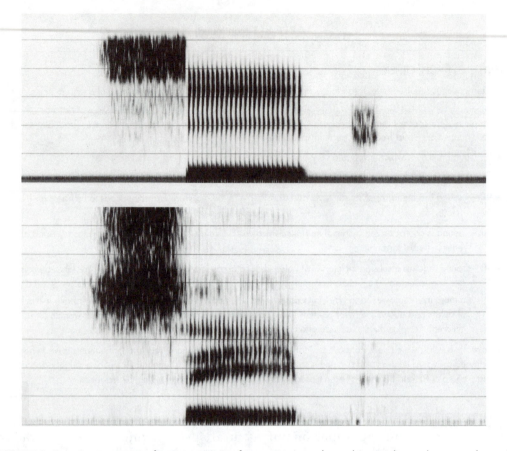

FIGURE 8-2. Spectrograms of two utterances of "seep." Lower channel: natural speech; upper channel: synthetic speech by the Klatt and Klatt (1990) synthesizer.

phase of [p], and from 590–680 are the values for the aspiration of [pʰ]. This gross segmentation is reflected in the source parameters, AV for voicing and AF for frication. Note that f0 is specified in tenths of hertz; the value 1000 means 100.0 Hz. FL for "flutter," better known as jitter, has been set to 20% during the vowel, producing the slight fluctuation in f0 during the middle part of the vowel, as shown in Figure 8–4, channel 4. Note that the parameters A2F through A6F are the amplitudes of the *parallel* resonators. These are used only when the source is frication, during the [s] and the aspiration. The aspiration of [p] has a fricative source (AF rather than AH), because the noise is generated partly at the lips, as well as at the glottis. Table 8–3 illustrates the

detailed consideration that must go into formant synthesis.

How good can formant synthesis be? Essentially, as good as one has patience to make it. If one starts with a spectrogram to match, for example, and specifies many parameters at each update, listening to the output occasionally and revising accordingly, a painstaking investigator can shape the output closer and closer to the target. Holmes (1973) managed to produce speech which listeners could not reliably distinguish from a natural recording. Two main sources of unnaturalness in synthetic speech are the lack of small variations in fundamental frequency and other parameters and the difficulty of creating a voice source which mimics that produced by the larynx, particularly during rapid changes in f0.

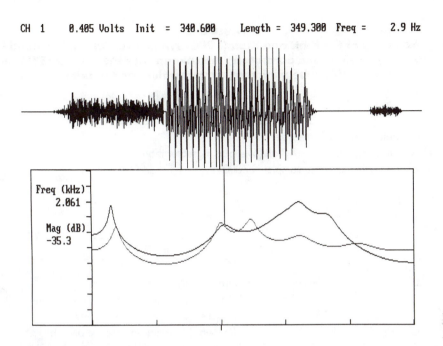

CH 1   0.405 Volts Init = 340.600   Length = 349.300 Freq =   2.9 Hz

Freq (kHz)
   2.061

Mag (dB)
  -35.3

FIGURE 8–3. Spectra of the vowel [i] shown in Figure 8–2. The lighter trace is for the natural speech. The cursor points to F2 in the synthetic speech (darker trace). The waveform above the spectra is of the synthetic speech, with the cursor at the position from which the spectrum was calculated.

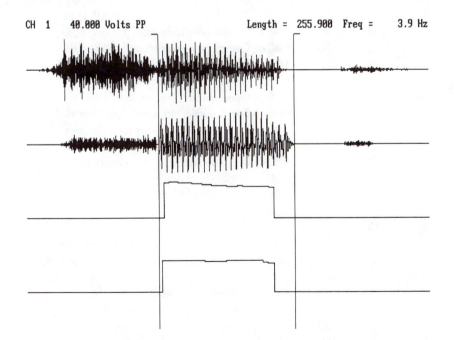

CH 1   40.000 Volts PP   Length = 255.900 Freq =   3.9 Hz

FIGURE 8–4. Waveforms and f0 contours of the utterances shown in Figure 8–2. Channels 1 and 3 are the waveform and f0 contour, respectively, of the natural speech.

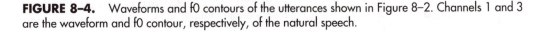

TABLE 8-2

The 60 parameters of the Klatt and Klatt (1990) synthesizer, as implemented by Sensimetrics. Each row is one parameter; the columns are the symbol (SYM); whether variable or constant (V/C); the minimum, current value, and maximum; and a description.

Synthesis specification for file: seep2.dat

KLSYN88a Laboratory Speech Synthesizer

Maximum output signal is −7.8 dB (overload if greater than 0.0 dB)

Total number of waveform samples = 7000

CURRENT CONFIGURATION:

60 parameters

SYM	V/C	MIN	VAL	MAX	DESCRIPTION
DU	C	30	700	5000	Duration of the utterance, in msec
UI	C	1	5	20	Update interval for parameter reset, in msec
SR	C	5000	10000	20000	Output sampling rate, in samples/sec
NF	C	1	5	6	Number of formants in cascade branch
SS	C	1	2	3	Source switch (1=impulse, 2=natural, 3=LF model)
RS	C	1	8	8191	Random seed (initial value of random # generator)
SB	C	0	1	1	Same noise burst, reset RS if AF=AH=0, 0=no, 1=yes
CP	C	0	0	1	0=Cascade, 1=Parallel tract excitation by AV
OS	C	0	0	20	Output selector (0=normal, 1=voicing source, . . .)
GV	C	0	60	80	Overall gain scale factor for AV, in dB
GH	C	0	60	80	Overall gain scale factor for AH, in dB
GF	C	0	70	80	Overall gain scale factor for AF, in dB
FO	V	0	1000	5000	Fundamental frequency, in tenths of a Hz
AV	V	0	60	80	Amplitude of voicing, in dB
OQ	v	10	50	99	Open quotient (voicing open-time/period), in %
SQ	v	100	200	500	Speed quotient (rise/fall time, LF model), in %
TL	v	0	0	41	Extra tilt of voicing spectrum, dB down @ 3 kHz
FL	V	0	0	100	Flutter (random fluct in f0), in % of maximum
DI	v	0	0	100	Diplophonia (alt periods closer), in % of max
AH	v	0	0	80	Amplitude of aspiration, in dB
AF	V	0	0	80	Amplitude of frication, in dB
F1	V	180	500	1300	Frequency of 1st formant, in Hz
B1	V	30	60	1000	Bandwidth of 1st formant, in Hz
DF1	v	0	0	100	Change in F1 during open portion of period, in Hz
DB1	v	0	0	400	Change in B1 during open portion of period, in Hz
F2	V	550	1500	3000	Frequency of 2nd formant, in Hz
B2	V	40	90	1000	Bandwidth of 2nd formant, in Hz
F3	V	1200	2500	4800	Frequency of 3rd formant, in Hz
B3	V	60	150	1000	Bandwidth of 3rd formant, in Hz
F4	v	2400	3250	4990	Frequency of 4th formant, in Hz
B4	v	100	200	1000	Bandwidth of 4th formant, in Hz
F5	v	3000	3700	4990	Frequency of 5th formant, in Hz

(continued)

TABLE 8–2 (continued)

SYM	V/C	MIN	VAL	MAX	DESCRIPTION
B5	v	100	200	1500	Bandwidth of 5th formant, in Hz
F6	v	3000	4990	4990	Frequency of 6th formant, in Hz (applies if NF=6)
B6	v	100	500	4000	Bandwidth of 6th formant, in Hz (applies if NF=6)
FNP	v	180	280	500	Frequency of nasal pole, in Hz
BNP	v	40	90	1000	Bandwidth of nasal pole, in Hz
FNZ	v	180	280	800	Frequency of nasal zero, in Hz
BNZ	v	40	90	1000	Bandwidth of nasal zero, in Hz
FTP	v	300	2150	3000	Frequency of tracheal pole, in Hz
BTP	v	40	180	1000	Bandwidth of tracheal pole, in Hz
FTZ	v	300	2150	3000	Frequency of tracheal zero, in Hz
BTZ	v	40	180	2000	Bandwidth of tracheal zero, in Hz
A2F	V	0	0	80	Amp of fric-excited parallel 2nd formant, in dB
A3F	V	0	0	80	Amp of fric-excited parallel 3rd formant, in dB
A4F	V	0	0	80	Amp of fric-excited parallel 4th formant, in dB
A5F	V	0	0	80	Amp of fric-excited parallel 5th formant, in dB
A6F	V	0	0	80	Amp of fric-excited parallel 6th formant, in dB
AB	v	0	0	80	Amp of fric-excited parallel bypass path, in dB
B2F	v	40	250	1000	Bw of fric-excited parallel 2nd formant, in Hz
B3F	v	60	300	1000	Bw of fric-excited parallel 3rd formant, in Hz
B4F	v	100	320	1000	Bw of fric-excited parallel 4th formant, in Hz
B5F	v	100	360	1500	Bw of fric-excited parallel 5th formant, in Hz
B6F	v	100	1500	4000	Bw of fric-excited parallel 6th formant, in Hz
ANV	v	0	0	80	Amp of voice-excited parallel nasal form., in dB
A1V	v	0	60	80	Amp of voice-excited parallel 1st formant, in dB
A2V	v	0	60	80	Amp of voice-excited parallel 2nd formant, in dB
A3V	v	0	60	80	Amp of voice-excited parallel 3rd formant, in dB
A4V	v	0	60	80	Amp of voice-excited parallel 4th formant, in dB
ATV	v	0	0	80	Amp of voice-excited par tracheal formant, in dB

Given the demands which they make on one's patience, formant synthesizers have been useful mainly in research, especially perceptual research comparing the effects of changing one or two parameters within a relatively small number of syllables. Clearly, setting 60 rather technical parameters every 5 ms is not a practical way of meeting the more commercial needs for speech synthesis, even with the aid of automatic interpolation. There certainly would have been no *Speak & Spell*™ if users had to know about formant frequencies and bandwidths! Conversely, however, there would have been no *Speak & Spell*™ or other practical synthesis if researchers using formant synthesizers had not painstakingly discovered the parameter settings which are now programmed into the commercial products.

Synthesis by Rule

A key step toward making synthesis of wider practical value is the realization that many parameters are roughly predictable over syllables, words, and utterances if one

TABLE 8–3

The specifications for the utterance "seep" shown in Figure 8-2. Each row describes one 5 ms section; the columns represent the 15 parameters which were varied to create that utterance. The parameters are described in the text.

Varied Parameters: time	F0	AV	FL	AF	F1	B1	F2	B2	F3	B3	A2F	A3F	A4F	A5F	A6F
0	1000	0	0	0	320	200	1390	80	2530	200	0	0	0	50	60
5	1000	0	0	3	319	196	1402	82	2538	204	0	0	0	50	60
10	1000	0	0	6	319	193	1415	84	2547	208	0	0	0	50	60
15	1000	0	0	10	319	190	1427	87	2555	212	0	0	0	50	60
20	1000	0	0	13	319	187	1440	89	2564	216	0	0	0	50	60
25	1000	0	0	16	319	184	1453	92	2573	220	0	0	0	50	60
30	1000	0	0	20	318	181	1465	94	2581	224	0	0	0	50	60
35	1000	0	0	23	318	178	1478	96	2590	228	0	0	0	50	60
40	1000	0	0	27	318	175	1490	99	2598	232	0	0	0	50	60
45	1000	0	0	30	318	172	1503	101	2607	236	0	0	0	50	60
50	1000	0	0	33	318	169	1516	104	2616	240	0	0	0	50	60
55	1000	0	0	37	317	165	1528	106	2624	244	0	0	0	50	60
60	1000	0	0	40	317	162	1541	109	2633	248	0	0	0	50	60
65	1000	0	0	43	317	159	1554	111	2642	252	0	0	0	50	60
70	1000	0	0	47	317	156	1566	113	2650	256	0	0	0	50	60
75	1000	0	0	50	317	153	1579	116	2659	260	0	0	0	50	60
80	1000	0	0	54	316	150	1591	118	2667	264	0	0	0	50	60
85	1000	0	0	57	316	147	1604	121	2676	268	0	0	0	50	60
90	1000	0	0	60	316	144	1617	123	2685	272	0	0	0	50	60
95	1000	0	0	60	316	141	1629	125	2693	276	0	0	0	50	60
100	1000	0	0	60	316	138	1642	128	2702	280	0	0	0	50	60
105	1000	0	0	60	315	134	1654	130	2710	284	0	0	0	50	60
110	1000	0	0	60	315	131	1667	133	2719	288	0	0	0	50	60
115	1000	0	0	60	315	128	1680	135	2728	292	0	0	0	50	60
120	1000	0	0	60	315	125	1692	138	2736	296	0	0	0	50	60
125	1000	0	0	60	315	122	1705	140	2745	300	0	0	0	50	60
130	1000	0	0	60	314	119	1718	142	2754	304	0	0	0	50	60
135	1000	0	0	60	314	116	1730	145	2762	308	0	0	0	50	60
140	1000	0	0	60	314	113	1743	147	2771	312	0	0	0	50	60
145	1000	0	0	60	314	110	1755	150	2779	316	0	0	0	50	60
150	1000	0	0	60	314	107	1768	152	2788	320	0	0	0	50	60
155	1000	0	0	60	313	103	1781	154	2797	324	0	0	0	50	60
160	1000	0	0	60	313	100	1793	157	2805	328	0	0	0	50	60
165	1000	0	0	60	313	97	1806	159	2814	332	0	0	0	50	60
170	1000	0	0	60	313	94	1819	162	2823	336	0	0	0	50	60
175	1000	0	0	60	313	91	1831	164	2831	340	0	0	0	50	60
180	1000	0	0	60	312	88	1844	167	2840	344	0	0	0	50	60
185	1000	0	0	60	312	85	1856	169	2848	348	0	0	0	50	60
190	1000	0	0	60	312	82	1869	171	2857	352	0	0	0	50	60
195	1000	0	0	60	312	79	1882	174	2866	356	0	0	0	50	60
200	1000	0	0	60	312	76	1894	176	2874	360	0	0	0	50	60
205	1000	0	0	60	311	72	1907	179	2883	364	0	0	0	50	60
210	1000	0	0	60	311	69	1919	181	2891	368	0	0	0	50	60
215	1000	0	0	60	311	66	1932	183	2900	372	0	0	0	50	60
220	1000	0	0	60	311	63	1945	186	2909	376	0	0	0	50	60

(continued)

TABLE 8–3 (continued)

Varied Parameters:														
time	F0	AV	FL	AF	F1	B1	F2	B2	F3	B3	A2F	A3F	A4F	A5F	A6F
225	1000	0	0	60	311	60	1957	188	2917	380	0	0	0	50	60
230	1000	0	0	60	310	57	1970	191	2926	384	0	0	0	50	60
235	1000	0	0	60	310	54	1983	193	2935	388	0	0	0	50	60
240	1000	0	0	60	310	51	1995	196	2943	392	0	0	0	50	60
245	1000	30	0	30	310	48	2008	198	2952	396	0	0	0	25	30
250	1000	60	20	0	310	45	2020	200	2960	400	0	0	0	0	0
255	1000	60	20	0	309	45	2021	200	2960	400	0	0	0	0	0
260	1000	60	20	0	309	45	2022	200	2960	400	0	0	0	0	0
265	1000	60	20	0	308	45	2023	200	2960	400	0	0	0	0	0
270	1000	60	20	0	308	45	2025	200	2960	400	0	0	0	0	0
275	1000	60	20	0	307	45	2026	200	2960	400	0	0	0	0	0
280	1000	60	20	0	307	45	2027	200	2960	400	0	0	0	0	0
285	1000	60	20	0	306	45	2028	200	2960	400	0	0	0	0	0
290	1000	60	20	0	306	45	2030	200	2960	400	0	0	0	0	0
295	1000	60	20	0	305	45	2031	200	2960	400	0	0	0	0	0
300	1000	60	20	0	305	45	2032	200	2960	400	0	0	0	0	0
305	1000	60	20	0	304	45	2033	200	2960	400	0	0	0	0	0
310	1000	60	20	0	304	45	2035	200	2960	400	0	0	0	0	0
315	1000	60	20	0	303	45	2036	200	2960	400	0	0	0	0	0
320	1000	60	20	0	303	45	2037	200	2960	400	0	0	0	0	0
325	1000	60	20	0	302	45	2039	200	2960	400	0	0	0	0	0
330	1000	60	20	0	302	45	2040	200	2960	400	0	0	0	0	0
335	1000	60	20	0	301	45	2041	200	2960	400	0	0	0	0	0
340	1000	60	20	0	301	45	2042	200	2960	400	0	0	0	0	0
345	1000	60	20	0	300	45	2044	200	2960	400	0	0	0	0	0
350	1000	60	20	0	300	45	2045	200	2960	400	0	0	0	0	0
355	1000	60	20	0	299	45	2046	200	2960	400	0	0	0	0	0
360	1000	60	20	0	299	45	2047	200	2960	400	0	0	0	0	0
365	1000	60	20	0	298	45	2049	200	2960	400	0	0	0	0	0
370	1000	60	20	0	298	45	2050	200	2960	400	0	0	0	0	0
375	1000	60	20	0	297	45	2051	200	2960	400	0	0	0	0	0
380	1000	60	20	0	297	45	2053	200	2960	400	0	0	0	0	0
385	1000	60	20	0	296	45	2054	200	2960	400	0	0	0	0	0
390	1000	60	20	0	296	45	2055	200	2960	400	0	0	0	0	0
395	1000	60	20	0	295	45	2056	200	2960	400	0	0	0	0	0
400	1000	60	20	0	295	45	2058	200	2960	400	0	0	0	0	0
405	1000	60	20	0	294	45	2059	200	2960	400	0	0	0	0	0
410	1000	60	20	0	294	45	2060	200	2960	400	0	0	0	0	0
415	1000	60	20	0	293	45	2061	200	2960	400	0	0	0	0	0
420	1000	60	20	0	293	45	2063	200	2960	400	0	0	0	0	0
425	1000	60	20	0	292	45	2064	200	2960	400	0	0	0	0	0
430	1000	60	20	0	292	45	2065	200	2960	400	0	0	0	0	0
435	1000	60	20	0	291	45	2067	200	2960	400	0	0	0	0	0
440	1000	60	20	0	291	45	2068	200	2960	400	0	0	0	0	0
445	902	60	20	0	290	45	2069	200	2960	400	0	0	0	0	0
450	900	60	20	0	290	45	2070	200	2960	400	0	0	0	0	0
455	888	60	20	0	290	46	2070	200	2960	400	0	0	0	0	0
460	877	60	20	0	290	48	2070	200	2960	400	0	0	0	0	0

(continued)

TABLE 8-3 (continued)

Varied Parameters:

time	F0	AV	FL	AF	F1	B1	F2	B2	F3	B3	A2F	A3F	A4F	A5F	A6F
465	866	60	20	0	290	50	2042	200	2885	400	0	0	0	0	0
470	855	60	20	0	290	52	2015	200	2811	400	0	0	0	0	0
475	844	60	20	0	290	53	1988	200	2737	400	0	0	0	0	0
480	833	60	20	0	290	55	1961	200	2662	400	0	0	0	0	0
485	822	52	20	0	290	57	1934	200	2588	400	0	0	0	0	0
490	811	45	20	0	290	59	1907	200	2514	400	0	0	0	0	0
495	800	37	20	0	290	60	1880	200	2440	400	0	0	0	0	0
500	790	30	0	0	290	60	0	0	0	0	0	0	0	0	0
505	780	22	0	0	290	60	0	0	0	0	0	0	0	0	0
510	770	15	0	0	290	60	0	0	0	0	0	0	0	0	0
515	760	7	0	0	290	60	0	0	0	0	0	0	0	0	0
520	750	0	0	0	290	60	0	0	0	0	0	0	0	0	0
525	692	0	0	0	290	60	0	0	0	0	0	0	0	0	0
530	634	0	0	0	290	60	0	0	0	0	0	0	0	0	0
535	576	0	0	0	290	60	0	0	0	0	0	0	0	0	0
540	519	0	0	0	290	60	0	0	0	0	0	0	0	0	0
545	461	0	0	0	290	60	0	0	0	0	0	0	0	0	0
550	403	0	0	0	290	60	0	0	0	0	0	0	0	0	0
555	346	0	0	0	290	60	0	0	0	0	0	0	0	0	0
560	288	0	0	0	290	60	0	0	0	0	0	0	0	0	0
565	230	0	0	0	290	60	0	0	0	0	0	0	0	0	0
570	173	0	0	0	290	60	0	0	0	0	0	0	0	0	0
575	115	0	0	0	290	60	0	0	0	0	0	0	0	0	0
580	57	0	0	0	290	60	0	0	0	0	0	0	0	0	0
585	0	0	0	0	290	60	0	0	0	0	0	0	0	0	0
590	0	0	0	16	200	60	1600	100	2360	170	50	50	0	0	0
595	0	0	0	33	200	60	1600	100	2360	170	50	50	0	0	0
600	0	0	0	50	200	60	1600	100	2360	170	50	50	0	0	0
605	0	0	0	50	200	60	1600	100	2360	170	50	50	0	0	0
610	0	0	0	50	200	60	1600	100	2360	170	50	50	0	0	0
615	0	0	0	50	200	60	1600	100	2360	170	50	50	0	0	0
620	0	0	0	50	200	60	1600	100	2360	170	50	50	0	0	0
625	0	0	0	50	200	60	1600	100	2360	170	50	50	0	0	0
630	0	0	0	50	200	60	1600	100	2360	170	50	50	0	0	0
635	0	0	0	50	200	60	1600	100	2360	170	50	50	0	0	0
640	0	0	0	50	200	60	1600	100	2360	170	50	50	0	0	0
645	0	0	0	50	200	60	1600	100	2360	170	50	50	0	0	0
650	0	0	0	45	200	60	1600	100	2360	170	50	50	0	0	0
655	0	0	0	30	200	60	1600	100	2360	170	50	50	0	0	0
660	0	0	0	25	200	60	1600	100	2360	170	50	50	0	0	0
665	0	0	0	20	200	60	1600	100	2360	170	50	50	0	0	0
670	0	0	0	15	200	60	1600	100	2360	170	50	50	0	0	0
675	0	0	0	10	200	60	1600	100	2360	170	50	50	0	0	0
680	0	0	0	0	200	60	1600	100	2360	170	50	50	0	0	0
685	0	0	0	0	0	0	0	0	0	0	0	0	0	0	0
690	0	0	0	0	0	0	0	0	0	0	0	0	0	0	0
695	0	0	0	0	0	0	0	0	0	0	0	0	0	0	0

knows the sequence of phonemes to be produced. Fundamental frequency declines slowly over utterances and rapidly at the end of a declarative sentence; vowels are lengthened before voiced consonants; vowels are nasalized before nasal consonants; low vowels are generally longer than high vowels: these are a few rules of thumb which are well-known bits of the phonology of English and other languages. Phonologists write such rules in precise forms, taking into account the effect of one upon another. If we can quantify those rules, we can automate much of the parameter-setting in synthesis. For example, How *much* longer are vowels before voiced consonants, and how does that factor interact with vowel height?

In such a system, the user might type in the sequence of phonemes in an utterance. The synthesizer would then start with a table of default values for each phoneme, for example, for each vowel, the duration, f0, and formant frequencies and bandwidths. It would then automatically tailor each of those values according to the context of each phoneme. The variety of rules which might be included, at least in principle, ranges from prosodic rules like "increase the duration and pitch change on the last stressed syllable in an utterance" to detailed acoustic specifications which are not found in phonology books, such as, "F2 changes toward a value of about 1800 Hz before alveolar consonants." Interestingly, one might seek to make the speech more natural by expanding this range of rules on both ends. At a higher level, one might try to formulate discourse rules, such as "increase the prominence (amplitude and duration) of a noun if this is the first time it has been mentioned in the discourse." At the other extreme, one might introduce small random fluctuations in fundamental frequency and amplitude during the longer syllables to simulate vocal jitter and shimmer.

Obviously, such a set of rules might be very formidable indeed, and even so

might not capture the subtle ways in which natural speech varies in relation to context at all linguistic levels. Nonetheless, speech researchers have created synthesis-by-rule programs which produce reasonably natural-sounding speech and yet operate rapidly on inexpensive hardware. That development has made possible the practical applications of synthesis, from toys to speech prostheses to reading machines.

Clearly, these applications depend on one more step, however. Most users cannot be expected to type in a representation of a string of phonemes. A reading machine must start with ordinary print. In virtually all of the practical applications, one prior translation is needed before synthesis by rule can operate: from ordinary spelling to a sequence of phonemes. Anyone acquainted with English spelling knows that for English, at least, such a translation is no trivial matter. However, with the aid of a built-in "dictionary," together with rules for words which are not in the dictionary, synthesizers can make this first translation. The result is reasonably natural-sounding speech, produced almost instantly from typed (or scanned) ordinary spelling!

One of the best commercial examples of such a synthesizer is DECtalk™, produced by Digital Equipment Corporation, and based on rules developed by Dennis Klatt. This device, first marketed in about 1983, takes ordinary spelling (from a keyboard, a computer file, or a scanner) as input and produces highly intelligible and reasonably natural English speech as output. It has seven built-in voices (three male, three female, and a child), plus one which the user can tailor to her needs, selecting 13 specifications ranging from sex and average pitch to head size and breathiness. Figure 8–5 is a flow chart, showing the sequence of operations by which DECtalk™ arrives at a pronunciation, taking account of punctuation as well as spelling.

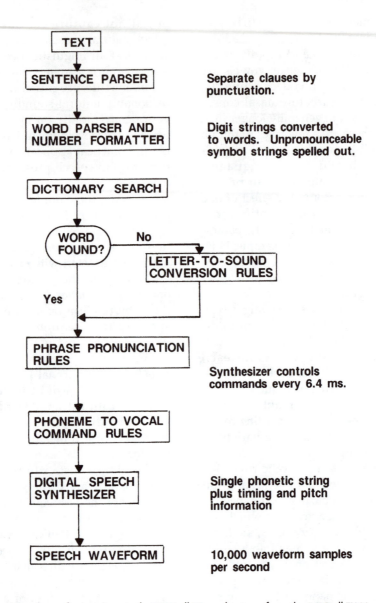

FIGURE 8–5. Flowchart of operations in the DECtalk™ synthesizer, from the DECtalk™ User Manual. The chart begins at the top with the input of standard spelling and ends with the production of synthetic speech.

Note that DECtalk™ searches its dictionary first and then applies its spelling-to-sound rules only to words not found there; thus the dictionary is a list of words with exceptional spellings. If a string of letters fails to match any word in its dictionary or its spelling-to-sound rules, DECtalk™ simply names the letters. If DECtalk's™ pronunciation is not satisfactory, the user may type in phonemic symbols instead of standard spelling. For example, DECtalk™ mispronounces *shoebench* as [ʃ ɔ b ɛ n t ʃ]. One solution is simply to hyphenate the word, but another is to replace the spelling with ['shuw-behnch]. What one cannot control with DECtalk™ is precisely what one *must* control with a formant synthesizer, namely the formant frequencies and bandwidths over time.

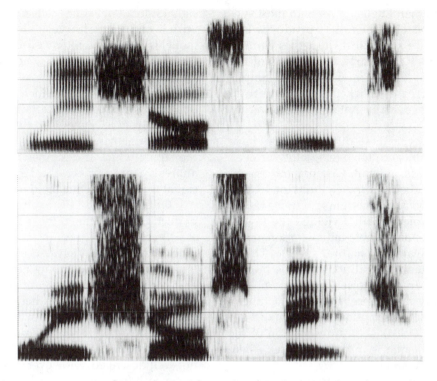

FIGURE 8–6. Spectrograms of two utterances of "We show speech." Lower channel: natural speech by an adult male; upper channel: synthetic speech by the DECtalk™ synthesizer.

Figure 8–6 shows two spectrograms of "We show speech," the upper one uttered by DECtalk™ from standard spelling and the lower one by an adult male speaker at approximately the same rate. The most obvious difference is in frequency range. DECtalk™ produces very little sound above 5 kHz (the scale of the spectrogram is 0 to 8 kHz), whereas the natural speech has a great deal of sound energy above 5 kHz in the three fricatives including the second part of [tʃ] in "speech." However, this restriction is of no consequence in commercial applications, especially over the standard telephone network, which transmits only up to about 3.3 kHz.

Note the extensive shaping of the second and third formants in DECtalk's™ utterance, not only in the glide [w] of "we," but also in transitions at the beginning of the vowels of "show" and "speech." These contrast with the minimally specified synthetic speech shown in

Figure 8–2. Note also that the duration of each segment closely resembles that in the natural speech at a similar overall rate. In both of these respects, DECtalk™ has taken the context of each phoneme into account.

There are also differences other than the frequency range that allow us to make inferences about DECtalk's™ built-in rules. The [p] in "speech" is considerably more aspirated in DECtalk's™ utterance than in the natural sample. DECtalk™ does know, however, that /p/ after initial /s/ is relatively unaspirated; it would produce /p/ in "peach" with much longer aspiration. Note also the falling f0 during the vowel of "speech," as shown by the distance between the vertical striations. Those striations become farther apart in DECtalk's™ production, but to a lesser degree than in the natural one. (One of DECtalk's™ weaker points is intonation in yes-no questions, which sounds more like

Swedish than English.) As with most synthetic speech, DECtalk™ produces less amplitude variation than this human speaker. Particularly at the ends of the vowels of "show" and "speech," amplitude decreases markedly in the natural speech, especially notable in the higher formants.

However, these differences may have little significance for intelligibility or even naturalness. Logan, Greene, and Pisoni (1989) studied the intelligibility of 10 synthesis-by-rule systems. DECtalk's™ default voice ("Paul") yielded the lowest error rate; on syllable-initial consonants, it was equivalent to natural speech. Under good listening conditions (words in context, low ambient noise), one rarely notices difficulty in comprehending DECtalk™. For further description of DECtalk,™ see Bruckert (1984). For a description of the rules built into its predecessor, see Allen, Hunnicutt, and Klatt (1987).

Considering that it produces its utterances almost instantaneously once it encounters a final punctuation mark (a period, question mark, or exclamation point), DECtalk's™ speech is audible testimony to the accomplishments of contemporary speech science. We should bear in mind that the recent achievements, such as Klatt's remarkable synthesizer and his detailed rules, are built upon fundamental understandings that have been developing for most of this century, such as the source-filter theory presented in Chapter 2. Progress in speech science has been additive and has sometimes surprised even those who take part in it.

Linear Predictive Synthesis

A third type of synthesis begins with linear predictive coding (LPC), which was described in Chapter 4. LPC *parameterizes* the speech signal; that is, it analyzes the complex, constantly changing speech signal into a few values called parameters, which change relatively slowly. The model is the source-filter view described in Chapter 2; the parameters which represent the signal are the frequencies and bandwidths of a set of filters which would produce that signal, given a certain excitation. This analysis is reversible; given an LPC analysis, one can produce (or synthesize) the signal which it describes. If the LPC analysis were perfect, the resynthesized signal would exactly match the original.

Of course, the LPC analysis is never perfect. For one thing, most LPC models are *all-pole* models, meaning that they provide for resonances only. As a result, they have difficulty in describing nasal and lateral sounds, which have antiresonances (zeroes) as well. For another, the model describes the filter but not the source; the glottal waveform in voiced speech and the noise source in fricatives are not well described. However, resynthesizing speech from an LPC analysis is at least a check on how good the analysis was.

If that were all it could do, linear predictive synthesis probably would not qualify for inclusion in this chapter. However, it has one additional feature which makes it interesting: having represented the speech signal as a small set of parameters, one can *edit* those parameters before resynthesizing. For instance, we can change the frequency or bandwidth of F1 independently of all other formants and then listen to the effect. We have no way of performing such an operation on the speech signal itself. We cannot edit one formant or ask a live talker to vary just F1! In a sense, LPC synthesis is like having a formant synthesizer which starts with an analysis of real speech, so that we do not have to build each signal from scratch. A typical experiment, for example, is to start with a recording of the vowel /i/; perform LPC analysis; then edit that analysis, moving F1 up and F2 down in ten steps; synthesize the resulting ten variants; and play them in random order for listeners, to determine at what point the /i/ begins to sound more like /e/ or /æ/.

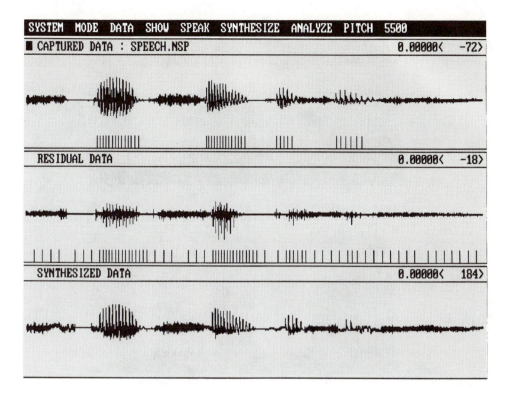

FIGURE 8–7. Three waveforms in display of ASL™, a program for LP analysis and synthesis. The phrase is "speech synthesis," spoken by an adult male. Upper channel: speech waveform; middle channel: residual signal; lower channel: synthesized speech.

As an example, we will use ASL™, an LPC analysis/synthesis program sold by Kay Elemetrics Corp. as an addition to their digital spectrograph and as part of a speech analysis program known as CSL™. Figure 8–7 is one of ASL's™ basic displays. The upper channel shows the waveform of the phrase "speech synthesis," spoken by a male talker. Under the voiced part of each syllable, a series of short vertical ticks marks the glottal periods. These ticks become farther apart during the last two syllables because f0 was falling at the end of the utterance. ASL™ can perform such an analysis of fundamental periods automatically and then the user can edit it if necessary. Its importance is that LPC analysis (and thus resynthesis) is more accurate if it is *pitch-synchronous*, that is, if (in the voiced portions only) the unit of analysis is a glottal period.

After a linear predictive analysis, there is a part of the signal which remains unaccounted for by the sequence of digital filters which the analysis has developed. This part is known as the *error* or *residual* signal. For our example utterance, the waveform of the residual signal is shown in the middle panel of Figure 8–7. Ideally, the residual should represent just the source: the glottal waveform and the noise excitation. The residual may be a very weak signal; its apparent amplitude has been normalized to fill the panel in Figure 8–7. However, it is evident that the residual in the voiced parts of syllables is not just a glottal waveform; it is too complex. In fact, listening to a residual signal, one may hear traces of the original vowels if all of the formant structure was not captured in the analysis.

Having done the LPC analysis, we can then resynthesize the signal. We have a

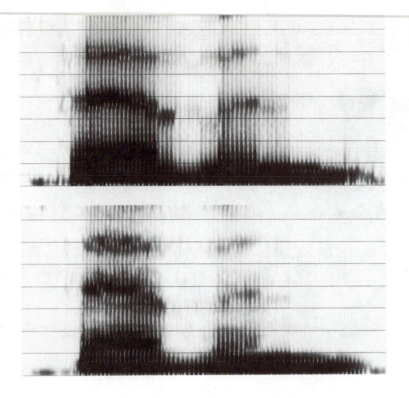

FIGURE 8–8. Spectrograms of two utterances of "seven." Lower channel: natural speech by an adult female; upper channel: that utterance after LP analysis and resynthesis.

choice of using or not using the residual signal to complete the synthesis. Using it means adding back that part of the signal which the analysis did not account for; the resulting synthesized signal should be identical to the original. We get excellent synthesis but a poor test of the analysis.

In this example, we did not use the residual. The lowest panel of Figure 8-7 shows the resulting synthesized utterance. Comparing the waveform to the original (top panel), one can see that it is different. In a general way, one can even see that the synthesized waveform plus the residual would more closely approximate the original.

Figure 8–8 is a spectrographic view of a similar comparison. The lower channel is a spectrogram of "seven," spoken by a female talker; the upper channel is that same utterance after LPC analysis and resynthesis without the residual. Note

that the formant structure of both vowels is rather well reproduced in the synthesis, but that there are difficulties at the transitions between the fricatives and the vowels. Such transitions are major changes, not only in the source, but also in the shape and resonance of the vocal tract. Because LPC analysis operates on frames (in this case, 20 ms long during the voiceless parts of the signal), it has difficulty in representing rapid transitions between voiceless and voiced speech.

ASL™ provides two modes in which the user can edit the analysis before synthesizing. Figure 8–9 shows the full-screen graphic display of an analysis of "spurious," spoken by a male talker. The top panel is the waveform, with glottal periods marked; the middle panel is the formant display; and the lowest panel is the f0 contour during the voiced part of the word.

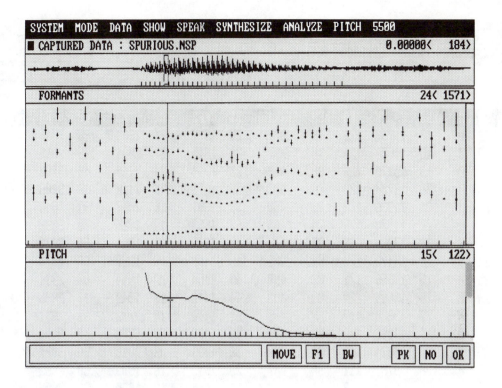

FIGURE 8–9. Formant display in ASL™ of "spurious," spoken by an adult male. Upper channel: speech waveform with fundamental periods marked by vertical ticks; middle channel: formants (horizontal lines) and bandwidths (vertical lines); lower channel: F0 contour.

In the middle panel, the short horizontal bars represent the formant center frequencies, and the vertical lines intersecting them represent bandwidths. One can readily track the first five formants during most of the voiced portion; during the fricatives, the formant frequencies change rapidly and the bandwidths are often wide, so that the vertical lines predominate. In this display, one can use a mouse to draw new formants or a new f0 contour for synthesis. An experienced user with a steady hand can create quite dramatic changes in the signal, although the results sometimes include noisy transitions or other unpredictable effects of interaction among these variables.

Figure 8–10 shows the numeric editor's display for the same utterance. Each row represents one analysis frame and each column one parameter. RES is the frame number (of the residual), PK stands for peak amplitude, LEN for the duration of the frame, B1 for the bandwidth of F1, and so on. Frame 26, just below the middle of the table, is marked by a box in the waveform. It is near the [r], so that F2 (highlighted in the table) is low, at 1442 Hz. The user can edit any of the parameters, taking advantage of interpolation to produce changes at linear and nonlinear rates. In this mode one has precise control over every aspect of a spoken utterance represented by LPC parameters. This degree of control is not practical for the commercial applications of speech synthesis, but it opens important doors for research. For example, if one suspected that the rate of formant transitions after stop consonants is an important part of what makes certain dysarthric speech difficult to comprehend (Kent et al., 1989),

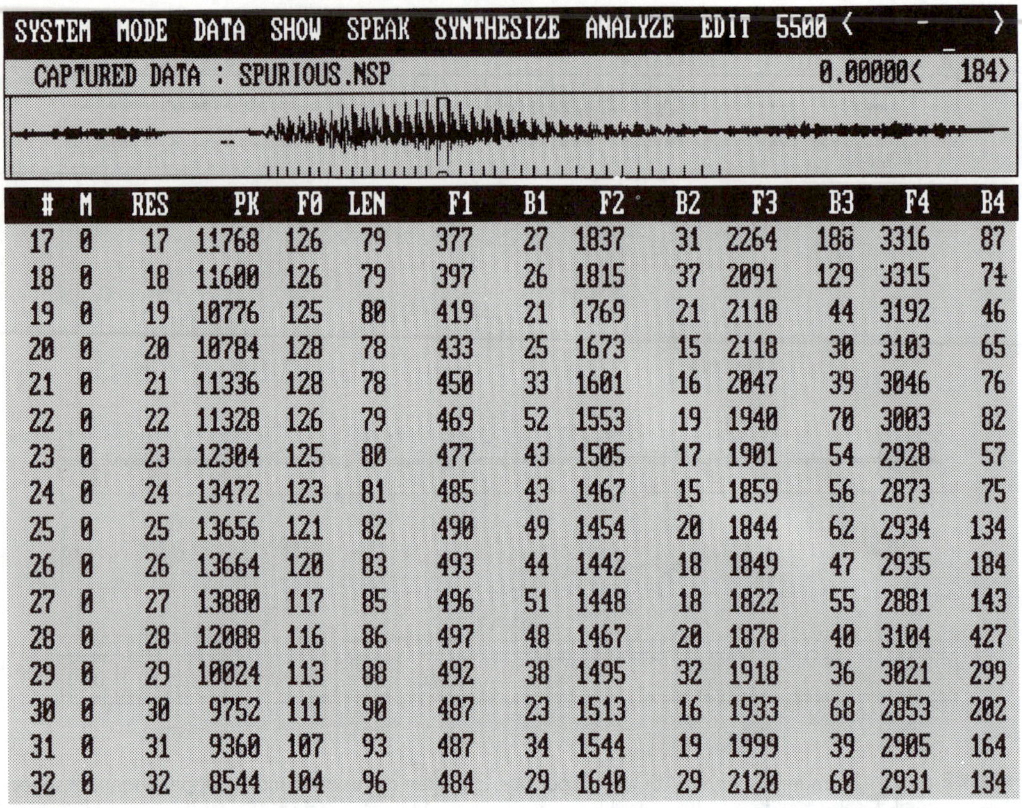

SYSTEM MODE DATA SHOW SPEAK SYNTHESIZE ANALYZE EDIT 5500 ‹ — ›
CAPTURED DATA : SPURIOUS.NSP   0.00000‹   184›

#	M	RES	PK	F0	LEN	F1	B1	F2	B2	F3	B3	F4	B4
17	0	17	11768	126	79	377	27	1837	31	2264	188	3316	87
18	0	18	11600	126	79	397	26	1815	37	2091	129	3315	74
19	0	19	10776	125	80	419	21	1769	21	2118	44	3192	46
20	0	20	10784	128	78	433	25	1673	15	2118	30	3103	65
21	0	21	11336	128	78	450	33	1601	16	2047	39	3046	76
22	0	22	11328	126	79	469	52	1553	19	1940	70	3003	82
23	0	23	12304	125	80	477	43	1505	17	1901	54	2928	57
24	0	24	13472	123	81	485	43	1467	15	1859	56	2873	75
25	0	25	13656	121	82	490	49	1454	20	1844	62	2934	134
26	0	26	13664	120	83	493	44	1442	18	1849	47	2935	184
27	0	27	13880	117	85	496	51	1448	18	1822	55	2881	143
28	0	28	12088	116	86	497	48	1467	20	1878	40	3104	427
29	0	29	10024	113	88	492	38	1495	32	1918	36	3021	299
30	0	30	9752	111	90	487	23	1513	16	1933	68	2853	202
31	0	31	9360	107	93	487	34	1544	19	1999	39	2905	164
32	0	32	8544	104	96	484	29	1640	29	2120	60	2931	134

FIGURE 8–10. Numeric editor display in ASL™ of the same utterance as in Figure 8–9. The rows are frames; the columns are results of the LPC analysis, including amplitude (PK), f0, the frame length (LEN), and formant frequencies and bandwidths (F1, B1, etc.).

one could edit just that characteristic and see what difference it makes. In a formant synthesizer, one has the same kind of control, but not starting with a parametric analysis of natural speech.

Conclusion

Current speech synthesis offers a panoply of options. One can start with ordinary English text, a sample of recorded speech to be edited, or a screen full of blank rows and columns to be filled in. The user may have no technical knowledge at all or an understanding of the acoustic structure of speech in immense detail. Instead of absolute limits, we face tradeoffs between time and degree of control.

In whatever form, speech synthesis today illustrates the idea that one truly understands a process only when one can reproduce it. That all of these types of synthesis can produce comprehensible speech must indicate that we understand a considerable part of the nature of speech — that they are all imperfect indicates that there is important work yet to be done.

References

Abberton, E. R. M., Howard, D. M., & Fourcin, A. J. (1989). Laryngographic assessment of normal voice: A tutorial. *Clinical Linguistics and Phonetics, 3,* 281–296.

Abramson, A. S. (1977). Laryngeal timing in consonant distinctions. *Phonetica, 34,* 295–303.

Adams, S. G. (1990). Rate and clarity of speech: An x-ray microbeam study. Unpublished doctoral dissertation, University of Wisconsin-Madison.

Al-Bamerni, A. (1975). An instrumental study of the allophonic variation of /l/ in RP. Unpublished master's dissertation, University College of North Wales, Bangor, England.

Allen, G. D., & Hawkins, S. (1980). Phonological rhythm: Definition and development. In G. H. Yeni-Komshian, J. F. Kavanagh, & C. A. Ferguson (Eds.), *Child phonology* (Vol. 1), (pp. 227–256). New York: Academic Press.

Allen, J., Hunnicutt, M. S., & Klatt, D. H. (1987). *From text to speech: The MITalk system.* Cambridge, England: Cambridge University Press.

Alwan, A. (1989). Perceptual cues for place of articulation for the voiced pharyngeal and uvular consonants. *Journal of the Acoustical Society of America, 86,* 549–556.

Assman, P., Nearey, T., & Hogan, J. (1982). Vowel identification: Orthographic, perceptual, and acoustic aspects. *Journal of the Acoustical Society of America, 71,* 975–989.

Atal, B. S., & Hanauer, S. L. (1971). Speech analysis and synthesis by linear prediction of the speech wave. *Journal of the Acoustical Society of America, 50,* 637–655.

Atal, B. S., Miller, J. L., & Kent, R. D. (Eds.) (1991). *Papers in speech communication: Speech processing.* Woodbury, NY: Acoustical Society of America.

Atal, B. S., & Schroeder, M. R. (1970). Adaptive predictive coding of speech signals. *Bell System Technical Journal, 49,* 1973–1986.

Badin, P., Perrier, P., Boe, L.-J., & Abry, C. (1990). Vocalic nomograms: Acoustic and articulatory considerations upon formant convergences. *Journal of the Acoustical Society of America, 87,* 1290–1300.

Baken, R. (1987). *Clinical measurement of speech and voice.* Boston: Little, Brown.

Baken, R. (1990). Irregularity of vocal period and amplitude: A first approach to the fractal analysis of voice. *Journal of Voice, 4,* 185–197.

Baken, R., & Daniloff, R. (Eds.) (1990). *Readings in clinical spectrography of speech.* San Diego: Singular Publishing Group.

Barry, W. (1979). Complex encoding in word-final voiced and voiceless stops. *Phonetica, 36,* 361–372.

Bauer, H. R., & Kent, R. D. (1986). Acoustic analysis of infant fricative and trill vocalizations. *Journal of the Acoustical Society of America, 81,* 505–511.

Baum, S. R., & Blumstein, S. E. (1987). Preliminary observations on the use of duration as a cue to syllable-initial fricative voicing in English. *Journal of the Acoustical Society of America, 82,* 1073–1077.

Beckman, M. E. (1986). *Stress and non-stress accent. Netherlands Phonetic Archives 7.* Dordrecht: Foris.

Beckman, M. E., & Edwards, J. (1991). Prosodic categories and duration control. *Journal of the Acoustical Society of America, 87* (Suppl. 1) S65.

Behne, D. (1989). Acoustic effects of focus and sentence position on stress in English and French. Unpublished doctoral dissertation, University of Wisconsin-Madison, Madison.

Behrens, S., & Blumstein, S. E. (1988). On the role of the amplitude of the fricative noise in the perception of place of articulation in voiceless fricative consonants. *Journal of the Acoustical Society of America, 84,* 861–867.

Bekesy, G. von (1960). *Experiments in hearing.* New York: McGraw-Hill.

Berg, J. W. van den (1955). Transmission of the vocal cavities. *Journal of the Acoustical Society of America, 27,* 161–168.

Bergem, D. R. van, Pols, L. C. W., & Koopmans-van Beinum, F. J. (1988). Perceptual normalization of the vowels of a man and a child in various contexts. *Speech Communication, 7,* 1–20.

Bernstein, L., Goldstein, M., & Mahshie, J. (1988). Speech training aids for profoundly deaf children. *Journal of Rehabilitation Research and Development, 27,* 53–62.

Black, J. W., Lashbrook, W., Nash, E., Oyer, H. J., Pedrey, C., Tosi, O. I., & Truby, H. (1973). Reply to "Speaker identification by speech spectrograms: Some further considerations." *Journal of the Acoustical Society of America, 54,* 535–537.

Bladon, A. (1983). Two-formant models of vowel perception: Shortcomings and enhancements. *Speech Communication, 2,* 305–313.

Bladon, R. A. W., & Fant, G. (1978). A two-formant model and the cardinal vowels. Royal Institute of Technology Speech Transmission Laboratory (Stockholm), *Quarterly Progress and Status Reports,* Vol. 1, 1–8.

Bless, D.M., Biever, D., & Shaikh, A. (1986). Comparisons of vibratory characteristics of young adult males and females. *Proceedings of International Conference on Voice,* Kurume, Japan, Vol. 2, 46–54.

Blumstein, S. E. (1986). On acoustic invariance in speech. In J. Perkell & D. H. Klatt (Eds.), *Invariance and variability in speech processes* (pp. 178–197). Hillsdale, NJ: Lawrence Erlbaum and Associates.

Blumstein, S. E., Isaacs, E., & Mertus, J. (1982). The role of the gross spectral shape as a perceptual cue to place of articulation in initial stop consonants. *Journal of the Acoustical Society of America, 72,* 43–50.

Blumstein, S. E., & Stevens, K. N. (1979). Acoustic invariance in speech production: Evidence from measurements of the spectral characteristics of stop consonants. *Journal of the Acoustical Society of America, 66,* 1001–1017.

Blumstein, S. E., & Stevens, K. N. (1980). Perceptual invariance onset spectra for stop consonants in different vowel environments. *Journal of the Acoustical Society of America, 67,* 648–662.

Bolt, R. H., Cooper, F. S., David, E. E., Denes, P. B., Pickett, J. M., & Stevens, K. N. (1970). Speaker identification of speech spectrograms: A scientist's view of its reliability for legal purposes. *Journal of the Acoustical Society of America, 47,* 597–612.

Bolt, R. H., Cooper, F. S., David, E. E., Denes, P. B., Pickett, J. M., & Stevens, K. N. (1973). Speaker identification by speech spectrograms: Some further observations. *Journal of the Acoustical Society of America, 54,* 531–534.

Bogert, B. P. (1953). On the bandwidth of the vowel formants. *Journal of the Acoustical Society of America, 25,* 791–792.

Bond, Z. S. (1977). Perception of anticipatory coarticulation for selected English consonants. *Journal of Phonetics, 5,* 313–316.

Brenner, M., & Shipp, T. (1988). Voice stress analysis. In *Mental-State Estimation 1987* (pp. 363–376). NASA Conference Publication 2504.

Bruckert, E. (1984). A new text-to-speech product produces human-quality voice. *Speech Technology,* January/February, 114–119.

Carlson, R., Fant, G., & Granstrom, B. (1975). Two-formant models, pitch and vowel perception. In G. Fant and M.A.A. Tatham (Eds.), *Auditory analysis and perception of speech* (pp. 55–82). London: Academic Press.

Carre, R., & Mrayati, M. (1990). Articulatory-acoustic-phonetic relations and modelling, regions and modes. In W. J. Hardcastle and A. Marchal (Eds.), *Speech production and speech modelling* (pp. 211–240). Dordrecht, Netherlands: Kluwer.

Chen, M. (1970). Vowel length variation as a function of the voicing of the consonant environment. *Phonetica, 22,* 129–159.

Chiba, T., & Kajiyama, M. (1946). *The vowel: Its nature and structure.* Tokyo: Phonetic Society of Japan.

Chistovich, L. A., & Lublinskaja, V. V. (1979). The 'centre of gravity' effect in vowel spectra and critical distance between the formants: Psychoacoustical study of the perception of vowel-like stimuli. *Hearing Research, 1,* 185–195.

Chistovich, L. A., Sheikin, R. L., & Lublinskaja, V. V. (1979). Centres of gravity and spectral peaks as the determinants of vowel quality. In B. Lindblom and S. Ohman (Eds.), *Frontiers of speech communication research* (pp. 143–158). London: Academic Press.

Clement, B. (1991). Relations between acoustic-phonetic information and consonant perception in normal-hearing listeners. Unpublished master's thesis, University of Wisconsin-Madison.

Cohen, A., Collier, R., & t'Hart, J. (1982). Declination: Construct or intrinsic feature of speech pitch? *Phonetica, 39,* 254–273.

Cole, R. A., & Scott, B. L. (1974). Toward a theory of speech perception. *Psychological Review, 81,* 348–374.

Collier, R., Bell-Berti, F., & Raphael, L. (1982). Some acoustic and physiological observations on diphthongs. *Language and Speech, 25,* 305–323.

Cooper, F. S., Delattre, P. C., Liberman, A. M., Borst, J. N., & Gerstman, L. J. (1952). Some experiments on the perception of synthetic speech sounds. *Journal of the Acoustical Society of America, 24,* 597–606.

Cooper, W. E., Ebert, R. R., & Cole, R. A. (1976). Perceptual analysis of stop consonants and glides. *Journal of Experimental Psychology: Human Perception and Performance, 2,* 92–104.

Craig, C. H., & Kim, B. W. (1990). Effects of time gating and word length on isolated word recognition performance. *Journal of Speech and Hearing Research, 33,* 808–815.

Crystal, T. H., & House, A. S. (1982). Segmental durations in connected speech signals: Preliminary results. *Journal of the Acoustical Society of American, 72,* 705–716.

Crystal, T. H., & House, A. S. (1988). A note on the durations of fricatives in American English. *Journal of the Acoustical Society of America, 84,* 1932–1935.

Dalby, J. M. (1986). *Phonetic structure of fast speech in American English.* Bloomington, IN: Indiana University Linguistics Club.

Dalston, R. (1975). Acoustic characteristics of English /w,r,l/ spoken correctly by young children and adults. *Journal of the Acoustical Society of America, 57,* 462–469.

Davis, S. (1976). Computer evaluation of laryngeal pathology based on inverse filtering of speech. Speech Communications Research Laboratory, Inc. (Santa Barbara, CA.) *SCRL Monograph No. 13.*

Delattre, P., Liberman, A. M., & Cooper, F. S. (1955). Acoustic loci and transitional cues for consonants. *Journal of the Acoustical Society of America, 27,* 769–774.

DiBenedetto, M.-G. (1989a). Vowel representation: Some observations on temporal and spectral properties of the first formant frequency. *Journal of the Acoustical Society of America, 86,* 55–66.

DiBenedetto, M.-G. (1989b) Frequency and time variations of the first formant: Properties relevant to the perception of vowel height. *Journal of the Acoustical Society of America, 86,* 67–78.

Diehl, R., McCusker, S., & Chapman, L. (1981). Perceiving vowels in isolation and in consonantal context. *Journal of the Acoustical Society of America, 69,* 239–248.

Dorman, M. F., Raphael, L. C., & Eisenberg, D. (1980). Acoustic for a fricative-affricate contrast in word-final position. *Journal of Phonetics, 8,* 397–405.

Dorman, M. F., Studdert-Kennedy, M., & Raphael, L.F. (1977). Stop consonant recognition: Release bursts and formant transitions as functionally equivalent, context-dependent cues. *Perception and Psychophysics, 22,* 109–122.

Dubno, J. R., & Levitt, H. (1981). Predicting consonant confusions from acoustic analysis. *Journal of the Acoustical Society of America, 69,* 249–261.

Edwards, A. D. N. (1991). *Speech synthesis: Technology for disabled people.* London: Paul Chapman Publishing Ltd.

Endres, W., Bambach, W., & Flosser, G. (1971). Voice spectrograms as a function of age, voice disguise, and voice imitation. *Journal of the Acoustical Society of America, 49,* 1842–1848.

Fallside, F., & Woods, W.A. (1985). *Computer speech processing.* Englewood Cliffs, NJ: Prentice-Hall.

Fant, G. (1960a). *Acoustic theory of speech production.* The Hague: Mouton.

Fant, G. (1960b). Descriptive analysis of the acoustic aspects of speech. *Logos, 5,* 3–17.

Fant, G. (1973). *Speech sounds and features.* Cambridge, MA: MIT Press.

Fant, G. (1975). Non-uniform vowel normalization. Royal Institute of Technology Speech Transmission Laboratory (Stockholm), *Speech Transmission Laboratory Quarterly Progress and Status Report, 2–3,* 1–9.

Farmer, A., & Lencione, R. (1977). An extraneous vocal behavior in cerebral palsied speakers. *British Journal of Disorders of Communication, 12,* 109–118.

Fischer-Jorgensen, E. (1954). Acoustic analysis of stop consonants. *Miscellanea Phonetica, 2,* 42–49.

Flanagan, J. L. (1972). *Speech analysis, synthesis and perception.* New York: Springer-Verlag.

Flanagan, J. L., and Rabiner, L. R. (1973). *Speech synthesis.* Stroudsburg, PA: Dowden, Hutchinson and Ross, Inc.

Forrest, K., Weismer, G., Milenkovic, P., & Dougall, R. N. (1988). Statistical analysis of word-initial voiceless obstruents: preliminary data. *Journal of the Acoustical Society of America, 84,* 115–123.

Fox, R. A. (1983). Perceptual structure of monophthongs and diphthongs in English. *Language and Speech, 26,* 21–60.

Fox, R. A. (1989). Dynamic information in the identification and discrimination of vowels. *Phonetica, 46,* 97–116.

Frisch, U., & Orszag, S. A. (1990, January). Turbulence: Challenges for theory and experiment. *Physics Today,* 24–32.

Fry, D. (1955). Duration and intensity as physical correlates of linguistic stress. *Journal of the Acoustical Society of America, 27,* 765–768.

Fry, D. B. (1977). *Homo loquens.* Cambridge, England: Cambridge University Press.

Fry, D. B. (1979). *The physics of speech.* Cambridge, England: Cambridge University Press.

Fry, D. B., Abramson, A. S., Eimas, P. D., & Liberman, A. M. (1962). The identification and discrimination of synthetic vowels. *Language and Speech, 5,* 171–189.

Fujimura, O. (1962). Analysis of nasal consonants. *Journal of the Acoustical Society of America, 34,* 1865–1875.

Gade, S., & Herlufsen, H. (1988). Windows to FFT analysis. *Sound and Vibration, 22,* 14–22.

Gates, S. (1989, February). Analog to digital converters in the laboratory. *Scientific Computing and Automation,* 49–56.

Gay, T. (1968). Effect of speaking rate on diphthong formant movements. *Journal of the Acoustical Society of America, 44,* 1570–1573.

Gerstman, L. (1968). Classification of self-normalized vowels. *IEEE Transactions on Audio and Electroacoustics, AU-16,* 78–80.

Giles, S.B. (1971). A study of articulatory characteristics of /l/ allophones in English. Unpublished doctoral dissertation, University of Iowa, Iowa City, Iowa.

Gordon-Salant, S. (1987). Effects of acoustic modification on consonant recognition by elderly hearing-impaired subjects. *Journal of the Acoustical Society of America, 81,* 1199–1202.

Gurlekian, J. A. (1981). Recognition of the Spanish fricatives. *Journal of the Acoustical Society of America, 70,* 1624–1627.

Haggard, M. (1973). Abbreviation of consonants in English pre- and post-vocalic clusters. *Journal of Phonetics, 1,* 9–24.

Haggard, M. P., Ambler, S., & Callow, M. (1970). Pitch as a voicing cue. *Journal of the Acoustical Society of America, 47,* 613–617.

Halle, M., Hughes, G. W., & Radley, J. P. (1957). Acoustic properties of stop consonants. *Journal of the Acoustical Society of America, 29,* 107–116.

Handel, S. (1989). *Listening: An introduction to the perception of auditory events.* Cambridge, MA: MIT Press.

Harris, K. (1958). Cues for discrimination of American English fricatives in spoken syllables. *Language and Speech, 1,* 1–17.

Hawkins, S., & Stevens, K. N. (1985). Acoustic and perceptual correlates of the non-nasal—nasal distinction for vowels. *Journal of the Acoustical Society of America, 77,* 1560–1575.

Heinz, J. M., & Stevens, K. N. (1961). On the properties of voiceless fricative consonants. *Journal of the Acoustical Society of America, 33,* 589–596.

Henton, C. G., and Bladon, R. A. W. (1985). Breathiness in normal female speech: Inefficiency versus desirability. *Language and Communication, 5,* 221–227.

Hermansky, H. (1990). Perceptual linear predictive (PLP) analysis of speech. *Journal of the Acoustical Society of America,* 1738–1752.

Hess, W. J. (1982). Algorithms and devices for pitch determination of speech signals. *Phonetica, 39,* 219–240.

Hogan, J. T., & Rozsypal, A. J. (1980). Evaluation of vowel duration as a cue for the voicing distinction in the following word-final consonant. *Journal of the Acoustical Society of America, 67,* 1764–1771.

Holbrook, A., & Fairbanks, G. (1962). Diphthong formants and their movements. *Journal of Speech and Hearing Research, 5,* 38–58.

Hollien, H. (1974). Peculiar case of "voiceprints." *Journal of the Acoustical Society of America, 56,* 210–213.

Hollien, H. (1980). Vocal indicators of psychological stress. In F. Wright, C. Bahn & R. W. Rieber (Eds.), *Forensic Psychology and Psychiatry. Annals of the New York Academy of Sciences, 347,* 47–72.

Holmberg, E. B., Hillman, R. E., & Perkell, J. S. (1988). Glottal air flow and pressure measurements for soft, normal and loud voice by male and female speakers. *Journal of the Acoustical Society of America, 84,* 511–529.

Holmes, J. N. (1973). Influence of glottal waveform on the naturalness of speech from a parallel formant synthesizer. *IEEE Transactions on Audio and Electroacoustics, AU-21,* 298–305.

House, A. S. (1961). On vowel duration in English. *Journal of the Acoustical Society of America, 33,* 1174–1178.

House, A. S., & Fairbanks, G. (1953). The influence of consonant environment upon the secondary acoustical characteristics of vowels. *Journal of the Acoustical Society of America, 25,* 105–113.

House, A. S., & Stevens, K. N. (1958). Estimation of formant bandwidths from measurements of the transient response of the vocal tract. *Journal of Speech and Hearing Research, 1,* 309–315.

Howell, P., & Rosen, S. (1983). Production and perception of rise time in the voiceless affricate/fricative distinction. *Journal of the Acoustical Society of America, 73,* 976–984.

Hughes, G. W., & Halle, M. (1956). Spectral properties of fricative consonants. *Journal of the Acoustical Society of America, 28,* 303–310.

Jenkins, J. (1987). A selective history of issues in vowel perception. *Journal of Memory and Language, 26,* 542–549.

Jenkins, J. J., Strange, W., & Edman, T. R. (1983). Identification of vowels in "vowelless" syllables. *Perception and Psychophysics, 34,* 441–450.

Johns-Lewis, C. (Ed.) (1986). *Intonation in discourse.* Beckenham, Kent, England: Croom Helm.

Jong, K. J. de (1991). The oral articulation of English stress accent. Unpublished doctoral dissertation, Ohio State University, Columbus, OH.

Jongman, A. (1989). Duration of frication noise required for identification of English fricatives. *Journal of the Acoustical Society of America, 85,* 1718–1725.

Jongman, A., & Blumstein, S. E. (1985). Acoustic properties for dental and alveolar stop consonants: A cross-language study. *Journal of Phonetics, 13,* 235–251.

Joos, M. (1948). Acoustic Phonetics. *Language Monographs,* No. 23 (Suppl. 24).

Kasuya, H., Ogawa, S., & Kikuchi, Y. (1986). An acoustic analysis of pathological voice and its application to the evaluation of laryngeal pathology. *Speech Communication, 5,* 171–181.

Kent, R. D. (in press). Phonological development as biology and behavior. In R.S. Chapman (Ed.), *Processes in language acquisition.* Chicago: Year Book Medical Publishers.

Kent, R. D. (1981). Sensorimotor aspects of speech development. In R. N. Aslin, J. R. Alberts, & M. R. Peterson (Eds.), *Development of perception: Psychobiological perspectives* (Vol. 1) (pp.161–189). New York: Academic Press.

Kent, R. D., Adams, S. G., & Turner, G. (in press). Models of speech production. In N.J. Lass (Ed.), *Principles of experimental phonetics.* New York: Academic Press.

Kent, R. D., Atal, B. S., & Miller, J. L. (Eds.)

(1991). *Papers in speech communication: Speech production.* Woodbury, NY: Acoustical Society of America.

Kent, R. D., & Bauer, H.R. (1985). Vocalizations of one-year-olds. *Journal of Child Language, 12,* 491–526.

Kent, R. D., & Burkhard, R. (1981). Changes in the acoustic correlates of speech production. In D. S. Beasley & G. A. Davis (Eds.), *Aging: Communication processes and disorders* (pp. 47–62). New York: Grune & Stratton.

Kent, R. D., & Forner, L. L. (1980). Speech segment durations in sentence recitations by children and adults. *Journal of Phonetics, 8,* 157–168.

Kent, R. D., Kent, J. F., Weismer, G., Sufit, R. L., Brooks, B. R., & Rosenbek, J. C. (1989). Relationships between speech intelligibility and the slope of second-formant transitions in dysarthric subjects. *Clinical Linguistics and Phonetics, 3,* 347–358.

Kent, R. D., Liss, J., & Philips, B. J. (1989). Acoustic analysis of velopharyngeal dysfunction in speech. In K. Bzoch (Ed.), *Communicative disorders related to cleft lip and palate,* Rev. Ed. (pp. 258–270). Boston: Little, Brown.

Kent, R. D., & Murray, A. D. (1982). Acoustic features of infant vocalic utterances. *Journal of the Acoustical Society of America, 72,* 353–365.

Kent, R. D., & Netsell, R. (1971). Effects of stress contrasts on certain articulatory parameters. *Phonetica, 24,* 23–44.

Kent, R. D., & Rosenbek, J. C. (1983). Acoustic patterns of apraxia of speech. *Journal of Speech and Hearing Research, 26,* 231–249.

Kewley-Port, D. (1983a). Time-varying features as correlates of place of articulation in stop consonants. *Journal of the Acoustical Society of America, 73,* 322–335.

Kewley-Port, D. (1983b). Measurement of formant transitions in naturally produced stop consonant-vowel syllables. *Journal of the Acoustical Society of America, 72,* 379–389.

Kewley-Port, D., Pisoni, D.B., & Studdert-Kennedy, M. (1983). Perception of static and dynamic acoustic cues to place of articulation in initial stop consonants. *Journal of the Acoustical Society of America, 73,* 1779–1793.

Kewley-Port, D., Watson, C.S., Elbert, M., Maki, D., & Reed, D. (1991). The Indiana Speech Training Aid (ISTRA) II: Training curriculum and selected case studies. *Clinical Linguistics and Phonetics, 5,* 38.

Klatt, D. H. (1974). Duration of [s] in English

words. *Journal of Speech and Hearing Research, 17,* 41–50.

Klatt, D. H. (1975). Voice onset time, frication and aspiration in word-initial consonant clusters. *Journal of Speech and Hearing Research, 18,* 686–706.

Klatt, D. H. (1976). Linguistic uses of segmental duration in English: Acoustic and perceptual evidence. *Journal of the Acoustical Society of America, 59,* 1208–1221.

Klatt, D. H. (1979). *Synthesis by rule of consonant-vowel syllables* (Speech Communication Group Working Papers No. 3, pp. 93–105). Cambridge, MA: MIT Press.

Klatt, D. H. (1980). Software for a cascade/parallel formant synthesizer. *Journal of the Acoustical Society of America, 67,* 979–995.

Klatt, D. H. (1987). Review of text-to-speech conversion for English. *Journal of the Acoustical Society of America, 82,* 737–793.

Klatt, D. H., & Klatt, L. C. (1990). Analysis, synthesis, and perception of voice quality variations among female and male talkers. *Journal of the Acoustical Society of America, 87,* 820–857.

Klingholz, F., Penning, R., & Liebhardt, E. (1988). Recognition of low-level alcohol intoxication from speech signal. *Journal of the Acoustical Society of America, 84,* 929–935.

Koenig, W. (1949). A new frequency scale for acoustic measurements. *Bell Laboratories Record, 27,* 299–301.

Koenig, W., Dunn, H. K., & Lacy, L. Y. (1946). The sound spectrograph. *The Journal of the Acoustical Society of America, 17,* 19–49. Reprinted in R. J. Baken & R. G. Daniloff (Eds.), *Readings in clinical spectrography of speech.* San Diego: Singular Publishing Group.

Kuehn, D. P., & Moll, K. L. (1972). Perceptual effects of forward coarticulation. *Journal of Speech and Hearing Research, 15,* 654–664.

Kurowski, K., & Blumstein, S. E. (1984). Perceptual integration of the murmur and formant transitions for place of articulation in nasal consonants. *Journal of the Acoustical Society of America, 76,* 383–390.

Ladefoged, P. (1975). *A course in phonetics.* New York: Harcourt, Brace, Jovanovich.

Lahiri, A., Gewirth, L., & Blumstein, S.E. (1984). A reconsideration of acoustic invariance for place of articulation in diffuse stop consonants: Evidence from a cross-language study. *Journal of the Acoustical Society of America, 76,* 391–404.

Landahl, K. H. (1980). Language-universal aspects of intonation to children's first sentences. *Journal of the Acoustical Society of America, 67* (Suppl. 1), S63.

Lang, G. F. (1987). Bits, bytes, baud, Bell and bull. *Sound and Vibration, 21,* 10–14.

LaRiviere, C., Winitz, H., & Herriman, E. (1975a). The distribution of perceptual cues in English prevocalic fricatives. *Journal of Speech and Hearing Research, 18,* 613–622.

LaRiviere, C., Winitz, H., & Herriman, E. (1975b). Vocalic transitions in the perception of voiceless initial stops. *Journal of the Acoustic Society of America, 57,* 470–475.

Lehiste, I. (1964). Acoustical characteristics of selected English consonants. *International Journal of American Linguistics, 30* (No. 3, Part 4).

Lehiste, I. (1967). *Readings in acoustic phonetics.* Cambridge, MA: M.I.T. Press.

Lehiste, I. (1970). *Suprasegmentals.* Cambridge, MA: MIT Press.

Lehiste, I. (1972). The timing of utterances and linguistic boundaries. *Journal of the Acoustical Society of America, 51,* 2018–2024.

Lehiste, I., & Peterson, G. E. (1961). Transitions, glides, and diphthongs. *Journal of the Acoustical Society of America, 33,* 268–277.

Lewis, D. (1936). Vocal resonance. *Journal of the Acoustical Society of America, 8,* 91–99.

Liberman, A. M., Cooper, F. S., Shankweiler, D.S., & Studdert-Kennedy, M. (1967). Perception of the speech code. *Psychological Review, 74,* 431–461.

Liberman, A.M., Delattre, P. C., & Cooper, F. S. (1952). The role of selected stimulus variables in the perception of unvoiced stop consonants. *American Journal of Psychology, 65,* 497–516.

Liberman, A. M., Delattre, P. C., Cooper, F. S., & Gerstman, L. J. (1954). The role of consonant-vowel transitions in the perception of the stop and nasal consonants. *Psychological Monographs, 68,* 1–13.

Liberman, A. M., Delattre, P. C., Cooper, F.S., & Gerstman, L.J. (1956). Tempo of frequency change as a cue for distinguishing classes of speech sounds. *Journal of Experimental Psychology, 52,* 127–137.

Lieberman, P. (1967). *Intonation, perception and language.* Cambridge, MA: MIT Press.

Lieberman, P. (1972). *Speech acoustics and perception.* Indianapolis: Bobbs-Merrill.

Lieberman, P., Katz, W., Jongman, A., Zimmerman, R., & Miller, M. (1985). Measures of the sentence intonation of read and spontaneous speech in American English. *Journal of the Acoustical Society of America, 77,* 649–657.

Lieberman, P., & Tseng, C. Y. (1981). On the fall of the declination theory: Breath-group versus "declination" as the base form for intonation. *Journal of the Acoustical Society of America, Suppl. 67,* S63.

Lindblom, B. E. F. (1963). Spectrographic study of vowel reduction. *Journal of the Acoustical Society of America, 35,* 1773–1781.

Lindblom, B. (1990). Explaining phonetic variation: A sketch of the H&H theory. In W.J. Hardcastle & A. Marchal (Eds.), *Speech production and speech modelling* (pp. 403–439). Amsterdam: Kluwer.

Lindblom, B. E. F., Lubker, J., & Pauli, S. (1977). An acoustic-perceptual method for the quantitative evaluation of hypernasality. *Journal of Speech and Hearing Research, 20,* 485–496.

Lindblom, B. E. F., & Sundberg, J. (1971). Acoustical consequences of lip, tongue, jaw and larynx movement. *Journal of the Acoustical Society of America, 50,* 1166–1179.

Lindblom, B., & Zetterstrom, R. (1986). *Precursors of early speech.* New York: Stockton Press.

Linggard, R. (1985). *Electronic synthesis of speech.* Cambridge, England: Cambridge University Press.

Lindqvist, J., & Sundberg, J. (1972). Acoustic properties of the nasal tract. *Phonetica, 33,* 161–168.

Lippmann, R. P. (1982). A review of research on speech training aids for the deaf. In N.J. Lass (Ed.), *Speech and language: Advances in basic research and practice* (pp. 105–133). New York: Academic Press.

Lisker, L. (1978). *Rapid vs. rabid:* A catalogue of acoustic features that may cue the distinction. Haskins Laboratories (New Haven, CT) *Status Report on Speech Research* (No. SR–54), pp. 127–132.

Lisker, L., & Abramson, A. S. (1964). A cross-language study of voicing in initial stops: Acoustical measurements. *Word, 20,* 384–422.

Lisker, L., & Abramson, A. (1971). Distinctive features and laryngeal control. *Language, 47,* 767–785.

Logan, J. S., Greene, B. G., and Pisoni, D. B. (1989). Segmental intelligibility of synthetic speech produced by rule. *Journal of the Acoustical Society of America, 86,* 566–581.

Lubker, J. F. (1979). Acoustic-perceptual methods for evaluation of defective speech. In N. J. Lass (Ed.), *Speech and language: Advances in basic research and practice,* Vol. 1, (pp. 49–87). New York: Academic.

Macchi, M. J. (1980). Identification of vowels spoken in isolation versus vowels spoken in consonantal context. *Journal of the Acoustical Society of America, 68,* 1636–1642.

Maeda, S. (1976). *A characterization of American English intonation.* Cambridge, MA: MIT Press.

Makhoul, J. (1975). Linear prediction: A tutorial review. *Proceedings of the IEEE, 63,* 561–580.

Malecot, A. (1956). Acoustic cues for nasal consonants: An experimental study involving a tape-splicing technique. *Language, 32,* 274–284.

Manrique, A. M. B. de (1979). Acoustic study of /i, u/ in the Spanish diphthongs. *Phonetica, 36,* 194–206.

Manrique, A .M. B., & Massone, M. I. (1981). Acoustic analysis and perception of Spanish fricative consonants. *Journal of the Acoustical Society of America, 69,* 1145–1153.

Matthei, E., & Roeper, T. (1983). *Understanding and producing speech.* Bungay, Suffolk, England: Chaucer Press.

McGovern, K., & Strange, W. (1977). The perception of /r/ and /l/ in syllable-initial and syllable-final position. *Perception and Psychophysics, 21,* 162–170.

Miller, J. D. (1984). Auditory processing of the acoustic patterns of speech. *Archives of Otolaryngology, 110,* 154–159.

Miller, J. D. (1989). Auditory-perceptual interpretation of the vowel. *Journal of the Acoustical Society of America, 85,* 2114–2134.

Miller, J. L., & Baer, T. (1983). Some effects of speaking rate on the production of /b/ and /w/. *Journal of the Acoustical Society, 73,* 1751–1755.

Miller, J. L., Kent, R. D., & Atal, B. S. (Eds.) (1991). *Papers in speech communication: Speech perception.* Woodbury, NY: Acoustical Society of America.

Miller, J. L., & Liberman, A. M. (1979). Some effects of later-occurring information on the perception of stop consonant and semivowel. *Perception and Psychophysics, 25,* 457–465.

Miller, R. L. (1959). Nature of the vocal cord wave. *Journal of the Acoustical Society of America, 31,* 667–677.

Miner, R., & Danhauer, J. L. (1977). Relation

between formant frequencies and optimal octaves in vowel perception. *Journal of the American Audiology Society, 2*, 162–168.

Mines, M., Hansen, B., & Shoup, J. (1978). Frequency of occurrence of phonemes in conversational English. *Language and Speech, 21*, 221–241.

Monsen, R. B., & Engebretson, A. M. (1983). The accuracy of formant frequency measurements: A comparison of spectrographic analysis and linear prediction. *Journal of Speech and Hearing Research, 26*, 89–97.

Moon, S. J., & Lindblom, B. (1989). Formant undershoot in clear and citation-form speech: A second progress report. Royal Institute of Technology Speech Transmission Laboratory (Stockholm) *Quarterly Progress and Status Reports*, (No.1), 121–123.

Moore, B. C. J. (1989). *An introduction to the psychology of hearing* (3rd Ed.). New York: Academic Press.

Murry, T., & Murry, J. (1980). *Infant communication: Cry and early speech*. Houston, TX: College-Hill Press.

Nartey, J. N. A. (1982). On fricative phones and phonemes: Measuring the phonetic differences within and between languages. *UCLA Working Papers in Phonetics* (Department of Linguistics, University of California at Los Angeles), No. 55.

Nearey, T. M. (1978). *Phonetic feature systems for vowels*. Indiana University Linguistics Club, Bloomington, IN.

Nearey, T. M. (1989). Static, dynamic, and relational properties in vowel perception. *Journal of the Acoustical Society of America, 85*, 2088–2113.

Noll, A. M. (1967). Cepstrum pitch determination. *Journal of the Acoustical Society of America, 41*, 293–309.

Nolan, F. (1983). *The phonetic bases of speaker recognition*. Cambridge, England: Cambridge University Press.

Nordstrom, P. -E., & Lindblom, B. (1975). A normalization procedure for vowel formant data. *Proceedings of the 8th International Congress of Phonetic Sciences*, Leeds, England.

Nyquist, H. (1928, April). Certain topics in telegraph transmission theory. *Transactions in Audio, Industrial and Electrical Engineering*.

O'Connor, J. D., Gerstman, L. J., Liberman, A. M., Delattre, P. C., & Cooper, F. S. (1957). Acoustic cues for the perception of initial /w, j, r, l/ in English. *Word, 13*, 24–43.

Ohde, R. N., & Sharf, D.J. (1977). Order effect of acoustic segments of VC and CV syllables on stop and vowel identification. *Journal of Speech and Hearing Research, 20*, 543–554.

Ohde, R. N., & Stevens, K. N. (1983). Effect of burst amplitude on the perception of the stop consonant place of articulation. *Journal of the Acoustical Society of America, 74*, 706–714.

Oller, D.K. (1986). Metaphonology and infant vocalizations. In B. Lindblom & R. Zetterstrom (Eds.), *Early precursors of speech* (pp. 21–35). Basingstoke: Macmillan.

O'Shaughnessy, D. (1987). *Speech communication: Human and machine*. Reading, MA: Addison-Wesley.

Paliwal, K. K., Lindsay, D., & Ainsworth, W. A. (1983). A study of two-formant models for vowel identification. *Speech Communication, 2*, 295–303.

Pentz, A., Gilbert, H. R., & Zawadski, P. (1979). Spectral properties of fricative consonants in children. *Journal of the Acoustical Society of America, 66*, 1891–1892.

Peters, H. F. M., Boves, L., & I. C. H. van Dielen (1986). Perceptual judgment of abruptness of voice onset in vowels as a function of the amplitude envelope. *Journal of Speech and Hearing Research, 51*, 299–308.

Peterson, G. E., & Barney, H. E. (1952). Control methods used in a study of vowels. *Journal of the Acoustical Society of America, 24*, 175–184.

Peterson, G. E., & Lehiste, I. (1960). Duration of syllable nuclei in English. *Journal of the Acoustical Society of America, 24*, 693–703.

Peturrson, M. (1972). Peut-on interpreter les donnees de la radiocinematographie en function du tube acoustique a section uniforme? *Travaux de l'Institut de Phonetique de Strasbourg*, No. 4.

Picheny, M. A., Durlach, N. I., & Braida, L. D. (1986). Speaking clearly for the hard of hearing. II: Acoustic characteristics of clear and conversational speech. *Journal of Speech and Hearing Research, 29*, 434–446.

Pickett, J. M. (1980). *The sounds of speech communication*. Baltimore: University Park Press.

Piir, H. (1983). Acoustics of the Estonian diphthongs. *Estonian Papers in Phonetics, 82–83*, 5–96.

Pinto, N. B., & Titze, I. R. (1990). Unification of perturbation measures in speech signals. *Journal of the Acoustical Society of America, 87*, 1278–1289.

Pisoni, D. B., & Martin, C. S. (1989). Effects of

alcohol on the acoustic-phonetic properties of speech: Perceptual and acoustic analyses. *Alcoholism: Clinical and Experimental Research, 13*, 577–587.

Polka, L., & Strange, W. (1985). Perceptual equivalence of acoustic cues that differentiate /r/ and /l/. *Journal of the Acoustical Society of America, 78*, 1187–1206.

Port, R. F., & Dalby, J. (1982). Consonant/vowel ratio as a cue for voicing in English. *Perception and Psychophysics, 32*, 141–152.

Potter, R., Kopp, G., & Green, H. (1947). *Visible speech.* New York: Van Nostrand Reinhold (Reprinted in 1966 by Dover Press, New York.)

Poza, F. (1974). Voiceprint identification: Its forensic application. Proceedings of the 1974 Carnahan Crime Countermeasures Conference, April 16–19, University of Kentucky, Lexington.

Price, P. J. (1989). Male and female voice source characteristics: Inverse filtering results. *Speech Communication, 8*, 261–278.

Prout, J. H., & Bienvenue, G. R. (1990). *Acoustics for you.* Melbourne, FL: Krieger.

Rakerd, B., & Verbrugge, R.R. (1985). Linguistic and acoustic correlates of the perceptual structure found in an individual differences scaling study of vowels. *Journal of the Acoustical Society of America, 77*, 296–301.

Raphael, L. (1972). Preceding vowel duration as a cue to the perception of the voicing characteristic of word-final consonants in English. *Journal of the Acoustical Society of America, 51*, 1296–1303.

Raphael, L. J., Dorman, M. F., Tobin, C., & Freeman, F. (1975). Vowel and nasal duration as cues to voicing in word-final consonants in American English. *Journal of the Acoustical Society of America, 51*, 1296–1303.

Read, C., Buder, E. H., & Kent, R. D. (1990). Speech analysis systems: A survey. *Journal of Speech and Hearing Research, 33*, 363–374.

Read, D., Buder, E. H., & Kent, R. D. (in press). Speech analysis systems: An evaluation. *Journal of Speech and Hearing Research.*

Read, C., & Schreiber, P. A. (1982). Why short subjects are harder to find than long ones. In E. Wanner & L. Gleitman (Eds.), *Language acquisition: The state of the art.* Cambridge, England: Cambridge University Press.

Recasens, D. (1983). Place cues for nasal conso-nants with special reference to Catalan. *Journal of the Acoustical Society of America, 73*, 1346–1353.

Reich, A. R., Moll, K. L., & Curtis, J. F. (1976). Effects of selected vocal disguises upon spectrographic speaker identification. *Journal of the Acoustical Society of America, 60*, 919–925.

Remez, R. E., Rubin, P. E., & Pisoni, D. B. (1983). Coding of the speech spectrum in three time-varying sinusoids. *Annals of the New York Academy of Sciences, 405*, 485–489.

Remez, R. E., Rubin, P. E., Pisoni, D. B., & Carrell, T. D. (1981). Speech perception without traditional speech cues. *Science, 212*, 947–950.

Ren, H. (1986). On the acoustic structure of diphthongal syllables. Unpublished doctoral dissertation, University of California at Los Angeles.

Repp, B. H., Liberman, A. M., Eccardt, T., & Pesetsky, D. (1978). Perceptual integration of acoustic cues for stop, fricative, and affricate manner. *Journal of Experimental Psychology: Human Perception and Performance, 4*, 621–637.

Repp, B. H., & Svastikula, K. (1988). Perception of the [m]-[n] distinction in VC syllables. *Journal of the Acoustical Society of America, 83*, 237–247

Robb, M. P., & Saxman, J. H. (1988). Acoustic observations in young children's non-cry vocalizations. *Journal of the Acoustical Society of America, 83*, 1876–1882.

Robb, M. P., Saxman, J. H., & Grant, A. A. (1989). Vocal fundamental frequency characteristics during the first two years of life. *Journal of the Acoustical Society of America, 85*, 1708–1717.

Rosen, S., & Howell, P. (1990). *Signals and systems for speech and hearing.* New York: Academic Press.

Schutte, H. K., & Miller, R. (1983). Differences in spectral analysis of trained and untrained voices. *NATS Bulletin, 40*, 22–23.

Schwartz, M. F. (1970). Duration of /s/ in /s/-plosive blends. *Journal of the Acoustical Society of America, 47*, 1143–1144.

Scully, C. (1987). Linguistic units and units of speech production. *Speech Communication, 6*, 77–142.

Shadle, C. H. (1990). Articulatory-acoustic relationships in fricative consonants. In W.J. Hardcastle & A. Marchal (Eds.), *Speech production and speech modelling* (pp. 187–209). Dordrecht, Netherlands: Kluwer.

Sharf, D. J., & Ohde, R. N. (1981). Physiologic,

acoustic and perceptual aspects of coarticulation: Implications for the remediation of articulatory disorders. In N.J. Lass (Ed.), *Speech and language: Advances in basic research and practice* (Vol. 5), pp. 153–247. New York: Academic Press.

Shinn, P. (1984). A cross-language investigation of the stop, affricate and fricative manner of articulation. Unpublished doctoral dissertation, Brown University, Providence, RI.

Shoup, J. E., & Pfeifer, L. L. (1976). Acoustic characteristics of speech sounds. In N.J. Lass (Ed.), *Contemporary issues in experimental phonetics* (pp. 171–224). New York: Academic Press.

Shriberg, L. D., & Kent, R. D. (1982). *Clinical phonetics*. New York: Wiley.

Slis, I. H., & Cohen, A. (1969). On the complex regulating the voiced-voiceless distinction. I. *Language and Speech, 1,* 80–102.

Sobell, L., & Sobell, M. (1972). Effects of alcohol on the speech of alcoholics. *Journal of Speech and Hearing Research, 15,* 861–868.

Soli, S. D. (1981). Second formants in fricatives: Acoustic consequences of fricative-vowel coarticulation. *Journal of the Acoustical Society of America, 70,* 976–984.

Sondhi, M. M. (1986). Resonances of a bent vocal tract. *Journal of the Acoustical Society of America, 79,* 1113–1116.

Sorensen, J. M., & Cooper, W. E. (1980). Syntactic coding of fundamental frequency in speech production. In R.A. Cole (Ed.), *Perception and production of fluent speech* (pp. 399–440). Hillsdale, NJ: Lawrence Erlbaum.

Stetson, R. H. (1928). *Motor phonetics. Archives Neerlandaises de Phonetique Experimental, 3.* 2nd ed. published at Amsterdam: North-Holland Publishing Co. (1951). Reprinted in J. A. S. Kelso & K. G. Munhall (Eds.), *R. H. Stetson's motor phonetics: A retrospective edition*. Boston: Little, Brown (1988).

Stevens, K. (1971). Airflow and turbulence noise for fricative and stop consonants: Static considerations. *Journal of the Acoustical Society of America, 50,* 1180–1192.

Stevens, K. N. (1972). The quantal nature of speech: Evidence from articulatory-acoustic data. In E.E. David, Jr., and P.B. Denes (Eds.), *Human communication: A unified view*. New York: McGraw-Hill.

Stevens, K. N. (1985). Spectral prominences and phonetic distinctions in language. *Speech Communication, 4,* 137–144.

Stevens, K. N. (1989). On the quantal nature of speech. *Journal of Phonetics, 17,* 3–45.

Stevens, K. N., & Blumstein, S. E. (1975). Quantal aspects of consonant production and perception: A study of retroflex stop consonants. *Journal of Phonetics, 3,* 215–233.

Stevens, K. N., & Blumstein, S. E. (1978). Invariant cues for the place of articulation in stop consonants. *Journal of the Acoustical Society of America, 64,* 1358–1368.

Stevens, K. N., & Blumstein, S. E. (1981). The search for invariant acoustic correlates of phonetic features. In P. Eimas and J. Miller (Eds.), *Perspectives in the study of speech* (pp. 1–38). Hillsdale, NJ: Lawrence Erlbaum.

Stevens, K. N., & House, A. S. (1955). Development of a quantitative description of vowel articulation. *Journal of the Acoustical Society of America, 27,* 484–493.

Stevens, K. N., & House, A. S. (1956). Studies of formant transitions using a vocal tract analog. *Journal of the Acoustical Society of America, 28,* 578–585.

Stevens, K. N., & House, A. S. (1961). An acoustic theory of vowel production and some of its implications. *Journal of Speech and Hearing Research, 4,* 303–320.

Strange, W. (1987). Evolving theories of vowel perception. *Journal of the Acoustical Society of America, 85,* 2081–2087.

Strange, W., Edman, T. R., & Jenkins, J. J. (1979). Acoustic and phonological factors in vowel identification. *Journal of the Acoustical Society of America, 65,* 643–656.

Strange, W., Verbrugge, R., Shankweiler, D., & Edman, T. (1976). Consonant context specifies vowel identity. *Journal of the Acoustical Society of America, 66,* 213–224.

Strevens, P. (1960). Spectra of fricative noise in human speech. *Language and Speech, 3,* 32–49.

Sundberg, J. (1977, March). The acoustics of the singing voice. *Scientific American,* 82–91.

Sundberg, J. (1987). *The science of the singing voice*. DeKalb, IL: Northern Illinois University Press.

Sundberg, J. (1991). *The science of musical sounds*. New York: Academic Press.

Sussman, H. M. (1989). Neural coding of relational invariance in speech: Human language analogs to the barn owl. *Psychological Review, 96,* 631–642.

Syrdal, A. K. (1984). Aspects of a model of the auditory representation of American English vowels. *Speech Communication, 4,* 121–135.

Syrdal, A. K., and Gopal, H. S. (1986). A perceptual model of vowel recognition based on the auditory representation of American English vowels. *Journal of the Acoustical Society of America, 79,* 1086–1100.

Tarnoczy, T. (1948). Resonance data concerning nasals, laterals and trills. *Word, 4,* 71–77.

Thorsen, N.G. (1985). Intonation and text in standard Danish. *Journal of the Acoustical Society of America, 77,* 1205–1216.

Titze, I. (1989). Physiologic and acoustic differences between male and female voices. *Journal of the Acoustical Society of America, 85,* 1699–1707.

Umeda, N. (1975). Vowel duration in English. *Journal of the Acoustical Society of America, 58,* 434–445.

Umeda, N. (1977). Consonant duration in American English. *Journal of the Acoustical Society of America, 61,* 846–858.

Umeda, N. (1982). Fundamental frequency decline is situation dependent. *Journal of Phonetics, 10,* 279–290.

Verbrugge, R. R., Strange, W., Shankweiler, D. P., & Edman, T. R. (1976). What information enables a listener to map a talker's vowel space? *Journal of the Acoustical Society of America, 60,* 198–212.

Villchur, E. (1965). *Reproduction of sound.* New York: Dover Publications.

Voss, R. J., & Clark, J. (1975). "1/f noise" in music and speech. *Nature, 258,* 317–318.

Walsh, T., Parker, F., & Miller, C.J. (1987). The contribution of rate of F1 decline to the perception of [+voice]. *Journal of Phonetics, 15,* 101–103.

Wardrip-Fruin, C. (1982). On the status of phonetic cues to phonetic categories: Preceding vowel duration as a cue to voicing in final stop consonants. *Journal of the Acoustical Society of America, 71,* 187–195.

Warren R. M. (1970). Perceptual restoration of missing speech sounds. *Science, 167,* 392–393.

Warren, R. M. (1976). Auditory illusions and perceptual processes. In N.J. Lass (Ed.), *Contemporary issues in experimental phonetics* (pp. 389–417). New York: Academic Press.

Weismer, G. (1979). Sensitivity of voice-onset time (VOT) to certain segmental features in speech production. *Journal of Phonetics, 7,* 197–204.

Weismer, G. (1984). Acoustic descriptions of dysarthric speech: Perceptual correlates and physiological inferences. In J.D. Rosenbek (Ed.), *Current views of dysarthria. Seminars in Speech and Language, 5,* 293–314. New York: Thieme-Stratton.

Whalen, D. H., Wiley, E. R., Rubin, P. E., & Cooper, F. S. (1990). The Haskins Laboratories' pulse code modulation (PCM) system. *Behavior Research Methods, Instruments, and Computers, 22,* 550–559.

Winitz, H., Scheib, M. E. & Reeds, J. A. (1972). Identification of stops and vowels for the burst portion of the /p,t,k/ isolated from conversational speech. *Journal of the Acoustical Society of America, 51,* 1309–1317.

Witten, I. H. (1982). *Principles of computer speech.* London: Academic Press.

Wolf, C. G. (1978). Voicing cues in English final stops. *Journal of Phonetics, 6,* 299–309.

You, H. - Y. (1979). An Acoustical and Perceptual Study of English Fricatives. Unpublished master's thesis, University of Edmonton, Edmonton, Canada.

Zue, V. (1976). Acoustic Characteristics of Stop Consonants: A Controlled Study. Unpublished doctoral dissertation, Massachusetts Institute of Technology, Cambridge, MA.

Zue, V. W., & Laferriere, M. (1979). Acoustic study of medial /t,d/ in American English. *Journal of the Acoustical Society of America, 66,* 1039–1050.

Zwicker, E., & Terhardt, E. (1980). Analytical expressions for critical-band rate and critical bandwidth as a function of frequency. *Journal of the Acoustical Society of America, 68,* 1523–1525.

Appendix A: Phonetic Symbols for Vowels and Consonants; Abbreviations Used in the Text

Table A–1
Symbols used for vowels of American English, by traditional articulatory categories.

	Front	Central	Back
High	i ɪ	ʊ	ʊ
Mid	e ɛ	ə	o ɔ
Low	æ	a	ɑ

Monophthongs

Example words containing these vowels in Northern Midwestern American English:

[i]:   beat

[ɪ]:   bit

[e]:   bait   [ə]:   about

[ɛ]:   bet   [a]:   (see below)

[æ]:   bat   [ɑ]:   pot

[u]:   boot

[ʊ]:   book

[o]:   boat

[ɔ]:   bought

Major diphthongs based on these nuclei are:

> Note: In this dialect, [a] does not occur as a monophthong, but occurs as the nucleus of two diphthongs.

aᶦ: bite

aᵁ : bout

ɔᶦ: boy

Rhotacized ("r-colored") vowels include [ɚ], a rhotacized schwa, as in father.

Table A–2. Symbols used for consonants of American English, by traditional articulatory categories.

	Bilabial	Labio-dental	Inter-dental	Alveo-lar	Retro-flex	Alveo-palatal	Velar	Glottal
Stop	p b			t d			k g	ʔ
Fricative		f v	θ ð	s z		ʃ ʒ		h
Affricate						tʃ dʒ		
Nasal	m		n				ŋ	
Liquid				l	r			
Glide	w					j	w	

Notes:

(1) Among the obstruents (the stops, fricatives, and affricates), the symbol on the left is for the voiceless sound while that on the right is for the voiced one.

(2) In other books, [h] is sometimes classified as a glide, approximant, or semivowel.

(3) [w] is labiovelar; that is, it is articulated at both places.

(4) [j] is actually palatal; in other American books, it is often written [y].

Example words containing these consonants in Northern Midwestern American English:

[p]:	pet, tip		[ʃ]:	ship, mesh
[b]:	bet, rib		[ʒ]:	measure, rouge
[t]:	tip, pet		[h]:	heat
[d]:	dip, bed			
[k]:	cap, back		[tʃ]:	church
[g]:	gap, bag		[dʒ]:	judge
[ʔ]:	"unh-unh" (negative)			
[f]:	fat, laugh		[m]:	mean, lamb
[v]:	vat, have		[n]:	near, win
[θ]:	thin, bath		[ŋ]:	sing
[ð]:	then, bathe			
[s]:	sip, less		[l]:	live, all
[z]:	zip, reds		[r]:	red, car
			[w]:	wet
			[j]:	yet

Table A-3.
Abbreviations used in this book.

Frequency:

Hz	hertz, or cycles per second
kHz	kilohertz (1000 hertz)
cps	cycles per second
f0	fundamental frequency
F1	first formant; F2 = second formant, and so forth

Time:

s	second
cs	centisecond (0.01 second)
ms	millisecond (0.001 second)
μs	microsecond (0.000001 second)

Amplitude:

dB	decibel
v	volt
mv	millivolt (0.001 volt)

Length:

m	meters
cm	centimeters (0.01 meter)
mm	millimeters (0.001 meter)
l	length

Speech sounds:

[p]	A phonetic symbol in brackets represents a phone, that is, a speech sound.
/p/	A phonetic symbol in slashes represents a phoneme, that is, a linguistically significant class of speech sounds.
IPA	The International Phonetic Alphabet

Acoustic analyses:

LPC	Linear predictive coding
FFT	Fast Fourier Transform
DFT	Discrete Fourier Transform

Digital Sampling:

A/D	analog to digital conversion or converter
D/A	digital to analog conversion or converter

Speed:

c	the speed of sound in air at sea level

Appendix B: Elementary Physics of Sound

Acoustics is the branch of physics that deals with sound. *Psychoacoustics* is the study of the psychological response to sound; it is a division of psychophysics, or the general study of psychological responses to physical stimuli. The study of speech acoustics has both a physical and psychophysical side. The physical side pertains to the physical structure of the sounds of speech. The psychophysical side is concerned with the perception of these sounds. A proper understanding of speech requires knowledge of both of these aspects of speech acoustics. A well-known riddle asks, "If a tree falls in the forest, but there is no one to hear it, did it make a sound?" Of course, the answer depends on the definition of terms. If *sound* is defined with respect to human perception, then no sound could be verified. But if *sound* is defined as a physical disturbance in the air, then sound must have occurred. A riddle more apropos to speech might be: "If speech is made visible as patterns on paper (or a video monitor), but no one hears it, is it really speech?"

Sound is vibration. Vibration is a repetitive to-and-fro motion of a body. Usually, we do not directly hear the actual vibrations in a sound source such as an engine, but rather we hear the vibrations that are propagated, or transmitted, in a medium like air. When we stand next to a humming machine, we hear the vibrations produced by the machine at a distance and air is the medium of propagation. Figure B-1 shows a simple physical arrangement to demonstrate the nature of

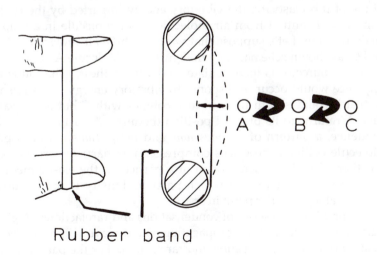

Rubber band

FIGURE B-1. Sound generation with a rubber band. When the band is plucked, it vibrates. As it does so, it causes a chain reaction of collisions for the adjacent air particles A, B, and C. Because air is elastic, each particle returns to its original position following the collision. Therefore, each particle moves in a to-and-fro manner.

215

sound. The sound source is a stretched rubber band that can be plucked to set it into vibration. The band undergoes a series of to-and-fro vibrations after it is plucked. The initial vibrations are of large amplitude, meaning that the to-and-fro swings have a relatively great motion. The amplitude diminishes until motion eventually stops altogether. The reduction in amplitude reflects *damping*, or the loss of energy. In the natural world, vibrations do not continue indefinitely after the energy source responsible for the vibration has ceased. Rather, vibrations die out. The rate at which they die out is a measure of damping, which is the rate at which energy is absorbed. When a coin is dropped on a hard tile floor, the sound seems to "ring" for a short time. When the coin is dropped on a sofa cushion, the sound is more like a dull thud that quickly dies out. The coin and tile combination produces a low rate of damping, so that sound energy continues for a time beyond the initial impact of the coin on the floor. Therefore, the coin rings. In contrast, the coin and cushion produce a sound that is quickly damped and we hear a thud.

How do we hear the vibrations of the rubber band in the example described earlier? To answer this question, we consider first the way in which the vibrating rubber band interacts with air molecules immediately adjacent to it. Air is made up of particles that move in response to applied energy. When the rubber band vibrates, its outward motion pushes against the adjacent air molecules, compressing them. If air were a rigid body, then the entire air mass would move back and forth with the rubber band, like a giant piston. But air is elastic, so that its molecules can move relative to one another, as though they were interconnected by tiny springs. Molecules that have been displaced tend to return to their original position. By virtue of this elasticity, the vibratory energy imparted by the rubber band is transmitted from air molecule to air molecule in a kind of chain reaction. Let's suppose that we have three air molecules, A, B, and C, as shown schematically in Figure B-1. Molecule A is closest to a sound source, B is intermediate, and C is farthest. The following sequence would occur in response to vibratory energy: A is pushed so that it collides with B. B in turn collides with C but at the same time A returns to its original position (because of elasticity). In this sequence, a pattern of *compressions* and *rarefactions* is developed. Molecule collision produces compression as particles are pressed together. But the return motion of a particle in the elastic medium produces a rarefaction in which particle density is momentarily reduced at a particular point in space.

Sound is thus a series of condensations and rarefactions. A given particle in the path of the propagating sound wave will be subjected to an impulse of condensation and rarefaction. For the particles A, B, and C introduced above, short time lags would occur between their motion: Molecule A moves first, then B, and then C. When we watch lightning and hear thunder, we have a common example of this time lag. We see the flash of lightning immediately because light travels very fast, at about 186,000 miles per second. But the accompanying sound of thunder reaches our ears after a delay, sometimes of several seconds, because sound moves more slowly through the air medium at about 600 miles per second. Sound travels slowly enough that we often hear evidence that the "sound barrier" has been broken. When a jet aircraft exceeds the speed of sound, we hear a sonic boom. The same thing happens when we crack a whip—the rapid movement of the end of the whip catches up with the sound wave and, in so doing, makes a small sonic boom.

What we hear as sound is the response of the human ear to vibrations in the surrounding medium, usually air, but, for example, which could be water if we are swimming. The ear detects particle excursions as small as 0.0001 inch. In fact, the sensitivity of the ear falls just short of responding to the random movements of air particles. Small pressure fluctuations in the air give rise to sound. These fluctuations move in a wave-like fashion, and sound is therefore described in terms of wave motion.

There are two major types of wave motion. Sound moves as a *longitudinal wave*, meaning that the particles move back and forth along the direction of the wave. Recall the particles A, B, and C described above: They moved in succession, to and fro, along the path of the sound wave. In contrast, the waves that are produced when a stone is dropped into the middle of a pond are *transverse waves*, in which the particles move up and down, or perpendicular to the advancing wave. The longitudinal wave of sound is not as easily seen as the transverse waves in a pool of water. However, the nature of the longitudinal wave of sound can be imagined with the demonstration illustrated in Figure B-2. This is a *Gedanken* (thought) experiment that would actually be very difficult to perform. Suppose that a pencil is attached to the tine of a tuning fork. When the tuning fork is struck to set it into vibration, the pencil at the end of the fork's tine will vibrate to and fro with the fork. The to-and-fro motion would be drawn by the pencil as a repeating motion, so that the pencil's line would be drawn on itself over and over again. Now if we smoothly pull the vibrating fork across the sheet of writing paper, the result

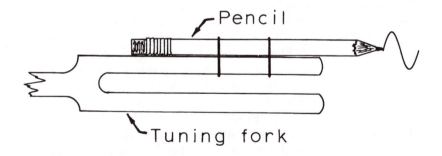

FIGURE B–2.   A *Gedanken* (thought) experiment to illustrate sinusoidal vibration. A pencil is attached to the tine of a tuning fork. When the tuning fork is struck, it vibrates a particular frequency. The idea of this illustration is that as the vibrating tuning fork with attached pencil is drawn across a piece of paper, a sinusoidal waveform would be traced out.

would be a pattern in which the to-and-fro motions appear as a line that smoothly varies up and down. Because the tuning fork vibrates at a single frequency, that is, it has a simple periodic to-and-fro motion, the pattern produced on paper takes the shape of a *sinusoid* (named for the sine function in geometry).

The graph shown in Figure B-3 is called a *waveform*, which is a graph of amplitude versus time. All sounds can be represented in a two-dimensional graph of amplitude and time. The waveform in Figure B-3 is especially important, because the sinusoid is a basic waveform that can be used as a kind of analysis unit. The idea is that all sounds can be decomposed into a number of sinusoidal components. To see how this is possible, we need to examine some features of the waveform and introduce some additional concepts.

One complete *cycle* of vibration of the tuning fork (a to-and-fro motion) is represented on the sinusoidal waveform as a sequence of up and down motion. The time required for this cycle is called the *period*. The frequency of vibration is measured as the number of cycles in a second (called hertz, abbreviated Hz). If a tuning fork vibrates at 256 Hz, it completes 256 cycles of vibration in one second. The period, or duration of one cycle, can be computed simply by dividing the number of cycles into one second. That is, the period is the reciprocal of frequency. The period of the 256 Hz tone is about 0.004 seconds, or 4 milliseconds (ms). The physical measure of frequency correlates highly with the perceptual phenomenon of pitch. A high-pitched sound has a high frequency, and a low-pitched sound has a low frequency. The range of frequencies that the human ear can detect is about 20–20,000 Hz, corresponding to a range of periods of 50 msec to 0.5 ms. Dogs and many other animals can hear an extended range of frequencies, which is why dogs can hear whistles that humans cannot. Sounds also vary in loudness. The primary physical correlate of loudness is amplitude. As amplitude of vibration increases, we tend to hear a louder sound.

The sound wave also can be represented spatially. Because sound propagates longitudinally, a cycle of vibration covers a certain distance in space. The distance is called a *wavelength* and is determined by dividing the speed of sound (about 1100 ft/s) by the frequency of the sound. A sound of low frequency has a long wavelength and a sound of high frequency has a short wavelength.

The sinusoid is an elemental waveform that is basic to acoustic analysis because various types of sounds can be analyzed into component sinusoids of specified frequency, amplitude, and phase. Frequency and amplitude already have been described as a measure of rate of vibration and a measure of the magnitude of excursion, respectively. Sounds of different frequency but same amplitude are illustrated as waveforms in Figure B-3a. Tones of different amplitudes but same frequency are illustrated in Figure B-3b. Phase specifies the time relationship among the components of a sound wave and is most effectively demonstrated with a *complex tone*, or a tone that is composed of two or more harmonics. Each harmonic is a sinusoid and the different harmonics are related as integer multiples. For

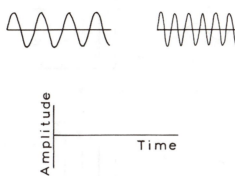

FIGURE B-3a.   Waveforms of sinusoids with same amplitude but different frequency (number of complete vibrations per unit of time, conventionally expressed as hertz (or number of cycles per second). The waveform at the left has a lower frequency than the one at the right.

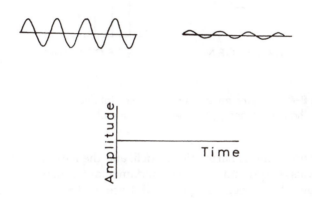

FIGURE B-3b.   Waveforms of sinusoids with same frequency but different amplitudes. The waveform at the left has a greater amplitude than the one at the right.

example, the third harmonic of a 100 Hz tone is a tone of 300 Hz (the harmonic number, 3, is multiplied by the fundamental, or lowest, tone).

We have seen that the waveform is a graph of amplitude versus time. It may be interpreted to reflect the displacement of an air molecule during sound propagation. An alternative way of viewing sound is the *spectrum*, which is a graph of amplitude versus frequency. The spectrum indicates the amplitude of each sinusoidal component in a sound. Figure B-4 shows several waveform and spectrum pairs. Note that a single sinusoid has one line in its spectrum because all of the sound energy is concentrated at one frequency. As more sinusoidal components are added, more lines appear in the spectrum. The most complex pattern in Figure B-4 resembles the sound of the human voice, that is, the sound generated by the vocal

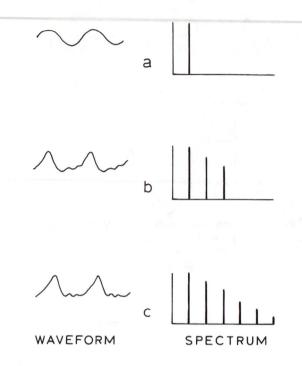

WAVEFORM   SPECTRUM

FIGURE B-4. Waveform and spectrum pairs: (a) sinusoid, (b) complex tone with three harmonics, and (c) complex tone with six harmonics.

folds. This sound is harmonically rich, and the harmonics are spaced at intervals corresponding to the fundamental frequency of vocal fold vibration. The spectra in Figure B-4 are all *line spectra*, so called because the spectra are composed of lines.

So far the discussion has been restricted to complex tones, or sounds having a harmonic composition. Harmonics are integer multiples. If the first harmonic is 100 Hz, then the second harmonic is 200 Hz, the third is 300 Hz, and so on. Sounds with harmonic structure are periodic, meaning that some basic vibratory pattern recurs repeatedly at a fixed interval. The fixed interval is the fundamental period, or the period of the lowest harmonic. In the example just cited, the fundamental period of a harmonic sequence of 100, 200, and 300 Hz would be 10 msec, the period of the lowest harmonic. But not all sounds in the world, or even in speech, are harmonic complexes. Many sounds are noiselike and do not have a regularly recurring pattern of vibration. Noise is much more random in its nature. This randomness is shown in Figure B-5 in both a waveform and spectrum. The waveform looks "noisy"—the amplitude varies with no detectable pattern. The spectrum shows that the noise is composed of energy at many different frequencies. This kind of spectrum is called a *continuous spectrum*.

The waveform and spectrum are alternative ways of representing a sound. The two representations are mathematically related by an operation called the *Fourier transform*. A spectrum is sometimes called a Fourier spectrum, and Fourier analysis is a very common type of spectral analysis. The basic objective of this spectral analysis is to convert the amplitude-by-time pattern of the waveform into an alternative pattern which reveals the amount of energy in the various sinusoidal components of the sound. Note that phase has been neglected in this simplified discussion. To make a waveform and spectrum completely interchangeable, phase information would have to be included with the spectral analysis. This information would describe the time relationships among the spectral components. Although phase cannot be neglected in the study of sound, phase generally is ignored in studies of speech acoustics because phase does not contribute critically to the perception of speech.

The unit of frequency measurement was defined as the hertz, which is a linear measure of frequency as the number of vibrations occurring in one second. But the human ear does not perceive pitch in a way that is linear in frequency. For example, on a piano keyboard, an equivalent increase in pitch is judged to occur in proceeding from middle C, to the next higher C, and so on. These intervals

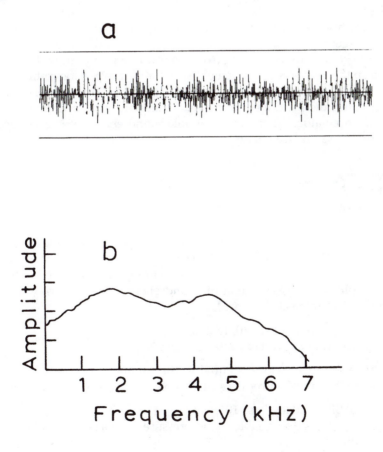

FIGURE B-5. Waveform and spectrum of noise. Note diffuse energy distribution in spectrum.

are called *octaves* and they correspond to multiplying the linear frequency values by two. If we go up one octave from 220, the corresponding linear frequency is 440 Hz.

To this point, the unit of amplitude measurement has been neglected. That neglect must now be remedied. Amplitude conceivably could be measured in terms of the actual excursions of molecules, but the measurement would be implausibly difficult for most applications. In addition, the human response to sound is such that loudness judgments change roughly with the logarithm of the actual physical changes in the signal. For example, with a base 10 logarithm, powers of ten would be represented with the log values of 0 for 1 or unity, 1 for a value of 10, 2 for a value of 100, 3 for a value of 1,000, and so on. Because the range of amplitudes to be considered in human hearing is vast, the logarithmic scale is convenient to represent this dimension of sound.

The unit typically used to measure sound energy is the *decibel*. The decibel has a rather complicated derivation, but the following sequence should help to clarify it.

The *decibel* is one tenth of a *bel*. Because the bel is too large to be a practical unit of measurement, the decibel (*deci* = one-tenth) is used instead.

The bel is a logarithm of a ratio. Recall that a logarithmic scale is advantageous because of the large range of sound amplitudes that need to be considered. Going from a linear to logarithmic scale helps to keep the numbers of convenient size, for example, a logarithm of 4 corresponds to a linear value of 10,000 (10 to the fourth power). The ratio enters the picture because sound energy is measured relative to a reference value. That is, the variable sound energy V is described relative to a standard energy S:

1 bel = log(base 10) V / S.

Because 1 bel (B) equals 10 decibels (dB),

10 dB = 1 B = log(base 10) V / S

and

1 dB = 10 log(base 10) V / S.

Both intensity and sound pressure are commonly used as the actual physical measurement of sound energy. For intensity measurement, or intensity level (IL),

1 dB IL = 10 log(base 10) Iv / Is,
where Iv is the variable intensity and Is is the standard intensity.

Because sound pressure is equal to the square of intensity, sound pressure level in dB introduces a factor of 2:

1 dB SPL = 20 log(base 10) Pv / Ps,
where Pv is the variable sound pressure and Ps is the standard sound pressure.

In this book, sound magnitude usually will be expressed in either dB intensity level or dB sound pressure level. Therefore, a spectrum of a sound will have the horizontal axis of frequency (in Hz or kHz, where k is a multiplier of 1,000) and a vertical axis of intensity or sound pressure level in dB. An interesting property of the logarithmic dB scale is that addition of dB values corresponds to multiplication of the original (antilog) values. This is a useful feature, as it simplifies some calculations in acoustics.

We have seen that sound is a wave phenomenon in which the vibratory energy is propagated in a medium. This wave property can be represented graphically as a waveform (amplitude of displacement versus time) or a wavelength (amplitude of displacement versus distance). One of the most useful ways to analyze sound is by means of the spectrum (energy versus frequency). A fundamental appeal of the spectrum is that even very complex sounds can be analyzed as a combination of elemental sounds, such as sinusoids. The Fourier spectrum accomplishes this kind of analysis, enabling us to describe various types of sounds in terms of their energy distributions across frequency. A general rule for relating waveform and spectral representations is as follows (assuming that the waveforms are plotted on the same time scale): The more peaked (sharp-cornered) the waveform, the greater the energy in the higher frequencies of the spectrum. This relation holds because sharp features in the waveform require high frequencies for their definition.

Speech sounds usually have energy distributed widely over frequency, but some energy regions are more important than others. Part of the goal of acoustic analysis of speech, then, is to determine how sounds differ in their spectra and to describe the most important spectral regions for each sound or sound class. The chapters in this book describe modern approaches to making speech visible, an enterprise that has occupied the labors of speech scientists for several decades. Almost a half-century ago, Potter, Kopp, and Green (1947) published a book, *Visible Speech*. The present book could be similarly subtitled and reports on about fifty years of progress in this quest.

Appendix C: Nonlinear Frequency Scales for Speech Analysis

The scales described in this section have been proposed as alternatives to linear frequency for the representation of speech sounds. A major argument for the use of these nonlinear frequency scales is that they come closer than a linear scale to the analysis performed by the ear. Although these nonlinear scales have been particularly important for vowels, they also can be used for consonants.

In each of the equations that follow, f designates a value of frequency. Equations are defined for mels, Barks, and Koenig values.

Technical mels (TM), were defined by Fant (1973),

$$TM = (1000 / \log 2) \log(f/1000 + 1)$$

The Bark transform (B for Bark), is calculated according to Zwicker and Terhardt's (1980) equation,

$$B = 13 \arctan (0.76f / 1000) + 3.5 \arctan (f / 7500)^2$$

Koenig values (K), from Koenig (1949) are calculated with the equations,

$$K = 0.002f \quad \text{for } 0 \leq f < 1000.$$
$$K = (4.5 \log f) - 11.5 \quad \text{for } 1000 < f \leq 10,000.$$

For a graphical comparison of these scales, see Miller (1989).

Glossary

This glossary defines selected terms encountered in digital signal processing and acoustic analysis. It is not an exhaustive glossary for all terms used in this book, but is an attempt to offer definitions for a number of important terms. It also includes some general computer terminology that is not discussed in this book but may be helpful to readers who use computer systems.

A/D converter: analog to digital converter; a hardware device that converts an analog (A) signal to a digital (D) form. The conversion process involves both **sampling** and **quantization** operations. A/D converters for microcomputers typically are expansion boards that fit into the computer.

Affricate: a speech sound that involves the two phases of a stop (vocal tract obstruction) and a prolonged frication.

Algorithm: a step-by-step procedure for solving a particular type of problem.

Allophone: a variant of a phoneme. The phoneme is a family of speech sounds that occur in various phonetic environments or that can be selected by a speaker without disturbing phonemic identity. For example, vowels in English can be either nasalized or not. The nasal allophone of a vowel is a variant produced with velopharyngeal opening. Most speakers produce nasalized vowels when they occur adjacent to nasal consonants. Similarly, many consonants can be produced with lip rounding when they occur adjacent to lip-rounded sounds.

Aliasing: artifacts or errors that arise during digitization because of the presence of sound energy in the analog signal at frequencies higher than one-half of the sampling frequency.

Amplifier: a device that increases the amplitude of a signal. Amplifiers are used to increase signal gain for purposes of recording, playback, or analysis.

Amplitude: the magnitude of displacement for a sound wave. The waveform of a sound is represented on a two-dimensional graph in which amplitude is plotted as a function of time. To a certain degree, amplitude of sound determines the perceived loudness of the sound.

Analog: a signal that has continuous variations in amplitude. The radiated sound-pressure waveform of speech is an analog signal because its amplitude varies continuously in time.

Antiformant: a transfer function property in which energy is not passed effectively; opposite in effect to a formant. Antiformants, or zeros, arise because of divided passages or constrictions in the vocal tract. The antiformant acts like a short circuit, trapping energy in the system.

ASCII: acronym for "American Standard Code for Information Interchange," a standard code for converting text to numbers.

Autocorrelation: an analytic procedure in which a signal is correlated with a time-shifted version of itself (auto = self). If the signal is periodic, the autocorrelation function will have a peak at the time-shift value corresponding to a fundamental period. If the signal is aperiodic, the autocorrelation function will not have conspicuous peaks at any time-shift value. Autocorrelation is sometimes used to determine the fundamental frequency of a speech signal.

Bandwidth: a measure of the frequency band of a sound, especially a resonance. Conventionally, bandwidth is determined at the half-power ("3 db down") points of the frequency response curve. That is, both the lower and higher frequencies that define the bandwidth are 3 db less intense than the peak energy in the band.

Bark scale: a nonlinear transformation of frequency that is thought to correspond to the analysis accomplished by the ear. The Bark scale is closely related to the concept of critical band in auditory perception.

Bit: a binary digit; the fundamental unit of information in a digital system. A bit has two possible values, conventionally expressed as 0 or 1.

Buffer: a memory (hardware device or a software routine) that temporarily holds a digital signal.

Burst: noise created during the release of a stop consonant.

Bus: a connecting system for the components of a microcomputer system. The type of bus determines the compatibility of add-in boards for a system.

Byte: a fundamental unit of storage in a digital computer; it is a collection of 8 bits, or binary decisions. An ASCII character is encoded as one byte.

Cepstrum: a Fourier transform of the power spectrum of a signal. The transform is described in terms of **quefrency** (note the transliteration from frequency), which has time-like properties. The cepstrum is used to determine the fundamental frequency of a speech signal. Voiced speech tends to have a strong cepstral peak, at the first **rahmonic** (note transliteration from harmonic).

Coarticulation: the phenomenon in speech in which the attributes of successive speech units overlap in articulatory or acoustic patterns. That is, one feature of a speech unit may be anticipated during production of an earlier unit in the string (anticipatory or forward coarticulation) or retained during production of a unit that comes later (retentive or backward coarticulation).

Command-driven: a computer program that requires the user to type in explicit commands (cf. menu-driven).

Coprocessor: an ancillary microchip added to a microcomputer to assist the microprocessor to perform specialized operations such as mathematics. A coprocessor can greatly increase the speed at which certain operations are performed.

Coupling: interaction between two or more systems; for example, oral-nasal coupling refers to the degree of interaction between the two resonating cavities. No coupling means no interaction.

CPU: acronym for central processing unit.

Damping: the rate of absorption of sound energy; related to bandwidth.

Dedicated processing: the use of a computer hardware system designed for one kind of application.

DFT: discrete Fourier transform; a Fourier transform that operates on digital (discrete) data, that is, sequences of numbers.

Diphthong: sound involving a gradual change in articulatory configuration from an onglide to offglide position. The usual phonetic symbol is a digraph, or combination of two symbols to represent the onglide and offglide portions.

Digital: a signal or message that is represented as discrete values (a sequence of numbers).

Digitization: the process of converting an analog signal to a digital form.

Direct memory access (DMA): a method by which primary memory can be read from or written to without use of the microprocessor. In speech applications, DMA permits the digital signal to be stored to the hard disk during the digitization process.

Display adapter: the hardware (board and monitor) that determines the display capabilities of a microcomputer system.

Driver: a computer program or subroutine that manages the communication with an input or output device.

EPROM: acronym for "erasable programmable read-only memory." EPROMS are microchips that store binary information indefinitely. They can be used to upgrade and expand the capabilities of a dedicated processor.

FFT: fast Fourier transform; an algorithm commonly used in microcomputer programs to calculate a Fourier spectrum. The FFT is a special type of DFT in which the number of points transformed is a power of 2. The number of points expresses the bandwidth of analysis; the higher the value, the narrower the bandwidth.

File header: the first few bytes of a data file; for speech analysis systems the file header typically specifies parameter settings such as sampling rate.

Filter: a hardware device or software program that provides a frequency-dependent transmission of energy. Commonly, a filter is used to exclude energy at certain frequencies while passing the energy at other frequencies, A low-pass filter passes the frequencies below a certain cut-off frequency; a high-pass filter passes the frequencies above a certain cut-off frequency; and a band-pass filter passes the energy between a lower and upper cut-off frequency.

Formant: a resonance of the vocal tract. A formant is specified by its center frequency (commonly called formant frequency) and bandwidth. Formants are denoted by integers that increase with the relative frequency location of the formants. F1 is the lowest-frequency formant, F2 is the next highest, and so on.

Formant synthesizer: a synthesizer that attempts to recreate the changing formants of speech. Typically, a formant synthesizer specifies the frequencies and bandwidths of a small number of formants at small intervals of time.

Fourier transform: a mathematical procedure that converts a series of values in the time domain (waveform) to a set of values in the frequency domain (spectrum). The spectrum is the Fourier transform of the spectrum.

Formant transition: a change in formant pattern, typically associated with a phonetic boundary; for example, the CV formant transition refers to formant pattern changes associated with the consonant-vowel transition.

Frame: a set of points taken as a single unit of analysis. Software that performs multiple operations over an extended set of data often performs the operations on successive frames or blocks of data. In speech analysis systems, the frame is the temporal interval in which operations are performed.

Frequency: the rate of vibration of a periodic event; for example, a periodic sound has a frequency measured as the number of cycles of vibration per second (expressed in hertz, Hz).

Frequency-domain operation: an operation that is performed in the frequency domain, for example, with a FFT or LPC spectrum.

Fricative: a speech sound characterized by a long interval of turbulence noise. Fricatives are often classified as **stridents** or **nonstridents**, depending on the degree of noise energy.

Function keys: the set of 10 or 12 keys on an IBM keyboard marked with F followed by a digit. These keys are used by some software programs.

Fundamental frequency: the lowest frequency (first harmonic) of a periodic signal. In speech, the fundamental frequency refers to the first harmonic of the voice. Fundamental frequency is the reciprocal of the fundamental period. Ideally, fundamental frequency is used to refer to a *physical* measure of the lowest periodic component of vocal fold vibration. *Pitch* should be used to indicate the perceptual phenomenon in which stimuli can be rated along a continuum of low to high. See **Pitch Determination Algorithm**.

Glide: a consonant sound that has a gradual (gliding) change in articulation reflected by a relatively long interval of formant-frequency shift.

Harmonic: an integer multiple of the fundamental frequency in voiced sounds. Ideally, the voice source can be conceptualized as a line spectrum in which energy appears as a series of harmonics.

I/O: abbreviation for input/output.

Interface: the communication scheme for the exchange of information between digital components.

Jitter: an index of instability in the laryngeal waveform, usually measured as the cycle-to-cycle variation in the fundamental period.

Kbyte: kilobyte; one thousand bytes.

Laminar flow: a type of air flow in which the air moves in smooth layers. Contrasts with **turbulence**.

LPC: linear predictive coding; a class of methods used to obtain a spectrum. Linear predictive coding uses a weighted linear sum of samples to predict an upcoming value.

Liquid: a cover term for the phonemes [l] and [r].

Machine speech recognition: the recognition of speech by a machine, especially a computer. Most of these systems attempt to determine the phonetic sequences or words of an input signal.

Mainframe: a large, powerful, general-purpose computer.

Mel: an auditory unit for the measurement of frequency. It follows certain nonlinear properties of the human perception of frequency.

Menu-driven: a program that presents a list of commands for user selection (cf. command-driven).

Microcomputer: a relatively small, freestanding computer system based on a microprocessor.

Microprocessor: microchip containing all the components of a central processing unit (CPU).

Mouse: an input device for a computer; it usually takes the form of a small hand-held box that is moved along a horizontal surface. Its position is echoed by a pointer on the computer screen.

Narrow-band analysis: an analysis in which the analyzing bandwidth is relatively narrow (such as 45 Hz in speech analysis). A narrow-band analysis is preferred when the interest is to increase frequency resolution, as in the analysis of harmonics for a man's voice.

Nasal: a speech sound that involves a nasal radiation of sound energy, either with or without an accompanying oral radiation.

Nasal formant: the low-frequency resonance associated with the nasal tract. For men's speech, the nasal formant has a frequency of less than 500 Hz.

Normalization: a correction for variance. **Speaker normalization** refers to the correction or scaling that reduces variability in acoustic measures such as formant frequencies. **Time normalization** refers to the correction or scaling that reduces variability in the durations of sound sequences.

Nyquist Sampling Theorem: this theorem states that a digital representation requires at least two sampling points for every periodic cycle in the signal of interest. Therefore, the sampling rate of digitization should be at least twice the highest frequency of interest in the signal to be analyzed. Unfortunately, the term *Nyquist Frequency* is inconsistently used. Some use it to indicate the highest frequency of interest in an analysis; other use it to refer to twice the highest frequency of interest, that is, to the sampling rate needed to prevent aliasing.

PC: abbreviation for personal computer. Originally used by IBM to refer to a particular design class of computers, but the term has been generalized to refer to similar computers made by other manufacturers.

Perturbation measures: indices of irregularity or instability, especially in the laryngeal waveform. The common measures of perturbation include **jitter, shimmer**, and **signal-to-noise ratio**.

Pitch Determination Algorithm (PDA) (also Pitch Extraction): a procedure used to extract the fundamental frequency of a speech signal. Although the term *pitch* strictly should be used to refer to a perceptual phenomenon, it is often used in speech analysis to refer to fundamental frequency.

Pixel: a single dot on a display; from *picture el*ement.

Preemphasis: in speech analysis, a filtering that boosts high-frequency energy relative to low-frequency energy. Because speech normally contains its strongest energy in the low frequencies, these frequencies would dominate analysis results if preemphasis were not performed.

Prevoicing: the onset of voicing before the appearance of a supraglottal articulatory event; for example, for stops, prevoicing means that voicing precedes the stop release. Also called voicing lead.

Quantization: the assignment of discrete values to the amplitude dimension of an analog signal. Quantization is the process by which a continuous variation in amplitude is represented as a sequence of discrete values. This process is necessary to represent the signal in a digital computer.

Quantization noise: a signal distortion that results from an inadequate number of quantization levels in digitizing a signal.

Radiation characteristic: the term in source-filter theory associated with the radiation of sound from the lips to the atmosphere. It is typically expressed as a 6 dB per octave increase in sound energy (hence, a high-pass filter).

Read-only memory (ROM): memory in a computer that can be read only, not altered by writing in new information or editing.

Real-time: an operation which takes no more time than the incoming signal itself.

Reynold's number: a dimensionless number that serves as an index of the development of turbulence.

Rounding: an articulatory description referring to the rounding (or protrusion) of the lips. As applied to vowels, rounding is associated with a lowering of the frequencies of all formants.

Sampling theorem: this theorem, developed by Nyquist, states that S samples per second are needed to represent a waveform with a bandwidth of S/2 Hz.

Segmentation: the delineation of successive sound segments in a speech signal. Typically, segmentation yields units such as phonemes, allophones, or some other phonetic segment.

Shimmer: an index of instability in the laryngeal waveform, usually measured as variation in the amplitude of successive glottal cycles.

Signal-to-noise ratio (S/N):   a measure of the ratio between signal energy and noise energy. In speech analysis, S/N usually refers to the periodic energy relative to noise energy.

Software: programs that run on computers. Software (computer instructions specified by a programmer) is opposed to hardware (the electronic components of a computer). A related term is firmware, which denotes programs that are not intended to be changed.

Source-filter theory: a theory of the acoustic production of speech that states that the energy from a sound source is modified by a filter or set of filters. For example, for vowels, the vibrating vocal folds usually are the source of sound energy and the vocal tract resonances (formants) are the filters.

Speaker normalization: a procedure that eliminates, or compensates for, interspeaker differences in some physical variable of speech; for example, speaker normalization of vowel formants refers to a procedure to minimize interspeaker variation in vowel formant frequencies.

Speaker recognition: the determination of a speaker who produced a given speech signal. Also called voice recognition.

Spectrogram: a pattern for sound analysis containing information on intensity, frequency and time. The typical spectrogram provides a three-dimensional display of time on the horizontal axis), frequency on the vertical axis, and intensity on the gray scale. A spectrogram can be printed as hard copy or displayed on a video monitor.

Spectrum: a graph showing the distribution of signal energy as a function of frequency; a plot of intensity by frequency.

Speech synthesis: the production of speech by artificial means; especially the generation of speech by computers or computer-controlled devices.

Spoiler: an obstacle in the path of air flow. In the production of fricative sounds, the upper and lower teeth may serve as spoilers.

Stop: a speech sound characterized by a complete obstruction of the vocal tract; usually followed by an abrupt release of air that produces a burst noise.

Stop gap: the acoustic interval corresponding to articulatory closure for a stop or affricate consonant; it is identified on a spectrogram as an interval of relatively low energy, conspicuously lacking in formant pattern or noise.

Strident: a fricative with an intense noise energy; also called a sibilant; /s/ and /ʃ/ are examples. The nonstrident fricatives have less energy; /θ/ is an example.

Time-domain operation: an operation that is performed in the time domain, for example, calculations performed with respect to the waveform of a sound.

Tongue advancement: an articulatory description referring to the relative position of the tongue in the anterior–posterior (front-back) dimension of the vocal tract. As applied to vowels, tongue advancement relates primarily to the relative frequency of F2, or to the frequency difference between F1 and F2. Front vowels tend to have relatively high F2 values and a relatively large value of the F2–F1 difference.

Tongue height: an articulatory description referring to the relative position of the tongue in the inferior–superior (low-high) dimension of the vocal tract. As applied to vowels, tongue height relates primarily to the relative frequency of F1; the higher the vowel, the lower F1 tends to be. Tongue height also varies with jaw position, such that high vowels tend to have a closed jaw position.

Turbulence: a condition of air flow in which eddies (rotating volume elements of air) are generated. This condition is associated with noise energy (hence we speak of *turbulence noise*). Turbulence contrasts with **laminar flow.**

Voice bar: a band of energy, typically reflecting the first harmonic of the voice source, that appears on a spectrogram; it is indicative of voicing.

Voice onset time (VOT): a measure of the time between a supraglottal event and the onset of voicing; for stops, VOT is the interval between release of the stop (usually determined acoustically as the stop burst) and the appearance of periodic modulation (voicing) for a following sound.

Waveform: a graph showing the amplitude versus time function for a continuous signal such as the acoustic signal of speech.

Wavelength: the distance that a periodic sound travels in one complete cycle. Wavelength = speed of sound/frequency.

Wide-band analysis: an analysis in which a relatively large analyzing bandwidth is used (such as 300 Hz in speech analysis). A wide-band analysis is preferred when the primary concern is to reveal formant pattern or to increase time resolution.

Window: a weighting function applied to a waveform so that its amplitude gradually increases and decreases; the window acts like an acoustic "lens" to focus the analysis on a representative part of the signal.

Subject Index